Rehabilitation Goal Setting

Theory, Practice and Evidence

REHABILITATION SCIENCE IN PRACTICE SERIES

Series Editors

Marcia J. Scherer, Ph.D.

President
Institute for Matching Person and Technology

Professor
Orthopaedics and Rehabilitation
University of Rochester Medical Center

Dave Muller, Ph.D.

Executive
Suffolk New College

Editor-in-Chief
Disability and Rehabilitation

Founding Editor
Aphasiology

Rehabilitation Goal Setting

Theory, Practice and Evidence

EDITED BY

Richard J. Siegert
AUT University, Auckland, New Zealand

William M. M. Levack
University of Otago, New Zealand

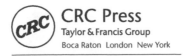

CRC Press
Taylor & Francis Group
Boca Raton London New York

CRC Press is an imprint of the
Taylor & Francis Group, an **informa** business

CRC Press
Taylor & Francis Group
6000 Broken Sound Parkway NW, Suite 300
Boca Raton, FL 33487-2742

First issued in paperback 2017

© 2015 by Taylor & Francis Group, LLC
CRC Press is an imprint of Taylor & Francis Group, an Informa business

ISBN-13: 978-1-4398-6329-9 (hbk)
ISBN-13: 978-1-138-07518-4 (pbk)

Library of Congress Cataloging-in-Publication Data

Rehabilitation goal setting : theory, practice, and evidence / editors, Richard J. Siegert and William M. M. Levack.
   p. ; cm. -- (Rehabilitation science in practice series)
   Includes bibliographical references and index.
   ISBN 978-1-4398-6329-9 (alk. paper)
   I. Siegert, Richard J., editor of compilation. II. Levack, William, editor of compilation. III. Series: Rehabilitation science in practice series.
   [DNLM: 1. Rehabilitation--methods. 2. Rehabilitation--psychology. 3. Evidence-Based Practice. 4. Goals. 5. Patient Outcome Assessment. WB 320]

RA975.5.R43
362.17'86--dc23
                                                  2014000461

Visit the Taylor & Francis Web site at
http://www.taylorandfrancis.com

and the CRC Press Web site at
http://www.crcpress.com

Contents

Section I Goal Theory in Rehabilitation

Section II Goal Setting in Clinical Practice

Section III   Specific Applications

Section IV   Conclusion

Foreword

A speciality is defined by specific knowledge and skills. Rehabilitation is, arguably, defined by three features. First, the process of rehabilitation is set within a holistic, biopsychosocial model of health and illness. Second, multidisciplinary teamwork is crucial, and single disciplines cannot deliver rehabilitation. And third, setting goals for patients is the central skill and process; without this skill, a clinician cannot deliver effective rehabilitation.

This book is, to the best of my knowledge, the first comprehensive scientifically based text to cover goal setting within the context of rehabilitation, and it is probably the first within the context of healthcare. Moreover it demonstrates, implicitly, the need to use the biopsychosocial model of illness that is exemplified by the World Health Organization's International Classification of Functioning, Disability and Health. It also, inevitably, considers how goal setting is a necessary part of multidisciplinary teamwork.

Rehabilitation is a process that aims to alter behaviour in the sense that it intends to change how a patient undertakes activities and/or change how others assist a patient in achieving his/her goals. This is why goal setting with a patient is so important – behaviour refers to actions that are undertaken to achieve some goal, be it immediate or long term. Therefore, the process of rehabilitation is centred on patient goals and patient activities.

One other group of medical specialities has a very similar focus – psychiatric or mental health services including those for people with learning disabilities. Although some services, possibly the majority in some countries, have adopted a very biological approach to psychiatric illness, the reality is that most clinical focus is on altering behaviour and helping people adapt and manage their long-term problems.

Consequently, this book should be read not only by anyone involved in any medical rehabilitation service but also by anyone involved in psychiatric and mental health services. Why?

Within the 19 chapters there is an extensive review of evidence about and discussion of the various theories that concern altering behaviour. This is all set in the general context of healthcare, although most of the original hypotheses and related evidence come from other spheres including management and sports sciences. The book draws upon a broad range of material, interpreting it in the particular context of rehabilitation.

There is also an extensive review of the evidence concerning the effectiveness of goal setting in improving the efficiency and effectiveness of rehabilitation. Most readers will not be surprised to learn that the evidence base is quite patchy and weak, although the evidence available certainly suggests that it is beneficial rather than harmful.

Recognizing the need for much more research, and recognizing that there are considerable challenges in undertaking this research, this book also discusses how the evidence base could be improved. The last chapter, which particularly discusses this, is based on the personal experience of the two editors. It should be read by anyone setting out to undertake research in this difficult field.

The book is also intended to help practicing clinicians and rehabilitation teams in their day-to-day work. The acronym most often associated with goal setting is SMART, and the authors agree with me that this is not necessarily a useful acronym. For a start, there is not even any agreement on what the letters stand for: is 'A' appropriate or achievable or attributable, and is 'M' measureable or meaningful?

Another commonly used acronym is GAS – goal attainment scaling – which refers to a method for scoring how well a person succeeds in achieving goals set. The process of using GAS probably increases patient engagement provided that it is not used to measure outcome at a group level or in relation to payment. Again, this process is discussed extensively in the book.

Within the book there are several discussions on the use of goal setting in different contexts, both clinical and cultural. For example, its application in people who have good cognition and communication is discussed, but also its application in people without full mental capacity such as children, or people with aphasia.

One interesting new idea is introduced – the importance of meaning in the process of setting goals. Although the ideas need further investigation and development, the central importance of meaning has been translated into a new acronym, MEANING. Although I have an intrinsic dislike of acronyms, this one avoids a simple letter-to-word translation and instead uses the acronym to propose an approach.

Another specific area that is discussed is the use of goal setting by patients who are taught self-management. This is likely to become increasingly important, and there is some evidence supporting its effectiveness, for example in people with chronic fatigue syndrome and other functional illnesses.

One very unusual aspect of this book, which is to be commended, is that it discusses the interaction between the goal setting process and ethical clinical practice. The first part of this discussion concerns a detailed description of one widely used approach to analysing ethical issues in any clinical practice, particularly relating this framework to rehabilitation practice.

I think that it is very important that all clinicians, and indeed all people working in healthcare, are familiar with an approach to analysing ethical issues. Even more important, all healthcare staff must be alert to the existence of the ethical dimension of each and every decision made about both individual patients and about services and groups of patients. This chapter should remind all readers of their responsibility.

However, the really interesting challenge is a claim that there is an ethical imperative to undertake goal setting with every patient (in rehabilitation). I would agree that there is a moral, professional requirement to establish with every patient what their wishes and expectations are; this is legally reinforced in many countries by statutes such as the Mental Capacity Act (2005) in England and Wales. I would also agree that without knowing these facts, any attempts to improve activities are likely to be less successful.

Nonetheless, I am less convinced that there is an additional moral imperative to engage the patient further in the goal-setting process. The authors may be correct, but I think at present we lack the evidence to support such a claim. I recommend each reader to read that chapter, especially its ending (see Chapter 4, Ethics and Goal Setting).

This book both excited and educated me from the moment I first read it. I had naively thought that I knew much about goal setting and had, in a rather self-centred way, considered that we at the Rivermead Rehabilitation Centre had developed the process not from scratch, but certainly from a low base. I now know that goal setting was being used well before I started in rehabilitation (in 1980), and I now know much more about its theoretical basis, its evidence base, and I have learned new ideas about its use.

I think that this book should be read by every team member from every involved profession – nurses, doctors, social workers, dieticians, physiotherapists, speech and language therapists, clinical psychologists, occupational therapists and so on.

Even more importantly, the people who manage rehabilitation services and the people who pay for rehabilitation services should also read this book. As professional managers, they will immediately recognize the process. On reading the book they will gain a useful insight into rehabilitation and, hopefully, they may well be able to help the clinical service improve still further in the process of goal setting.

Derick Wade
Oxford, United Kingdom

Editors

Richard J. Siegert, BSc, PGDipPsych (Clin), MSocSci, PhD, professor of psychology and rehabilitation, Person Centred Research Centre, School of Rehabilitation and Occupation Studies, Auckland University of Technology, Auckland, New Zealand. Richard trained in clinical psychology and completed his PhD in psychology at Victoria University of Wellington. He has worked clinically in forensic, mental health and neurology settings. Richard has lectured in psychology at Victoria University of Wellington and in rehabilitation at the University of Otago, Wellington, New Zealand, and also at King's College London in the Department of Palliative Care, Policy and Rehabilitation. Richard's research interests include neuropsychology, neurological rehabilitation, psychology applied to rehabilitation and psychometrics. He is an author of 90 peer-reviewed journal articles, 4 invited articles, 6 book chapters and a popular undergraduate rehabilitation textbook. With his colleague Lynne Turner-Stokes, he recently completed a longitudinal study of community rehabilitation services for people with complex neuro-disability in London. Richard's current interests include the application of mindfulness techniques for people with neurological conditions and outcome measurement in neuro-rehabilitation.

William M.M. Levack, BPhty, MHealSc (Rehabilitation), PhD, associate dean for research and postgraduate studies, and senior lecturer in rehabilitation, University of Otago, Wellington, New Zealand. William is a registered physiotherapist who trained at the University of Otago. He began his career working in services providing rehabilitation for age-related, neurological, and respiratory conditions, before moving to help establish a new branch of private residential rehabilitation service for people with acquired brain injury. William returned to the public health system to work as the physiotherapy team leader for Wellington Public Hospital, managing a team of 30 physiotherapists and support staff. In 2003, William was employed as a lecturer in the University of Otago, teaching interdisciplinary, postgraduate courses in rehabilitation by distance, and in 2008 he completed his PhD. William's research interests include goal theory, patient engagement in rehabilitation and inter-professional rehabilitation processes. His current research projects include work on the development of a clinical measure of loss and reconstruction of self-identity after traumatic brain injury, qualitative research into the barriers and facilitator of access to evidence-based rehabilitation and the use of kinetic video games as a form of therapeutic exercise for people with chronic respiratory disease.

Contributors

Stephen Ashford, HCPC (Physiotherapy), MCSP, BSc (Hons), PGCert (Non-Med. Prescribing), PGCertEd, MSc, PhD, clinical lecturer and consultant physiotherapist, Regional Rehabilitation Unit, North West London Hospitals NHS Trust and Department of Palliative Care, Policy and Rehabilitation, Cicely Saunders Institute, King's College London, UK. In 2003, Stephen became a clinical specialist and research physiotherapist at the Regional Rehabilitation Unit and Honorary Research Fellow, Department of Palliative Care, Policy and Rehabilitation, King's College London. He earned his PhD at King's College London investigating the measurement of arm function following focal interventions for spasticity. In 2012, he became consultant physiotherapist and, in 2013, NIHR clinical lecturer and is undertaking further investigations into focal spasticity and measurement of outcome. Stephen completed a postgraduate certificate in non-medical prescribing in 2013 at London Southbank University. He has published a number of peer-reviewed papers in the rehabilitation literature as well as book chapters and clinical guideline contributions. Stephen's ongoing research includes investigation of the use of goal attainment scaling alongside standardized outcome measures. He published a seminal paper on the use of goal attainment scaling for spasticity management using botulinum toxin, which has led to a wide uptake of this approach in clinical practice.

Bronwyn Davidson, BSpThy, PhD, associate professor in speech pathology, Department of Audiology and Speech Pathology, Melbourne School of Health Sciences, The University of Melbourne, Australia. Bronwyn has extensive clinical and academic experience in speech-language pathology and stroke rehabilitation, having worked in Australia, New Zealand, and the United Kingdom. In 2004, she completed her doctoral studies on the impact of aphasia on the everyday communication of older Australians and worked as an academic at the University of Queensland before taking up her current appointment as associate professor in speech pathology at The University of Melbourne in 2011. Bronwyn has a special interest in clinical research into interventions that address social interaction for people with aphasia and on the impact of communication disability on friendships. Her current research activities are with the Centre for Clinical Research Excellence in Aphasia Rehabilitation in Australia.

Sarah G. Dean, CPsychol, MCSP, BSc (Jt Hons), Grad DipPhys, MSc, PhD, senior lecturer in health services research, Institute of Health Research, University of Exeter Medical School, University of Exeter, Exeter, UK. Sarah trained to be a physiotherapist at Guy's Hospital after completing her first degree in psychology and physical education. She worked clinically in both the National Health Service (United Kingdom) and private sector, specializing in musculoskeletal rehabilitation, particularly exercise therapy for sports injuries and cardiac rehabilitation. During this time, she also trained and competed as an international athlete in the 400 m hurdles. She lectured in physiotherapy for nearly nine years at the University of Southampton, completing her PhD in health psychology during this time. Sarah then went to work in New Zealand as a senior lecturer in rehabilitation at the University of Otago, Wellington, as part of the inter-professional rehabilitation research and distance teaching unit. In 2009, Sarah returned to the United Kingdom to take up her current post as part of the Peninsula Collaboration for Leadership in Applied Health Research and Care (PenCLAHRC). Sarah's research interests include applying psychology to rehabilitation medicine, including goal setting, and facilitating adherence to exercise therapy for people with long-term conditions such as stroke, low back pain and urinary incontinence, as well as assessing fidelity to intervention delivery by health professionals. Sarah also leads the PenCLAHRC clinical decision making (putting evidence into practice) teaching workshops. A recently published textbook captures much of Sarah's approach to rehabilitation research and teaching – she is the lead editor of *Interprofessional Rehabilitation: A Person-Centred Approach*, published in 2012.

Diane Dixon, BA (Hons), BSc (Hons), PhD, reader in psychology and health psychologist, School of Psychological Sciences and Health, University of Strathclyde, Glasgow, UK. Diane originally trained as a pharmacologist, gaining her PhD in 1989. She subsequently retrained as a psychologist and now works as an academic health psychologist. Her research is in health psychology and health services research. She works on physical disability and on the development and evaluation of interventions for people with physical illnesses and those receiving medical and surgical interventions. She has particular interests in chronic pain, musculoskeletal conditions and stroke. Her theoretical interests are in the measurement of disability, in the explanation of activity limitations, the application of theory to the behaviour of individuals and the integration of theoretical models of disability derived from disparate academic disciplines.

Emmah Doig, BOccThy (Hons), PhD, postdoctoral research fellow, School of Health & Rehabilitation Sciences, University of Queensland, Australia. Since graduating from the University of Queensland in 1999, Emmah began her career as an occupational therapist in a large metropolitan hospital, working with people with stroke and acquired brain injury within acute care, inpatient and outpatient rehabilitation. Emmah then travelled to the United Kingdom where she worked in the inpatient rehabilitation unit and acute stroke unit at the Regional Neurological Rehabilitation Unit at Homerton Hospital. Upon returning to Australia, in conjunction with a colleague, Emmah established RehABIlity Acquired Brain Injury Services, which specializes in providing occupational therapy rehabilitation and case management services to people with acquired brain injury living in the community. Emmah completed her PhD in 2010 and is currently a postdoctoral research fellow funded by the National Health and Medical Research Council as part of the Moving Ahead Centre of Research Excellence in traumatic brain injury recovery. Emmah's research to date has focused on brain injury rehabilitation and has investigated occupation-based rehabilitation, the influence of rehabilitation context on outcomes, client-centred goal planning, community-based rehabilitation and the assessment of post-traumatic amnesia and disorders of consciousness.

Jennifer Fleming, BOccThy (Hons), PhD, conjoint associate professor, School of Health & Rehabilitation Sciences, University of Queensland, and Occupational Therapy Department, Princess Alexandra Hospital, Brisbane, Australia. Jennifer is an occupational therapist with 25 years' experience working and researching in the area of brain injury rehabilitation across the continuum from acute care to community rehabilitation. She completed her PhD in 1987 with the support of the Menzies Research Scholarship, and since 2001 she has been working in a conjoint research appointment with the University of Queensland and the Princess Alexandra Hospital in Brisbane, Australia. In 2012, Jennifer became a chief investigator on a Centre for Research Excellence in traumatic brain injury recovery funded by the National Health and Medical Research Council. Jennifer's research focuses on psychosocial aspects of brain injury rehabilitation including the transition from hospital to home, the role of environmental factors, lifetime care and support and cognitive rehabilitation – in particular the assessment and treatment of impaired self-awareness and prospective memory. Her work draws upon both qualitative and quantitative approaches to examine the effectiveness of rehabilitation processes including goal planning, the provision of feedback and group therapy. Jennifer has published her work in more than 130 journal articles and book chapters, and supervised 16 PhD students and many more occupational therapists conducting clinical research projects.

Krys Galama, BS OTR, unit manager, Revant Revalidatie Centrum Breda, Brabantlaan, Breda, the Netherlands. Krys is an occupational therapist who trained at the University of Puget Sound. She has worked in the field of children's rehabilitation her entire career, first as an occupational therapist and the past 11 years as unit manager of the children's department, managing a team of 55 health professionals and support staff.

Jan Willem Gorter, MD, PhD, FRCPC, associate professor and director of CanChild Centre for Childhood Disability Research, and paediatric physiatrist, Department of Pediatrics, McMaster University, Hamilton, Ontario, Canada. Jan Willem is a registered physiatrist who trained at the University of Amsterdam, Utrecht University Medical Center, and Rehabilitation Center De Hoogstraat in Utrecht, the Netherlands. He has a special clinical and research interest in outcome measurement in paediatric rehabilitation. He has led clinics for children and teenagers with developmental disabilities and their families at McMaster Children's Hospital since 2008. Since the International Classification of Functioning, Disability and Health (ICF) publication in 2001, the ICF concepts and framework have been reflected in Jan Willem's clinical activities, research and teaching. His research focuses on the themes of family (environmental factors) and function (activities and participation), with a special interest in transitions from adolescence to adulthood and in physical fitness and active lifestyles. Jan Willem has been involved in a range of applications of the ICF, from linking items of outcome measures in rehabilitation to the ICF items to interdisciplinary teaching. Jan Willem works with a number of undergraduate and graduate students at several universities in Canada and the Netherlands. He has published extensively in international peer-reviewed journals and book chapters.

Lenore A. Hawley, MSSW, LCSW, CBIST, private practice psychotherapist; research clinician, Research Department, Craig Hospital, Englewood, Colorado. Lenore has worked with individuals with brain injury and their families for over 30 years as a therapist, program developer and researcher. She is a licensed clinical social worker and a certified brain injury specialist trainer. Lenore has specific clinical expertise in group therapy, social competence and self-advocacy. She is the author of *A Family Guide to the Head Injured Adult*, editor and co-author of *Self Advocacy for Independent Life* and co-author of *Group Interactive Structured Treatment – GIST: For Social Competence*. Lenore is a research clinician at Craig Hospital in Englewood, Colorado. She has served as co-investigator on a research study showing the efficacy of the GIST intervention, and is currently co-director of intervention, training and dissemination on a U.S. Department of Defense multi-site grant investigating the effectiveness of the GIST intervention. She is also a principal investigator on a study investigating the effect of volunteer activity on psychological well-being for individuals with traumatic brain injury, and on a study of self-advocacy skills for individuals with brain injury and their families. Lenore provides group therapy for civilians with brain injury, as well as for soldiers and veterans with brain injury and post-traumatic stress disorder through her private practice.

Deborah Hersh, BSc (Hons), MSc (human communication), PhD, lecturer in speech pathology, School of Psychology and Social Science, Edith Cowan University, Australia.

Deborah qualified as a speech pathologist in 1989 and then worked in London for three years with adult and paediatric caseloads across a range of clinical settings. In 1993, after the completion of her MSc in human communication from University College London, she moved to Adelaide and continued her clinical work in adult acute care, outpatients, rehabilitation and community settings. In 1995, Deborah started the Talkback Group Program for Aphasia and established the Talkback Association for Aphasia in 1999. Between 1999 and 2002, Deborah studied at Flinders University for her PhD, exploring experiences of treatment termination in chronic aphasia. She has worked as a postdoctoral research fellow for the University of Queensland on an NHMRC-funded project grant looking at person-centred goal setting in aphasia rehabilitation. Deborah has presented and published in the areas of discharge practice, professional client relationships, clinical ethics, qualitative research approaches in speech pathology, group work for chronic aphasia and goal setting in aphasia rehabilitation. She is currently involved in research on how people with aphasia interact with nursing staff on acute wards, and the experiences of Indigenous Australians with acquired communication disorders.

Tami Howe, BEd, MHSc, PhD, senior lecturer in speech-language pathology, Department of Communication Disorders, University of Canterbury, Christchurch, New Zealand. Tami has worked in the field of speech-language pathology for several years in Canada, New Zealand, and Australia. After completing a PhD and a postdoctorate at the University of Queensland, she was employed as a lecturer in the Department of Communication Disorders at the University of Canterbury. Tami's research interests include goal setting in aphasia rehabilitation and exploring how people with aphasia and their family members live with the communication disorder, particularly in relation to social participation and accessibility.

Stephen Jacobs, BA, DipTchg, PhD, senior lecturer in clinical leadership and change management, School of Nursing, Faculty of Medical and Health Sciences, University of Auckland, and co-director of the Institute of Healthy Ageing, Waikato District Health Board, New Zealand. Stephen earned a PhD in medicine, developing a process to assist planners and funders to design, implement, performance-manage and evaluate health services for older people. His main focus now is working to assist nurses to develop and exercise clinical leadership and change management skills, and researching how organizational management can best support nurses at the point of care to be highly effective health professionals. Stephen worked with the New Zealand Ministry of Health from 2000 to 2006 – with the Disability Services Directorate, the Health of Older People team, and the Primary Health Care team. From 1995 to 2000, Stephen was manager of WesleyCare, a provider of community and residential services for older people. Prior to that he was a family therapist and counsellor for the Department of Social Welfare, the Family Court, the Ministry of Justice, and in non-government organizations dealing mainly with family violence and sexual abuse. He has also been a primary and secondary school teacher.

Fiona Jones, DipPhysiotherapy, PGCertEd, MSc, PhD, reader in rehabilitation, Faculty of Health, Social Care and Education, St. George's University of London and Kingston University, UK. Fiona is a state-registered physiotherapist, qualifying in London, United Kingdom, and has worked mainly in acute neurosciences and community neurorehabilitation during her clinical career. She was part of a team which set up one of the first specialist community stroke teams in the United Kingdom. After completing an MSc in clinical neurosciences at the University of Surrey, she made the transition into lecturing, starting in a post at the University of Brighton. Fiona has taught in subjects relating to neurorehabilitation and rehabilitation of older people since 1997. She moved to St. George's University of

London and Kingston University in 2002, where she continued teaching and set up a new MSc course in rehabilitation. Fiona completed her PhD in 2005 and has since developed her research interest in self-management after stroke. Fiona is the founder of the Bridges stroke self-management programme and leads on a number of research projects including studies exploring professional attitudes to self-management programmes in stroke and factors influencing sustainability of using programmes within rehabilitation. In 2009, Fiona received the Life After Stroke Award for excellence from the UK Stroke Association, and in 2011, she was made a fellow of the UK Chartered Society of Physiotherapists.

Nicola M. Kayes, BSc, MSc (Hons), PhD, senior lecturer, Centre for Person Centred Research, School of Rehabilitation and Occupation Studies, Auckland University of Technology, Auckland, New Zealand. Nicola graduated with her master's degree in health psychology from the University of Auckland in 2000 and her PhD from Auckland University of Technology (AUT) in 2011. She has been working in the Health and Rehabilitation Research Institute at AUT University since 2005 as part of the Centre for Person Centred Research where she contributes to both research and teaching in her role as senior lecturer and co-lead of the centre's engagement, health and rehabilitation research cluster. Nicola's research predominantly explores the intersection between health psychology and rehabilitation and in particular how drawing on psychology may enhance what we do as rehabilitation practitioners. Her key research interests include exploration of factors influencing engagement in rehabilitation (including the role that practitioners play); the development of novel strategies for engagement and supporting people to live well with chronic conditions, exploring how we can facilitate practitioners to integrate new ways of working into practice, and the development of outcome measures responsive to what matters most to patients undergoing rehabilitation.

Paula Kersten, BSc, PGCert, MSc, PhD, associate professor in rehabilitation, Centre for Person Centred Research, School of Rehabilitation and Occupation Studies, Auckland University of Technology, Auckland, New Zealand. Paula is a UK-registered physiotherapist who originally trained in the Netherlands in 1988. She completed her PhD in 1999 and has worked in academia ever since. In 2011, she joined AUT University as an associate professor in rehabilitation. There, she is also the deputy director of the Centre for Person Centred Research at the School of Rehabilitation and Occupation Studies. Her research interests focus on (1) the evaluation of new ways of working in rehabilitation and (2) the development and evaluation of meaningful outcomes in rehabilitation. Her recent work includes a feasibility study of mentoring support for people with a traumatic brain injury and a multi-centre randomized controlled trial to assess the effectiveness of a group-based cognitive behavioural approach to managing fatigue in people with multiple sclerosis. Paula is the research lead for the Centre for Person Centred Research Outcomes Research Cluster. The cluster aims to further the science of outcomes measurement through methodological research, build research capacity, and support clinicians and service leads in the use and interpretation of their outcomes data. This work has included detailed investigations of commonly used measurement tools such as the visual analogue scale, the Western Ontario and McMaster Universities Arthritis Index and the Strengths and Difficulties Questionnaire.

Marjolijn Ketelaar, PhD, is associate professor at the Brain Center Rudolf Magnus and Center of Excellence for Rehabilitation Medicine, University Medical Center Utrecht and De Hoogstraat, Utrecht, the Netherlands. She is the programme leader of a research group focusing on rehabilitation research in paediatrics and supervises a number of PhD and MSc students. Marjolijn has a background as a human movement scientist, VU Amsterdam. She completed her PhD at the Faculty of Social Science at the University of Utrecht in 1999, with a thesis on functional therapy for children with cerebral palsy. She is a partner of NetChild, Network for Childhood Disability Research in the Netherlands (www.netchild.nl), and an international collaborator of CanChild, Centre for Childhood Disability Research, Canada (www.canchild.ca). Her research interests include family-centred services and functional therapy approaches for children with disabilities, with a focus on optimizing participation of children with cerebral palsy and their families. She strongly believes in collaboration with families, clinicians and service providers in all stages of the research cycle to optimize relevance and usefulness of research and has great interest in research on knowledge translation and how research findings can be used in clinical practice.

Eline Lindeman, MD, PhD, was an excellent physiatrist and professor in rehabilitation medicine at the Center of Excellence for Rehabilitation Medicine, University Medical Center Utrecht and Rehabilitation Center De Hoogstraat. She made an significant contribution to rehabilitation throughout her working life. Prof. Dr. Eline Lindeman passed away on 27 September 2012.

Kathryn M. McPherson, BA (Hons), DipHV, RN, RM, FAFRM (Hons), PhD, professor of rehabilitation (Laura Fergusson Chair), director of the Centre for Person Centred Research in the Health and Rehabilitation Research Institute, School of Rehabilitation and Occupation Studies, Auckland University of Technology, Auckland, New Zealand. Subsequent to training as a nurse in Australia, Kath completed midwifery and a diploma in health visiting in Edinburgh, Scotland. She completed her psychology honours degree at the Open University (United Kingdom) before undertaking her PhD at the University of Edinburgh, graduating in 1998. She joined AUT University in Auckland, New Zealand, in late 2004, developing a successful teaching and research programme with her colleagues. Kath has authored/co-authored over 150 peer-reviewed publications. She works in partnership with a number of government organizations in New Zealand as well as with other health and social service organizations throughout the country to improve rehabilitation services. Kath's research focuses on developing a better understanding of, and response to, what matters most to clients and their families. Her recent projects include clinical trials of new approaches to goal setting, living well with a long-term condition, measuring what matters, quality of care, informing rehabilitation by psychological approaches, engagement in rehabilitation and enhancing understanding of theory in rehabilitation.

Thorsten Meyer, Dipl-Psych, PhD, Dr. habil, professor of rehabilitation research, Integrative Rehabilitation Research Unit, Institute for Epidemiology, Social Medicine and Health Systems Research, Hannover Medical School, Hannover, Germany. Thorsten completed a degree as a psychologist at Christian-Albrechts University of Kiel, Germany, and initially worked at a social psychiatry research group in Justus Liebig University Giessen (under Prof. Michael Franz). There he was involved in studies analysing effects of health care and social reforms for severely mentally ill people and dealt with issues of quality of life in schizophrenia. He earned his PhD at Christian-Albrechts University of Kiel with a thesis on perceptions of persons with schizophrenia on quality of life. In 2003, he started as a research assistant at the University of Luebeck, Germany (under Prof. Heiner Raspe), where he was involved in research on medical rehabilitation and priority setting and taught medical students in evidence-based and social medicine. He finished his habilitation in health services research in 2011. After one year as a group leader at the Swiss Paraplegic Research in Nottwil, Switzerland, Thorsten became a professor of rehabilitation research at the Institute for Epidemiology, Social Medicine and Health Systems Research, Hannover Medical School, Germany. Thorsten's research interests include variation of quality in rehabilitation care, priority setting in health care, epidemiology of functioning and health care, conceptual issues in rehabilitation, subjective experiences of health and rehabilitation care, quality of life and health status questionnaires, assessment of change and service user involvement in research.

Jody K. Newman, CCC-SLP, private practice speech–language pathologist; research clinician, Research Department, Craig Hospital, Englewood, Colorado. Jody is a speech-language pathologist who has been working with individuals with brain injury for over 30 years. She also has experience working with individuals with spinal cord injury. Since 1998, she has worked at Craig Hospital in Englewood, Colorado, first in the Speech–Language Department and currently in the Research Department. She is the co-author of *Group Interactive Structured Treatment – GIST: For Social Competence* and was a co-investigator on a research study showing the efficacy of the GIST intervention. She is currently co-director of Intervention, Training and Dissemination on a U.S. Department of Defense multi-site grant on social competence, studying the effectiveness of the GIST intervention. Jody has particular interest and experience in the areas of mild brain injury, social competence and contextualized cognitive treatment for individuals with brain injuries and other neurological disorders. In her private practice, Jody provides individual and group therapy for civilians, soldiers and veterans with brain injuries.

Christine O'Connell, BA, MSc (Neuroscience), trainee clinical psychologist, Canterbury Christchurch University, Kent, UK. Christine has been a trainee clinical psychologist at Canterbury Christchurch University, Kent, since September 2013. After completing her BA in psychology in 2009, Christine began her career working on a research study at King's College London which examined the community services that people with long-term neurological conditions receive. Following this, she completed her MSc in cognitive and clinical neuroscience at Goldsmith's University of London in 2012. Her thesis examined self-perception in children and adolescents with psychopathic traits. Christine then began to work with children and adolescents with neurological conditions and mental health problems in both clinical and research settings at Great Ormond Street Hospital in London.

Anand D. Pandyan, BEng, PhD (BioEng), professor of rehabilitation technology, School of Health and Rehabilitation and Institute for Science and Technology in Medicine, Keele University, Keele, Staffordshire, UK. Anand is a bioengineer with a special interest in neurological rehabilitation and applied clinical research. He completed his doctoral training at the Bioengineering Unit, University of Strathclyde, Glasgow, and has nine years of postdoctoral experience. Anand currently teaches a variety of courses at the School of Health and Rehabilitation at Keele University, both at postgraduate and undergraduate levels. Anand is interested in research methods; measurement in neurological rehabilitation (specifically non-invasive measurement of impairment and activity aimed at elucidating pathophysiology of common impairments); modelling the relationship between impairment, function and quality of life; motor control; muscle structure and function; and electrical stimulation. His current research interests focus on (1) developing a better understanding of the pathophysiological basis of spasticity and its impact on people with upper motor neurone lesions, (2) exploring the mechanisms for disordered motor control following stroke and cerebral palsy, (3) identifying the therapeutic benefits (and mechanism of action) of electrical stimulation, (4) exploring the impact of long-term antispasticity treatment and (5) exploring the impact of exercise on motor recovery, independence and well-being.

John G.M. Parsons, BSc (Hons) Physiotherapy, PGDipHSc, MSHc (Hons), PhD, lecturer in rehabilitation, School of Nursing, Faculty of Medical and Health Sciences, University of Auckland, and Clinical Lead (Rehabilitation), The Institute of Healthy Ageing, Waikato District Health Board, New Zealand. John is a physiotherapist and a senior lecturer at the Applied Ageing Research Group at the University of Auckland and clinical lead (rehabilitation) at the Institute of Health Ageing, Waikato District Health Board, New Zealand. He has established a solid research platform that concentrates on independence and physical function among older people and those with long-term conditions. John has advised both within New Zealand and internationally on the development of services for older people and is an invited expert to the development of clinical guidelines and protocols in a number of countries (Denmark, Australia and Singapore). Furthermore, John has been active in delivering training and providing support to clinical staff (both registered and unregulated) related to the implementation of rehabilitative strategies to maximize independence among frail older people across primary, secondary and tertiary care both in New Zealand and Australia.

Matthew J.G. Parsons, BSc (Hons), MSc, PhD, professor in gerontology, School of Nursing, Faculty of Medical and Health Sciences, University of Auckland, and The Institute of Healthy Ageing, Waikato District Health Board, New Zealand. Matthew holds the Chair of Gerontology which is a joint appointment between the University of Auckland and Waikato District Health Board. He holds a PhD and a master's in gerontology from the Institute of Gerontology, King's College London. He has won over $12 million in external research funds and has countless papers, conference proceedings and media presentations to his name. He works closely with a number of health boards and health organizations in New Zealand, Australia and the United Kingdom. He has a special interest in community-based services for older people and has established and evaluated multiple services across several countries.

Neil Pickering, BA, MA, MPhil, PhD, senior lecturer, Bioethics Centre, University of Otago, Dunedin, New Zealand. Neil is a philosopher by inclination, and focuses primarily on conceptual questions in the philosophy of psychiatry, in which he has a number of articles and a book published. His role at the University of Otago includes teaching on various aspects of ethics to health science undergraduates in medicine, dentistry, pharmacy, physiotherapy and dietetics. He has often spoken at conferences and training programmes to groups of health professionals, including nurses, midwives, duly authorized officers, general practitioners and members of ethics committees. He has served on the University of Otago Human Research Ethics Committee, the New Zealand Health Research Council Ethics Committee (including a period as chair), and has recently joined the National Ethics Advisory Committee (advising the New Zealand Minister of Health).

E. Diane Playford, MB BS, MRCP (UK), MD, FRCP (London), reader in neurological rehabilitation, UCL Institute of Neurology, University College London, UK. Diane is a consultant neurologist whose undergraduate training took place at the Medical College of St Bartholomew's Hospital, London, UK. She trained in neurology at the Atkinson Morley Hospital, Charing Cross Hospital and at the National Hospital for Neurology and Neurosurgery where she was lecturer and senior registrar in the neurological rehabilitation unit. Her first consultant post was in Derby, where she was also senior lecturer in rehabilitation medicine. In 1999, she moved back to London to take up a consultant post in neurology leading the neurological rehabilitation service and a senior lecturer post at the Institute of Neurology. Diane's research interests include rehabilitation processes, interventions and outcomes. Her current research projects include upper limb rehabilitation after stroke and vocational rehabilitation for people with multiple sclerosis and brain injury.

Nadine J. Pohontsch, PhD (Dr. rer. hum. biol.), research associate and lecturer, Department of Primary Medical Care, University Medical Center Hamburg-Eppendorf, Germany. Nadine works as a researcher and lecturer in the Department of Primary Medical Care at the University Medical Center Hamburg-Eppendorf in Hamburg, Germany, where she also heads the Qualitative Methods work group. Nadine trained as a psychologist and graduated from the Free University Berlin in 2006. She completed her PhD while working as a research assistant at the Department of Social Medicine at the University of Luebeck, Germany. Here, her studies focused on rehabilitation, employing mainly qualitative research methods. The topics included rehabilitation goals, rehabilitation for middle-aged patients, and interface management in rehabilitation services. Currently, Nadine's research interests centre on rehabilitation, primary medical care, patient participation and dementia. Her projects include the development of quality indicators in health care (using as an example the participation of patients with heart failure), the reduction of avoidable hospital admission for people with dementia and the prevention of inappropriate medications for elderly patients.

Alexandra Rauch, PT, BSc (Applied Health Sciences), MPH, researcher at the Chair for Public Health and Health Care Research in the Department of Medical Informatics, Biometry and Epidemiology, Research Unit for Biopsychosocial Health, Ludwig-Maximilians-University, Munich, Germany; lecturer in applied sciences. Alexandra is a registered physiotherapist who trained at the School for Physiotherapy at the Ludwig-Maximilian University, Munich, Germany. In the beginning of her career she worked in inpatient and outpatient rehabilitation facilities, specializing in the treatment of cardiovascular, musculoskeletal and neurological conditions. After eight years of practice she became a lecturer in physiotherapy at the Ludwig-Maximilian University in Munich, Germany. During this time, she also studied applied health sciences at the University for Applied Sciences in Magdeburg, Stendal, Germany. Following this, she moved to Switzerland to work at Swiss Paraplegic Research, Nottwil. Here she researched the implementation of the ICF into rehabilitation practice and studied physical activity in persons with spinal cord injury. During this time, she also studied public health at the universities of Bern, Basel and Zürich, Switzerland, and gained her master's degree in 2012. Since 2012, she has been working to finish her PhD at Ludwig-Maximilian University. Alexandra's research interests include the implementation of the ICF in various areas and settings of rehabilitation and the area of health behaviour in persons with disabilities. Her current projects include healthcare research on the implementation of the ICF Core Set for hand conditions in the German accident hospitals and investigation of the determinants for physical activity in persons with spinal cord injury. She also continues to work as a lecturer in physiotherapy and rehabilitation.

Sheeba Rosewilliam, MSc (Physiotherapy), lecturer in physiotherapy, College of Life and Environmental Sciences, University of Birmingham, Birmingham, UK. Sheeba is a physiotherapist who completed her undergraduate physiotherapy training in Christian Medical College, Vellore, India. She completed her master's in physiotherapy at Dr. MGR Medical University, Chennai, India, in 2001. After several years of experience working as a physiotherapist, she began teaching physiotherapy at universities in India, where she worked until 2004. She began her research career in Keele University, United Kingdom, where she worked on a clinical trial investigating the effects of electrical stimulation on the severely disabled stroke patients. Following this, she began work as lecturer at the University of Birmingham. Between 2004 and 2008, she worked on developing therapy protocols for the standardization of treatment for stroke patients based on local practice. Her research has also included further investigations of electrical stimulation of upper limb after stroke, a study of people's experiences of living with disability in the West Midlands of the United Kingdom and investigations of goal setting for stroke rehabilitation. The latter of these research topics is currently the subject of her PhD, which she is completing at the University Hospital of Birmingham.

Carolyn A. Roskell, MCSP, MSc, PhD, lecturer in physiotherapy, School of Sport, Exercise and Rehabilitation Sciences, University of Birmingham, Birmingham, UK. Carolyn is a registered physiotherapist who initially worked for a number of years specializing in cardiorespiratory physiotherapy in the United Kingdom and South Africa. She has worked in physiotherapy education for 25 years, most recently specializing in professionalism and professional development in health care. Carolyn has worked for the University of Birmingham since 1999 teaching on undergraduate and postgraduate programmes for healthcare professionals. She completed her PhD on the professional identity of cardiorespiratory physiotherapy in 2006. Carolyn's research interests include professional development in health-care professionals, both pre- and post-registration, with a particular focus on the development of patient-centred care and professional identity. Her current research projects include work exploring service user perspectives on the care received from allied health professionals and enhancing nursing and physiotherapy students' capabilities to deliver patient-centred care.

Anke Scheel-Sailer, MD, specialist in physical and rehabilitation medicine, general medicine, psychosocial and psychosomatic medicine and internal medicine, Consultant Rehabilitation Quality Management Research, Swiss Paraplegic Centre, Nottwil, Switzerland. Anke finished her studies of medicine at the University of Witten/Herdecke, Germany. She worked in different clinics to improve her knowledge in the field of internal, general, surgical, psychiatrics and rehabilitation medicine. Her first scientific work was accompanied by Prof. Dr. Aldgridge concerning the personal development and the effectiveness of art therapies for patients with spinal cord injury, a qualitative research of 21 patients during first rehabilitation. She received the Ludwig Goodman Prize for special work in the field of spinal cord injury in 2002. Since 2006, she has been working at the Swiss Paraplegic Centre in Nottwil, and since April 2013, she has been leading the Department of Rehabilitation Quality Management Research. Anke's research focuses on the implementation of the ICF, rehabilitation, functional training (also specialized for children and youth with spinal cord injury) and pressure ulcers. Other research topics of interest to Anke are quality management in rehabilitation, including autonomy and decision making, goal setting and application of comprehensive rehabilitation concepts. She also lectures at the University of Lucerne as a part of the Master of the Health Sciences programme.

Lesley Scobbie, BScOT, MSc (psychology and health), clinical research fellow, Nursing, Midwifery and Allied Health Professional Research Unit, Department of Nursing, Midwifery and Health, University of Stirling, Scotland, UK. Lesley qualified with a BSc in occupational therapy in 1989 and has worked as practitioner both in the United Kingdom and United States. Her 20 years of clinical practice focused mainly on multidisciplinary stroke rehabilitation in both hospital and community settings. In 2001, she completed an MSc in psychology and health, and since 2005, she has been working as clinical researcher at the University of Stirling. Her research interests include the improvement of patient outcomes through evidence-based practice. She has a particular interest in the application of theory to evidence-based goal setting within rehabilitation. She is currently a doctoral training fellow funded by the Chief Scientist Office, Edinburgh.

Sue Sherratt, BA, GCTT, BA (speech pathology and audiology) Hons, PhD, researcher and clinician in speech-language pathology, School of Health and Rehabilitation Sciences, University of Queensland, Australia. Sue graduated with a first class honours double degree in speech pathology and audiology in 1989 and has a further bachelor's degree in linguistics, psychology and African languages. She has worked within both private and public health settings, predominantly with adults with communication and swallowing disorders. Her PhD, completed in 2001 at University College London (United Kingdom), investigated the effects of age, socioeconomic status and right brain damage on discourse. She has been employed as a researcher, lecturer and clinical educator at the University of Newcastle. She has also completed an NHMRC-funded postdoctoral fellowship at the University of Queensland examining person-centred goal setting in rehabilitation with people with aphasia, their family members and their clinicians. Sue has presented and published widely in discourse, goal setting, aphasia rehabilitation groups, humour within therapy groups, therapeutic relationships, ethical misconduct, qualitative research, team communication and design cognition. Her current research includes a longitudinal study of recovery in people with aphasia, stroke narratives, emotional growth following aphasia and changing healthcare organizations.

Duco Steenbeek, MD, PhD, paediatric physiatrist, Departments of Physical Medicine and Rehabilitation, Revant Rehabilitation Centre Breda, and Department of Physical Medicine and Rehabilitation, Leiden Universital Medical Center, the Netherlands. Duco is a registered paediatric physiatrist at the Leiden University Medical Center in the Netherlands. He is employed as a lecturer in the University of Leiden and he has several teaching posts for medical students, specialty trainees and MSc students at the Leiden University Medical Center. He is a partner of NetChild, Network for Childhood Disability Research in the Netherlands (www.netchil.nl). From 2002 to 2013, he was affiliated with Revant Rehabilitation Centre Breda, the Netherlands. Between 2002 and 2010 he worked on his dissertation, studying goal attainment scaling in paediatric rehabilitation practice as used by the interdisciplinary paediatric rehabilitation team in the centre. In 2010, he completed his PhD at the Utrecht University in the Netherlands. In 2011, a practical Dutch manual on goal attainment scaling was published based on the method as studied in his thesis.

Lynne Turner-Stokes, BA (Oxon), MA (Oxon), ARCM, MBBS (London), DM (Oxon) FRCP, consultant in rehabilitation medicine, professor of rehabilitation, and director, Regional Rehabilitation Unit, Northwick Park Hospital and Department of Palliative Care and Rehabilitation Medicine, Cicely Saunders Institute, King's College London, UK. Lynne trained in general medicine, rheumatology and rehabilitation, at Oxford and then University College London. She directs the Regional Rehabilitation Unit at Northwick Park Hospital. This rehabilitation unit provides a tertiary specialist inpatient and community outreach service for younger adults with severe complex neurological disabilities, mainly following acquired brain injury. It also provides the central focus for the network of services for this group within the northwest (NW) Thames area in London, United Kingdom. As Herbert Dunhill Chair of Rehabilitation, she leads a two-site department of academic rehabilitation linking the NW Thames regional network of specialist rehabilitation services with the Department of Palliative Care and Policy and Rehabilitation at King's College London. Lynne has 157 published articles in peer-reviewed journals.

She has a special interest in outcomes measurement in rehabilitation and in developing evidence-based standards and guidelines to improve the quality of rehabilitation medicine in the United Kingdom. She is director of the UK Rehabilitation Outcomes Collaborative – a national database which gathers data on needs, inputs and outcomes for all inpatient specialist rehabilitation units in England. A particular focus for research and development has been the application of goal attainment scaling and other person-centred measures to complement standardized outcome measurement systems.

Lesley Wiart, BScPT, MScPT, PhD, clinical assistant professor, Department of Physical Therapy, Faculty of Rehabilitation Medicine, University of Alberta, and clinical outcomes site lead, Glenrose Rehabilitation Hospital, Edmonton, Alberta, Canada. Lesley is a paediatric physical therapist with clinical experience working with children with motor disabilities in a tertiary rehabilitation centre and in school settings. She completed her PhD in rehabilitation science in the Faculty of Rehabilitation Medicine at the University of Alberta, Canada, in 2008. Her main research interests are family experiences with rehabilitation, including goal-setting processes, and how those experiences can inform clinical practice in paediatric rehabilitation settings. She is also interested in how therapists can enhance meaningful participation of children and youth with motor disabilities in their communities.

Linda Worrall, BSpThy, PhD, professor of speech pathology, School of Health and Rehabilitation Sciences, University of Queensland, Brisbane, Australia. Linda is a speech pathologist who researches rehabilitation of aphasia after stroke and has been a co-director of the Communication Disability Centre since 1997. She has applied the WHO ICF to research in a range of disabilities, but has a particular interest in aphasia rehabilitation. In 2009, she was awarded a five-year NHMRC Centre of Clinical Research Excellence in Aphasia Rehabilitation and leads the national research effort towards developing an Australian Aphasia Rehabilitation Pathway.

Abbreviations

BCT   Behaviour change technique
BoNT   Botulinum neurotoxin
C-COGS   Client-Centredness of Goal-Setting Scale
CDSM   Chronic disease self-management
COPM   Canadian Occupational Performance Measure
FAM   Functional Assessment Measure
FIM   Functional Independence Measure
G-AP   Goal setting and action planning
GAS   Goal Attainment Scaling
GIST   Group Interactive Structured Treatment
GMT   Goal Management Training
GST   Goal-setting theory
ICF   International Classification of Functioning, Disability and Health
ICF-CY   ICF-Child and Youth version
IPP   Individual program plan
MDT   Multidisciplinary team
MRC   Medical Research Council
OECD   Organization for Economic Co-operation and Development
PEDI   Pediatric Evaluation of Disability Inventory
PEGS   Perceived Efficacy and Goal-Setting System
PRPP   Perceive, Recall, Plan and Perform system
RAP   Rehabilitation Activities Profile
RCP   Royal College of Physicians
RCT   Randomized controlled trial
ReACH   Rehabilitation at community and home
RLGQ   Rivermead Life Goals Questionnaire
SADI   Self-Awareness of Deficits Interview
SF-36   Short Form-36
SIGA   Self-Identified Goal Assessment
SOC   Selective optimization and compensation
SORT   Strategies to optimize recovery
TARGET   Towards Achieving Realistic Goals in Elders Tool
TBI   Traumatic brain injury
WHO   World Health Organization
ZOE   Zielorientierte Ergebnismessung (trans. goal-oriented outcome assessment)

Acronyms

The acronyms 'SMART' and 'RUMBA' are also referred to throughout this book. Note: these are not abbreviations, but memory aids used to help remember key components of goal planning promoted by various authors. Interpretations of these acronyms differ.

One typical interpretation of the 'SMART' acronym is that it stands for specific, measurable, achievable, relevant, and time-limited goals (see Chapter 6 for many other interpretations of this acronym). Similarly, 'RUMBA' has been said to stand for relevant, understandable, measurable, behavioural, and achievable. A new acronym, 'MEANING', is also introduced in Chapter 6 of this book.

Section I

Goal Theory in Rehabilitation

1

Challenges in Theory, Practice and Evidence

William M.M. Levack and Richard J. Siegert

CONTENTS

> ... the only truly serious goals in life are learning to love other people and acquiring knowledge.
>
> **Rinpoche (2002, p. 24)**

1.1 Why a Book on Goal Setting in Rehabilitation?

The idea for writing a book on goal setting in rehabilitation grew out of our shared experiences as academics teaching postgraduate health professionals about goal setting in rehabilitation. Having worked as clinicians – one in physiotherapy (WL) and the other in clinical neuropsychology (RS) – we were both used to being part of interdisciplinary teams that *did goal setting*. However, our experience of having to actually teach health professionals about goal setting in a postgraduate programme (and one which prided itself on being *evidence based* nonetheless) led us to realize that goal setting, this emperor of rehabilitation, had no clothes.

Indeed, the more we read and searched the literature for robust evidence on the effectiveness of goal setting in rehabilitation or even a sound theory to explain how it worked and why it might be effective, the more sceptical we grew. Even the *truths* that we had been taught in our own training, such as the notion that goals should be simple, measurable, achievable, realistic and time limited (i.e. SMART), seemed to be more an act of faith than based upon any firm evidence or explicit, well-constructed theories specific to the rehabilitation context.

However, at the same time, we were struck by the fact that everywhere you looked in rehabilitation, people were busy practising goal setting both as individual therapists and as coordinated teams. Furthermore, presentations and publications on goal setting seemed to be proliferating in rehabilitation, both in conferences and journals. As researchers ourselves, we found it difficult to find a plausible control condition to compare with goal setting, because all rehabilitation services seemed to be already using goal setting in one form or another. And therein lay the puzzle that intrigued us – namely, that the self-evident usefulness of goal setting in clinical rehabilitation seemed to belie the need for robust evidence or theory to underpin it. Indeed, it is difficult to imagine delivering rehabilitation in the current day without incorporating goal setting of some kind.

So the idea for a book on rehabilitation goal setting arose from a combination of our mutual enthusiasm for goal setting as a valued clinical tool and our shared dissatisfaction with its scientific basis. We believe that if rehabilitation, as a clinical discipline, is to continue to advance and compete with other parts of the health sector for limited resources, it must be theoretically rich and have a strong evidence base. We argue that it is the integration of clinical practice with intellectually rigorous theory *development* and methodologically rigorous theory *testing* that makes the discipline scientifically based, hence the name we chose for this book – *Rehabilitation Goal Setting: Theory, Practice and Evidence*. This title reflects three strands running throughout this book: the *theories* that underpin goal setting, the different approaches to the *practice* of goal setting in the clinic and community and the *evidence* that provides the empirical foundation for rehabilitation as a profession. It is these three strands that we aimed to bring together in a single volume.

Another aim was to provide a snapshot of the *state of the art* of rehabilitation goal setting in the early twenty-first century, to provide a resource for clinicians and researchers interested in this area of practice – for we are certain that goal setting will be a focus of clinical practice and research in rehabilitation for a long time to come. Interestingly, goal setting has not always featured as such a central part of rehabilitation practice, and in the next section, we trace the rise in its prominence throughout the late twentieth century.

1.2 Origins and Development of Goal Setting in Rehabilitation

There is general agreement that goal setting is a hallmark of contemporary rehabilitation and that skills in goal setting characterize those health professionals who work in this field (Barnes & Ward, 2000; Playford et al., 2000; Wade, 2009). Goal setting is considered part of *best practice* in rehabilitation and features in rehabilitation textbooks, journals and guidelines. Yet as far as we can tell, goal setting was largely ignored or unknown in the academic rehabilitation literature until the late 1960s. This is not to say that skilful clinicians were not setting goals with patients before that time, but simply that as a process, technique or method for providing rehabilitation services to people with impairment or disabilities, there seems to have been little or no formal recognition of goal setting in rehabilitation curricula, journals or texts.

The origins of contemporary rehabilitation in the Western world can be dated back to the early 1900s, with the growth of a collective sense of social obligation to address the needs of war veterans, injured workers and children with disabilities, particularly with regard to their economic productivity and independence (Kessler, 1965; Swan, 1964). For example, Gritzer and Arnold (1985) have detailed how the specialties of orthopaedic surgery, physiotherapy and occupational therapy grew rapidly with the entry of the United States into the First World War. In comparison, the process of goal setting did not appear in the literature on rehabilitation until the late 1960s and did not really gain prominence until the 1980s. One of the earliest and most influential references to a structured approach for goal setting was a paper by Kiresuk and Sherman (1968), which described the development of goal attainment scaling (GAS) for mental health service evaluation. Within 10 years, this tool had been applied to over 90 studies, and not just within mental health rehabilitation, although its popularity was associated with 'several modifications in and deviations from the original Kiresuk and Sherman GAS model' (Cytrynbaum, Ginath, Birdwell, & Brandt, 1979, p. 34).

Despite its almost immediate popularity, GAS did not completely dominate the rehabilitation literature, and commentaries on other approaches to goal setting in clinical rehabilitation began to appear. In the nursing literature through the late 1960s and early 1970s, several authors began linking the establishment and documentation of individualized patient goals to nurse care plans (Cross & Parsons, 1971; Little & Carnevali, 1967; Sutaria, 1975; Wagner, 1969; Zimmerman & Gohrka, 1970). Around this time, nursing literature was beginning to make a distinction between identifying the objectives (or *goals*) of interventions and the tasks required to achieve those objectives (Sutaria, 1975; Wagner, 1969; Zimmerman & Gohrka, 1970). These publications, however, were not specific to clinical rehabilitation or chronic condition management and were instead presented as approaches relevant to all areas of nursing practice.

One notable example of a sophisticated theoretical approach to goal setting in clinical practice is the goal attainment theory developed and researched by King (1971, 1981). This theory has been particularly influential within nursing since the late 1970s (Alligood & Marriner, 2010; Fewster-Thuente & Velsor-Friedrich, 2008; Fredenburgh, 1993; Kline, Scott, & Britton, 2007). King's goal attainment theory places emphasis on the negotiation and attainment of goals in a clinical context, which is viewed as an open system framework. Within King's goal attainment theory, nursing is presented as a major component in the larger health system, with a key part of this role being the interpersonal processes involved in nurses' interactions with their patients. However, it is our impression that while this one notable contribution to the goal-setting literature from the nursing profession most probably had some influence on medicine and the allied health disciplines, it did not feature significantly in the interprofessional rehabilitation literature.

The development of clinical rehabilitation during the 1970s was also associated with a growing concern regarding the participation of patients in clinical decision making. Advocacy for the involvement of patients in goal selection, which was not apparent in earlier publications, including Kiresuk and Sherman's (1968) GAS paper, began to emerge. For example, by the mid-1970s, Becker, Abrams, and Onder (1974) had suggested that processes for enhancing patient participation in goal setting might improve adherence to treatment regimes, while Trieschmann (1974) linked patient participation in goal setting to ethical obligations such as working towards outcomes that were individually meaningful and valued by patients.

Importantly, during the 1970s, researchers were beginning to empirically test specific hypotheses regarding the benefits of goal setting in clinical practice. Cross and Parsons (1971) conducted a small randomized controlled trial (RCT) testing the hypothesis that if patients were directed to try to achieve goals related to selection of healthy foods from hospital menus, they would show greater change in clinically desired dietary behaviour than patients who were provided with just education or those provided with no additional intervention. However, this study concluded that while patient education had a statistically significant effect on adherence to clinically recommended dietary behaviour (at least in the short term), the addition of prespecified goals regarding daily food choices provided no further clinical benefit (Cross & Parsons, 1971).

Later in the 1970s, LaFerriere and Calsyn (1978) and Hart (1978) had more success demonstrating a link between goal setting and improvements in patient outcomes in populations of people with mental health disabilities. Both groups of authors used RCT methods to test the application of modified approaches to GAS, which involved patient participation in the selection and monitoring of goals (Hart, 1978; LaFerriere & Calsyn, 1978). Hart reported that regular discussion with patients about their progress towards individualized goals resulted in statistically significant improvements in goal achievement when compared to a control group receiving similar interventions and similar involvement in initial goal selection, but no further involvement in monitoring or evaluation of goal attainment. LaFarriere and Calsyn's study concluded that when compared to a group of control patients who received no structured goal setting, people with mental health disabilities participating in GAS as part of their therapy had more positive outcomes in terms of standardized measures of anxiety, self-esteem and depression. In their paper, LaFerriere and Calsyn began to cautiously speculate about the relationship between collaborative approaches to goal setting in clinical settings and motivation to change, suggesting that this motivation may arise from clients having 'an opportunity to determine the direction of therapy' (p. 280).

Despite the foundation provided by publications such as those described earlier, by the end of the 1970s, goal setting was still considered a relatively new concept in rehabilitation. For example, in 1978, Gaines noted that while goal-oriented treatment plans were increasingly emphasized within state and federal guidelines for occupational therapy in the United States, 'the requisite skills (had) only recently been included in occupational therapy curricula' (Gaines, 1978, p. 512). Similarly, textbooks on clinical rehabilitation still often omitted mentioning goal setting at all. For example, Howard Rusk, who has been called the 'father of rehabilitation medicine' (Kottke & Knapp, 1988, p. 4), published the fourth edition of his textbook on clinical rehabilitation in 1977 and did not mention any structured approach to integrating the assessment or setting of goals into therapeutic activities or even the need for such considerations (Rusk, 1977).

From the 1980s onwards, however, *goal setting* or *goal planning* started becoming an increasingly common component of rehabilitation programmes. Indeed any obvious trends in the literature on goal setting during this period become more difficult to determine because of the sheer number of publications on the topic. Moreover, by 1999, a postal survey conducted on behalf of the British Society for Rehabilitation Medicine identified that the majority of rehabilitation services in the United Kingdom included goal setting in their team processes on a routine basis. The survey also reported that patients and their family/carers were actively involved in the goal-setting process *wherever possible* (Turner-Stokes, Williams, Abraham, & Duckett, 2000, pp. 473–474), indicating the strength of belief regarding the importance of goal setting in rehabilitation practice.

From the mid-1990s to the present day, there has been a proliferation of papers advocating new or modified approaches to goal setting. Today, when considering how to undertake goal setting in rehabilitation, clinicians can select from a wide range of potential approaches including

- GAS (Kiresuk & Sherman, 1968)
- Canadian Occupational Performance Measure (COPM) (Pendleton & Schultz-Krohn, 2005; Phipps & Richardson, 2007; Trombly, Radomski, Trexel, & Burnet-Smith, 2002; Wressle, Eeg-Olofsson, Marcusson, & Henriksson, 2002; Wressle, Lindstrand, Neher, Marcusson, & Henriksson, 2003)

- *SMART* goal planning* (Barnes & Ward, 2000; Mastos, Miller, Eliasson, & Imms, 2007; McLellan, 1997; Monaghan, Channell, McDowell, & Sharma, 2005; Schut & Stam, 1994)
- *RUMBA* goal planning, an acronym said to stand for goals which are *r*elevant, *u*nderstandable, *m*easurable, *b*ehavioural and *a*chievable (Barnett, 1999)
- Self-identified goal assessment (SIGA) (Melville, Baltic, Bettcher, & Nelson, 2002)
- Goal management training (GMT) (Levine et al., 2000)
- The Rivermead life goals questionnaire (RLGQ) and approaches to goal planning from Rivermead Rehabilitation Centre (McGrath & Davis, 1992; McGrath, Marks, & Davis, 1995; Nair & Wade, 2003; Wade, 1999a)
- Approaches to goal planning from the Wolfson Neurorehabilitation Centre (McMillan & Sparkes, 1999)
- Contractually organized goal setting (Powell, Heslin, & Greenwood, 2002)
- Collaborative goal technology (Clarke, Oades, Crowe, & Deane, 2006)
- Progressive Goal Attainment Programme (Sullivan, Adams, Rhodenizer, & Stanish, 2006)
- Patient-centred functional goal planning (Randall & McEwen, 2000)
- Goal setting based on the Patient Goal Priority Questionnaire or Patient Goal Priority List (Åsenlöf & Silijebäck, 2009)
- The TARGET approach to goal setting, an acronym for *Towards Achieving Realistic Goal for Elders Tool* (Parsons & Parsons, 2012)

Along with this great diversity of approaches evident in current rehabilitation practice, some other trends that we have observed in the recent literature include the following:

1. Increasing recognition that goal-setting practice can and must differ from one clinical environment to another (e.g. Playford et al., 2000).
2. Increasing evidence that goal-setting practice in the *real world* of rehabilitation does not always match the ideology, idealism or rhetoric being promoted. For example, patients are not always involved in goal setting to the degree that health professional believe they should be, with complex organizational and sociological issues impeding on implementation of the ideology of person-centred goal setting (e.g. Baker, Marshak, Rice, & Zimmerman, 2001; Barnard, Cruice, & Playford, 2010; Brown et al., 2013; Levack, Dean, Siegert, & McPherson, 2011; Nijhuis et al., 2008; Parry, 2004).
3. The emergence of interest in theory-based research on goal setting in rehabilitation (Scobbie, Wyke, & Dixon, 2009; Siegert, McPherson, & Taylor, 2004; Siegert & Taylor, 2004).

However, while goal setting and research on goal setting has flourished in rehabilitation, opinions still vary considerably over exactly how it should be practised (Playford, Siegert,

---

* To our knowledge, the first published reference to *SMART* goals in health science literature was by Schut and Stam (1994), but the earliest ever published version of *SMART* goals appeared in a management journal 13 years prior to this (Doran, 1981). If you search the Internet for the origins of the SMART acronym however, you will find that its full history is somewhat unclear.

Levack, & Freeman, 2009). In the next section, we briefly summarize the major ways that approaches to goal setting, as presented in the current literature, can differ from one another.

1.3 Major Differences in Approaches to Goal Setting

While the different approaches to goal setting frequently include a number of common features such as the need for goals to be measurable or the need for patients to be involved in goal selection, few features are common to all recommended approaches. Goals arising from the COPM, for example, do not necessarily need to be measurable in the same way that, say, SMART goals or GAS goals need to be measurable because outcomes with the COPM are evaluated by a patient's self-rating of their own performance and satisfaction with respect to their goals on separate 10-point scales (Law et al., 2005). Indeed, most approaches to goal setting in rehabilitation differ on a number of variables including:

1. The professional group (or groups) intended to use the approach
2. The intended patient population for the approach
3. The process by which goals are selected
4. The recommended characteristics of the goals set
5. The recommended content of goals set (i.e. what is considered an acceptable topic for a goal)
6. The intended purpose or function of using the approach

1. *Professional group*: Some of the published approaches to goal setting are intended for use in an *interdisciplinary* context (Barnes & Ward, 2000; McMillan & Sparkes, 1999; Schut & Stam, 1994; Wade, 1999a), while others are presented as profession specific. The COPM (Carswell et al., 2004) and the SIGA (Melville et al., 2002) were designed for use by occupational therapists. The COPM in particular was developed initially as a measurement tool, to assist occupational therapists with implementation of the Canadian Model of Occupational Performance in their clinical practice (Carswell et al., 2004), and later described as an approach to goal setting (Pendleton & Schultz-Krohn, 2005; Phipps & Richardson, 2007; Sewell, Singh, Williams, Collier, & Morgan, 2005; Trombly et al., 2002). The emphasis on occupational therapy is reflected in the recommended content of goals resulting from the COPM, with a requirement that goals fit within specific occupational domains (in particular, self-care, productivity and leisure). Instructions regarding the use of the COPM discourage the selection of goals that relate solely to impairments of body structure or body function (Law et al., 2005). Similarly, Randall and McEwen (2000) described an approach to goal setting tailored specifically for use by physiotherapists.

2. *Patient population*: GMT is an example of an approach to goal planning that has been designed specifically for use with people rehabilitating from brain injury (Levine et al., 2000). The aim of GMT is to teach people with brain injury to compensate for disorganized behaviour resulting from goal neglect (a cognitive impairment associated with frontal lobe damage). GMT therefore focuses mainly on problems with executive functioning (Alfonso, Caracuel, Delgado-Pastor, & Verdejo-García,

2011; Levine et al., 2000, 2011; van Hooren et al., 2007). Bergquist and Jacket (1993) also described an approach to goal setting that addresses the perceived needs of people with traumatic brain injury. Their approach, however, focused on assisting patients with brain injury to acknowledge and address impaired self-awareness. Other published papers have described goal-setting approaches that have been tailored for different populations of people: for example, those with stroke (Wade, 1999a), spinal injury (Kennedy, Walker, & White, 1991) and mental health illnesses (Clarke et al., 2006; MacPherson, Jerrom, Lott, & Ryce, 1999).

3. *Goal-setting process*: There is considerable variation across recommended approaches to goal setting in terms of the process by which goals are set. For example, for approaches that emphasize person-centredness in goal setting, such as the COPM and SIGA, patient involvement in goal selection is considered an integral part (Carswell et al., 2004; Melville et al., 2002). For other approaches, patient involvement in goal selection may be considered desirable but not necessarily essential (Conneeley, 2004; Rockwood, Joyce, & Stolee, 1997), and alternatives (such as family involvement in goal selection) may be recommended in circumstances where patients are unable to independently participate in the goal selection process (Law et al., 2005; Randall & McEwen, 2000; Wade, 1999b).

   For approaches to goal setting that centre on enhancing teamwork, greater levels of consultation with multiple parties are often advised, with formal meetings to coordinate information and perspectives from the various health professionals, family members and other stakeholders involved (McGrath et al., 1995; McMillan & Sparkes, 1999; Wade, 1999a). In contrast to this, there is some suggestion that for particular types of goal setting in particular contexts, having an authority figure (e.g. a health professional) select a goal on behalf of a third party (e.g. a patient) can have positive effects in terms of that person's effort and attention resulting in higher levels of performance on selected tasks (Gauggel & Hoop, 2004).

4. *Recommended characteristics of a goal*: Different authors emphasize different features when describing what might constitute a *good* goal. The GAS approach requires stated goals to be objective so that a third party (a health professional) can judge whether the patient has reached a prespecified level of goal achievement (Bovend'Eerdt, Botell, & Wade, 2009; Turner-Stokes, 2008). As mentioned previously, such operationalization of the goal itself is not required in the COPM because patients self-rate their outcomes on a separate 10-point scale (Law et al., 2005).

   Other recommended characteristics of goals, according to various authors, include (but are not limited to) the following: specific, realistic or achievable, relevant to the patient, motivating, challenging or difficult, written in language understood by the patient, time limited or time specific and/or broken down into short- and long-term goals. We can also add to this a whole range of other factors that could possibly influence the process or outcome of goal setting: the impact of leadership styles on goal setting within team contexts, the impact of different types of feedback on future goal-oriented behaviour (e.g. positively framed vs. negatively framed feedback; written/visual feedback vs. informal/oral feedback), the impact of making public statements of commitments to goals in group situations versus keeping goals private, and so forth.

   It is interesting to note that even within specific, named approaches to goal planning, there can be lack of agreement regarding the key features of what should constitute a *good* rehabilitation goal. For example, while the *SMART* approach to goal planning is commonly promoted in the rehabilitation literature (Barnes & Ward, 2000; Mastos et al., 2007; Monaghan et al., 2005; Schut & Stam, 1994), there appears to be a diverse number of interpretations about precisely what this acronym stands for. Schut and Stam (1994) have stated that the *SMART* acronym refers to goals that are *s*pecific, *m*otivating, *a*ttainable, *r*ational and *t*imed. Alternatively, McLellan (1997) used this acronym to emphasize that goals should be *s*pecific, *m*easurable, *a*ctivity-related, *r*ealistic and *t*ime specific, while Barnes and Ward (2000) preferred *s*pecific, *m*easurable, *a*chievable, *r*elevant and *t*ime limited. Almost every year, a slightly different version of the SMART acronym seems to get published. In Marsland and Bowman's (2010) recent version, the *A* in SMART referred to *activity-based*, while the *R* referred to *review*.

5. *Recommended content of goals*: While some authors place no restrictions on the preferred subject of rehabilitation goals, others are quite explicit about what rehabilitation goals should be about. Randall and McEwen (2000), for instance, recommended that all goals set by physiotherapists focus on what they call 'functional limitations and disabilities that are individually meaningful to patients' (p. 1198), specifically excluding impairments of body structure and body function from being the 'measured goals of therapy' (p. 1198). Similarly, as mentioned earlier, the COPM requires the content of goals to be on topics relating to specific occupational domains: self-care, productivity and leisure (Law et al., 2005). Likewise, Marsland and Bowman (2010) recommended restricting the subject of goals to activities that people wish to be able to perform.

6. *Purpose or function of using the approach*: Goal setting is used in rehabilitation for a number of very different purposes. Our own initial review identified four main purposes: goal setting can be used for (1) improving clinical outcomes, (2) evaluating outcomes, (3) enhancing patient/client autonomy and (4) meeting contractual, legislative or professional requirements (Levack, Dean, Siegert, & McPherson, 2006). Regarding the first of these purposes, there are a range of hypothesized ways that rehabilitation goals, or the process of goal setting, could function to improve clinical outcomes. These include improving the patients' *motivation* to engage and work hard in therapeutic activities, improving *teamwork* within interprofessional rehabilitation teams (improving communication and collaboration within teams and providing a shared direction), assisting patients to *psychologically adapt* to newly acquired disability, enhancing the *specificity of training* of therapy (e.g. focusing therapy on stair climbing in people who need to be able to navigate steps in order to safely return home after a hospital admission) and enhancing the working relationship between patients, families and health professional (e.g. through development of a shared language and shared understanding of a health condition) (Levack, Dean, Siegert et al., 2006; Levack, Dean, McPherson, & Siegert, 2006).

1.4 Definitions of Some Key Terms

Sixteen years ago, Professor Derick Wade noted that the problem for rehabilitation was the lack of any accepted or consistent vocabulary for talking about goal setting in rehabilitation (Wade, 1998). It is our impression as regular readers of the goal setting literature that things have not improved a great deal since then. It is important therefore to consider some of the major terms used in the field and to offer some working definitions from the outset. This issue of terminology and nomenclature in goal setting has important implications because of the interprofessional nature of rehabilitation. For example, rehabilitation has drawn heavily upon psychology for theoretical models to understand and justify goal setting despite the fact that the very word *goal* can have quite a different meaning in the two disciplines.

In their benchmark review of the psychology literature on goals, Austin and Vancouver (1996) defined goals as 'internal representations of desired states, where states are broadly construed as outcomes, events, or processes' (p. 338). In other words, a goal is a mental representation, something that cannot be directly observed and that exists only in the mind or neural networks of an individual. This is obviously not a very useful definition of a goal for a busy team of health professionals working with individual patients who are trying to rebuild their lives after disabling illnesses or injury.

Recently, for the purposes of a Cochrane review, we developed revised definitions of the key terms used in rehabilitation goal setting (Levack et al., 2012). These definitions are presented in Box 1.1. We do not offer these definitions lightly, as others have provided working definitions of the terms *goals* and *goal setting* in the past (Playford et al., 2000; Randall & McEwen, 2000; Wade, 1998). However, we believe these revised definitions provide a necessary refinement of the way certain terms should be conceptualized in rehabilitation. Underpinning our thinking here are several principles. First, we argue there is a need to make a distinction between goal terminology within a rehabilitation context and the way these terms are used in other contexts (such as the psychology literature,

---

BOX 1.1 DEFINITIONS OF KEY TERMS

Rehabilitation goal:

A desired future state to be achieved by a person with a disability as a result of rehabilitation activities. Rehabilitation goals are actively selected, intentionally created, have purpose and are shared (where possible) by the people participating in the activities and interventions designed to address the consequence of acquired disability.

Goal setting or goal planning:

The establishment or negotiation of rehabilitation goals.

Goal pursuit:

Activities beyond the selection of rehabilitation goals that are implemented in order to enhance the level of goal attainment or to maximize a person's likelihood of achieving a particular rehabilitation goal. These activities include (but are not limited to) the following: development of a plan or strategy to achieve stated rehabilitation goals, provision of explicit feedback (oral or written) on a person's progress towards their rehabilitation goals and use of strategies to maintain or enhance commitment to set goals (such as peer discussion of progress towards an individual's rehabilitation goals or use of posters and electronic diaries reminding people about their rehabilitation goals).

which takes a much broader perspective on which might be considered a *goal*). As a consequence, we provide a definition of the term *rehabilitation goal* and not a definition of the term *goal*, and we have couched this definition within the context of clinical practice in a rehabilitation environment.

Second, while we have endeavoured to incorporate within these definitions common features of the concepts of *goals* and *goal setting* as they are usually understood in rehabilitation, we have kept these definitions sufficiently open as to exclude value judgements regarding the *right* way of setting goals. For instance, within our definition of the term *rehabilitation goal*, we have been intentionally circumspect regarding the level of patient involvement in selection of those goals, acknowledging the reality that in some clinical contexts such patient involvement is not always possible, even if it is desirable. Likewise, we have not included within our definition the requirement for rehabilitation goals to be objective or measurable, as it is possible that these characteristics are not essential features of all forms of rehabilitation goal setting. Some types of goals, those to do with spiritual health or interpersonal relationships, for instance, are not immediately conducive to quantification.

Third, within our definitions, we have differentiated between the concepts of *goal setting* and *goal pursuit*. Goal-related activities in rehabilitation span the whole continuum of service delivery from admission, to implementation of treatment, to evaluation of progress and outcome. It is important to make a distinction between those activities that come nearer the start of the rehabilitation process (the negotiation and selection of goals for intervention) and those activities related to the application of goals for the purposes of rehabilitation planning, coordination of team work and engagement of people with disabilities and their families in the delivery of rehabilitation interventions.

There are two other terms related to goal setting in rehabilitation that are common in the literature, but which we have chosen not to define. These are the terms *short-term goal* and *long-term goal* (sometimes also called *proximal* and *distal* goals). We have chosen not to define these terms because they are used by several of the authors in the present text in different ways and their precise definition can vary depending on the type of goal setting used and the context. For example, the phrase *long-term goal* can mean very different things in an inpatient setting compared to an outpatient setting. It can refer to goals set for review at a particular time frame (e.g. after 3 months), a goal to be achieved by discharge from a particular service, a goal set at particularly high level of abstraction (e.g. a *life goal*) or some combination of all of these. Hence, we will not define these terms here and will instead leave the details of these definitions up to individual rehabilitation services to best meet their local purpose.

1.5 Basic Introduction to Goal Setting

This book contains a number of detailed discussions of different ways to undertake goal setting and many challenges as to what might be considered the status quo of goal setting in everyday, mainstream rehabilitation practice. For the novice reader, some of this content may appear far more complex than is easily applied to his or her clinical work. The following, therefore, is a brief description of one pragmatic method for the selection and documentation of rehabilitation goals that can be used by any health professional in pretty much any context. This is goal setting without the bells and whistles!

As stated in our definition, rehabilitation goals describe a desired future state to be achieved by a person with a disability as a result of rehabilitation activities. Because we, as rehabilitation clinicians, are most interested in how to help people function meaningfully in the world, rehabilitation goals typically are set at the level of activities they might be able to do (e.g. dressing oneself, walking to the bus stop, kicking a ball with school friends, writing a shopping list) or life roles that they might be able to participate in (e.g. returning to live at home with one's spouse and returning to work). In general, these goals are formulated by the rehabilitation team in negotiation with their patients, with involvement of the significant other people in their lives (e.g. family members, friends, employers) where appropriate.

Goal formulation is usually preceded by clinical assessment of patients (e.g. assessment of health status, pathology, functional abilities and limitations) and information gathered about their usual life contexts (e.g. their living or working environments, their personal values, their degree of expectation and motivation). This information is used by the rehabilitation professionals to predict what might be a reasonable range of outcomes to work towards, so that they can discuss with the patient what they might be able offer in terms of therapy.

If the period of therapy is anticipated to be long and the intervention complex, rehabilitation professionals may discuss with patients the setting of one or two goals to be achieved by the end of the duration of formal rehabilitation (i.e. *long-term goals*), with other shorter-term goals representing the necessary steps to achieve along the way. While, as mentioned previously, the *topic* of goals is selected on the basis of what is likely to be most meaningful to the individual patient, rehabilitation goals themselves are usually converted into some type of standardized format according to the rehabilitation teams' preferences. Often this involves making the goal more objective or fit with what the clinicians believe they can provide. For example, if an elderly woman after internal fixation of a fractured neck of femur states that her goal is to 'make my leg strong again', her health professional may ask: 'what do you want to be able to do once your leg is strong again?' The answer to this question (the activity the person ultimately wants to return to performing) might then become the subject of the goal setting, rather than the goal simply being about restoration of muscle strength.

Importantly, for any rehabilitation team, there is a strong need to make a distinction between rehabilitation goals that will be achieved as a result of therapy and the clinical tasks that the health professionals will undertake in order to achieve those goals. While this is a very basic requirement, it is a common mistake made by health professionals who have had little training in rehabilitation goal setting. For instance, one easy error to make when developing a goal plan would be to state that one rehabilitation goal is 'to complete a home visit within three weeks from admission'. In an inpatient environment, this is an activity that the rehabilitation team *knows* will occur, because it is something they are required to do prior to discharging the patient from their service. It is a *task* for the clinical team, not a rehabilitation goal as described in our aforementioned definition.

One simple method for formulating rehabilitation goals that addresses this problem and which provides a standardized method for teams to follow when developing rehabilitation plans is that provided by Randall and McEwen (2000). While Randall and McEwen's approach to goal setting was written primarily with a physical therapy audience in mind, it is a method which can be easily adapted for use by other health professionals and one that we recommend beginning with when running introductory workshops on goal setting for health professionals new to clinical rehabilitation.

Randall and McEwen (2000) recommended that all documented goals should include information to answer the following five questions: who, will do what, under what conditions, how well and by when? According to these authors, the 'Who?' of the goal should always be the patient. (This goes a long way to addressing the error of health professionals documenting clinical tasks rather than goals when formulating rehabilitation plans.) The question 'Will do what?' refers to the activity or health state that the patient will be to be able to carry out or achieve on completion of therapy. The question 'Under what conditions?' provides an opportunity to include information about the environmental context under which the activity is to be performed. For example, the objective of achieving independence with wheelchair mobility is quite different if referring to mobilizing within a well-designed rehabilitation hospital than if referring to mobilizing outside on city streets. The documented rehabilitation goal should make these kinds of details explicit.

The quality of performance expected from patients is captured by the question: 'How well?' For instance, this might refer to the speed of performance, or the number of attempts permitted, or the degree of additional assistance required (from another person or from assistive technology) before successful completion of the task is possible. Finally, the question 'By when?' refers to a time frame within which the goal is to be reached (or re-evaluated).

To illustrate how this approach can be applied to goals relevant to the work of a range of different members of an interprofessional team, a case study with hypothetical examples of rehabilitation goals is presented in Table 1.1. Please note: this table is not intended as a

TABLE 1.1

Case Study Example of Basic Rehabilitation Goals

Background

Paul is a 68-year-old man who suffered a dense stroke affecting the right side of his brain. On admission to the rehabilitation unit, Paul's main problems include being unable to sit on the edge of his bed unaided and being unable to stand, wash or dress without the assistance of two people. Paul has had some problems with urinary incontinence, but this seems to be mainly due to his problems with mobility and a reluctance to ask for help. He also has had difficulty with swallowing and is on thickened fluids to prevent aspiration. Furthermore, his recent stroke has motivated him to quit smoking, and he wants to get help for this while still in the hospital.

Breakdown of goals

Profession	Who?	Will Do What?	Under What Conditions?	How Well?	By When?
Nursing	Paul	Be continent	With assistance of one nurse to access the toilet	Without any episodes of accidental wetting	Within 2 weeks
Physiotherapy	Paul	Walk 20 m	Indoors	With assistance of one person for balance	Within 4 weeks
Occupational therapy	Paul	Dress his upper and lower body	Using a handrail to help with standing	Independently	Within 2 weeks
Speech–language therapy	Paul	Drink	Thin fluids	Without any episodes of choking	Within 4 weeks
Social worker/ counsellor	Paul	Quit smoking	With the aid of nicotine patches	With no relapses	By 4 weeks

Formulation of Paul's initial goals for his rehabilitation plan

- Paul will be fully continent, with no episodes of wetting, with assistance to access the toilet as needed, within 2 weeks.
- Paul will walk 20 m indoors, with the assistance of one person for balance, within 4 weeks.
- Paul will dress both his upper and lower body independently, using a handrail to help with standing, within 2 weeks.
- Paul will be able to drink thin fluids without any episodes of choking within 4 weeks.
- Paul will quit smoking with the aid of nicotine patches, with no smoking relapses for 4 weeks.

format for documenting goals in rehabilitation plans. Indeed, ideally rehabilitation goals in an interprofessional rehabilitation plan ought to be shared by all members of the clinical team rather than allocated to individual professional groups. However, we have included this table just to show how different types of goal can be constructed following the format outlined by Randall and McEwen (2000).

1.6 Overview of the Book

In the 19 chapters comprising this book, we hope that the reader will find a rich and comprehensive range of topics on goal setting in rehabilitation. While the various contributing authors have been ultimately responsible for the content of their respective chapters, as editors, we have strived to produce a text with certain features that we consider will reflect important characteristics of rehabilitation itself. First, as highlighted at the beginning of this chapter, we aimed to write a book that emphasizes the theory, the practice and the research on rehabilitation goal setting and the integration of these three components. In this regard, some chapters are more concerned with one or other of these three topics. Increasingly in rehabilitation, we are seeing theory-driven research and greater emphasis on translating research findings into everyday clinical practice. We hope that this book will further progress this trend.

Second, we have attempted to produce a book in which the contributors reflect the interprofessional nature of modern rehabilitation. The contributors include representatives from neurology, nursing, occupational therapy, physiotherapy, psychology, rehabilitation medicine and speech–language therapy. Third, the book reflects the international nature of rehabilitation with contributors from Australia, Canada, Germany, Great Britain, New Zealand, Switzerland and the United States. Fourth, the book represents the diverse range of conditions that require rehabilitation and the importance of rehabilitation throughout the human lifespan. Thus, along with chapters on goal setting for people after traumatic brain injury and stroke, there are two chapters on goal setting with children and one on older adults receiving community-based homecare.

The fifth characteristic of modern rehabilitation goal setting reflected in this book is the sheer diversity of its application. As we are sure you will agree upon reading this text, rehabilitation goal setting should no longer be considered one beast – that there is only one *right* way of setting goals in rehabilitation. Instead the plurality of approaches to goal setting is evident throughout. Readers, we hope, will find they can be selective when taking content from this book – that they can learn from the knowledge provided by the authors of this text to implement an evidenced-based, theory-rich approach to goal setting specifically tailored to meet the needs of the people in their own rehabilitation practice.

References

Alfonso, J. P., Caracuel, A., Delgado-Pastor, L. C., & Verdejo-García, A. (2011). Combined goal management training and mindfulness meditation improve executive functions and decision-making performance in abstinent polysubstance abusers. *Drug and Alcohol Dependence*, 117(1), 78–81.

Alligood, M. R., & Marriner, T. A. (Eds.). (2010). *Nursing theorists and their work* (7th ed.). Maryland Heights, MO: Mosby/Elsevier.

Åsenlöf, P., & Silijebäck, K. (2009). Goal priority questionnaire is moderately reproducible in people with persistent musculoskeletal pain. *Physical Therapy, 89*, 1226–1234.

Austin, J. T., & Vancouver, J. B. (1996). Goal constructs in psychology: Structure, process and content. *Psychological Bulletin, 120*(3), 338–375.

Baker, S. M., Marshak, H. H., Rice, G. T., & Zimmerman, G. J. (2001). Patient participation in physical therapy goal setting. *Physical Therapy, 81*(5), 1118–1126.

Barnard, R. A., Cruice, M. N., & Playford, E. D. (2010). Strategies used in the pursuit of achievability during goal setting in rehabilitation. *Qualitative Health Research, 20*(2), 239–250.

Barnes, M. P., & Ward, A. B. (2000). *Textbook of rehabilitation medicine.* Oxford, U.K.: Oxford University Press.

Barnett, D. (1999). The rehabilitation nurse as educator. In M. Smith (Ed.), *Rehabilitation in adult nursing practice* (pp. 53–76). Edinburgh, Scotland: Churchill Livingstone.

Becker, M. C., Abrams, K. S., & Onder, J. (1974). Goal setting: A joint patient-staff method. *Archives of Physical Medicine & Rehabilitation, 55*, 87–89.

Bergquist, T. F., & Jacket, M. P. (1993). Awareness and goal setting with the traumatically brain injured. *Brain Injury, 7*, 275–282.

Bovend'Eerdt, T. J. H., Botell, R. E., & Wade, D. T. (2009). Writing SMART rehabilitation goals and achieving goal attainment scaling: A practical guide. *Clinical Rehabilitation, 23*, 352–361.

Brown, M., Levack, W., McPherson, K. M., Dean, S. G., Reed, K., Weatherall, M., & Taylor, W. J. (2013). Survival, momentum, and things that make me 'me': Patients' perceptions of goal setting after stroke. *Disability & Rehabilitation,* [Early Online], 1–7.

Carswell, A., McColl, M. A., Baptiste, S., Law, M., Polatajko, H., & Pollock, N. (2004). The Canadian Occupational Performance Measure: A research and clinical literature review. *The Canadian Journal of Occupational Therapy, 71*(4), 210–222.

Clarke, S. P., Oades, L. G., Crowe, T. P., & Deane, F. P. (2006). Collaborative goal technology: Theory and practice. *Psychiatric Rehabilitation Journal, 30*(2), 129–136.

Conneeley, A. L. (2004). Interdisciplinary collaborative goal planning in a post-acute neurological setting: A qualitative study. *British Journal of Occupational Therapy, 67*(6), 248–255.

Cross, J. E., & Parsons, C. R. (1971). Nurse-teaching and goal-directed nurse-teaching to motivate change in food selection behavior of hospitalized patients. *Nursing Research, 20*(5), 454–458.

Cytrynbaum, S., Ginath, Y., Birdwell, J., & Brandt, L. (1979). Goal attainment scaling: A critical review. *Evaluation Quarterly, 3*(1), 5–40.

Doran, G. (1981). There's a S.M.A.R.T way to write management's goals and objectives. *Management Review, 70*(11), 35–36.

Fewster-Thuente, L., & Velsor-Friedrich, B. (2008). Interdisciplinary collaboration for healthcare professionals. *Nursing Administration Quarterly, 32*(1), 40–48.

Fredenburgh, L. (1993). *The effect of mutual goal setting on stress reduction in the community mental health client* (Master's thesis). D'Youville College, New York, NY.

Gaines, B. J. (1978). Goal-oriented treatment plans and behavioural analysis. *American Journal of Occupational Therapy, 32*(8), 512–516.

Gauggel, S., & Hoop, M. (2004). Goal-setting as a motivational technique for neurorehabilitation. In W. M. Cox & E. Klinger (Eds.), *Handbook of motivational counseling* (pp. 493–456). West Sussex, U.K.: John Wiley & Sons.

Gritzer, G., & Arluke, A. (1985). *The making of rehabilitation: A political economy of medical specialization, 1890–1980.* Berkeley, CA: University of California Press.

Hart, R. R. (1978). Therapeutic effectiveness of setting and monitoring goals. *Journal of Consulting and Clinical Psychology, 46*(6), 1242–1245.

Kennedy, P., Walker, L., & White, D. (1991). Ecological evaluation of goal planning and advocacy in a rehabilitation environment for spinal cord injured people. *Paraplegia, 29*, 197–202.

Kessler, H. H. (1965). Rehabilitation: Prospect and retrospect. *Rehabilitation Literature, 26*(6), 162–168.

King, I. M. (1971). *Toward a theory for nursing: General concepts of human behavior.* New York, NY: Wiley.

King, I. M. (1981). *A theory for nursing: Systems, concepts, process.* New York, NY: Wiley.

Kiresuk, T., & Sherman, R. (1968). Goal attainment scaling: A general method for evaluating community health programs. *Community Mental Health Journal, 4,* 443–453.

Kline, K. S., Scott, L. D., & Britton, A. S. (2007). The use of supportive-educative and mutual goal-setting strategies to improve self-management for patients with heart failure. *Home Healthcare Nurse, 25*(8), 502–510.

Kottke, F. J., & Knapp, M. E. (1988). The development of physiatry before 1950. *Archives of Physical Medicine & Rehabilitation, 69 Spec,* 4–14.

LaFerriere, L., & Calsyn, R. (1978). Goal attainment scaling: An effective treatment technique in short-term therapy. *American Journal of Community Psychology, 6*(3), 271–282.

Law, M., Baptiste, S., Carswell, A., McColl, M. A., Polatajko, H., & Pollock, N. (2005). *Canadian occupational performance measure* (4th ed.). Ottawa, Ontario, Canada: CAOT Publications ACE.

Levack, W. M. M., Dean, S., Siegert, R. J., & McPherson, K. M. (2006). Purposes and mechanisms of goal planning in rehabilitation: The need for a critical distinction. *Disability & Rehabilitation, 28*(12), 741–749.

Levack, W. M. M., Dean, S. G., McPherson, K. M., & Siegert, R. J. (2006). How clinicians talk about the application of goal planning to rehabilitation for people with brain injury-variable interpretations of value and purpose. *Brain Injury, 20*(13–14), 1439–1449.

Levack, W. M. M., Dean, S. G., Siegert, R. J., & McPherson, K. M. (2011). Navigating patient-centered goal setting in inpatient stroke rehabilitation: How clinicians control the process to meet perceived professional responsibilities. *Patient Education & Counseling, 85*(2), 206–213.

Levack, W. M. M., Siegert, R. J., Dean, S. G., McPherson, K., Hay-Smith, E. J. C., & Weatherall, M. (2012). Goal setting and activities to enhance goal pursuit for adults with acquired disabilities participating in rehabilitation. *Cochrane Database of Systematic Reviews,* Issue 4, Art. No.: CD009727. doi:10.1002/14651858.CD009727

Levine, B., Robertson, I. H., Clare, L., Carter, G., Hong, J., Wilson, B. A., … Stuss, D. T. (2000). Rehabilitation of executive functioning: An experimental–clinical validation of goal management training. *Journal of the International Neuropsychological Society, 6*(3), 299–312.

Levine, B., Schweizer, T. A., O'Connor, C., Turner, G., Gillingham, S., Stuss, D. T., … Robertson, I. H. (2011). Rehabilitation of executive functioning in patients with frontal lobe brain damage with goal management training. *Frontiers in Human Neuroscience, 5,* 9.

Little, D., & Carnevali, D. (1967). Nursing care plans: Let's be practical about them. *Nursing Forum, 6*(1), 61–76.

MacPherson, R., Jerrom, B., Lott, G., & Ryce, M. (1999). The outcome of clinical goal setting in a mental health rehabilitation service: A model for evaluating clinical effectiveness. *Journal of Mental Health, 8*(1), 95–102.

Marsland, E., & Bowman, J. (2010). An interactive education session and follow-up support as a strategy to improve clinicians' goal-writing skills: A randomized controlled trial. *Journal of Evaluation in Clinical Practice, 16,* 3–13.

Mastos, M., Miller, K., Eliasson, A. C., & Imms, C. (2007). Goal-directed training: Linking theories of treatment to clinical practice for improved functional activities in daily life. *Clinical Rehabilitation, 21,* 47–55.

McGrath, J. R., & Davis, A. M. (1992). Rehabilitation: Where are we going and how do we get there? *Clinical Rehabilitation, 6,* 225–235.

McGrath, J. R., Marks, J. A., & Davis, A. M. (1995). Towards interdisciplinary rehabilitation: Further developments at Rivermead Rehabilitation Centre. *Clinical Rehabilitation, 9,* 320–326.

McLellan, D. L. (1997). Introduction to rehabilitation. In B. A. Wilson & D. L. McLellan (Eds.), *Rehabilitation studies handbook* (pp. 1–20). Cambridge, U.K.: Cambridge University Press.

McMillan, T. M., & Sparkes, C. (1999). Goal planning and neurorehabilitation: The Wolfson Neurorehabilitation Centre approach. *Neuropsychological Rehabilitation, 9*(3/4), 241–251.

Melville, L. L., Baltic, T. A., Bettcher, T. W., & Nelson, D. L. (2002). Patients' perspectives on the self-identified goals assessment. *American Journal of Occupational Therapy, 56*(6), 650–659.

Monaghan, J., Channell, K., McDowell, D., & Sharma, A. (2005). Improving patient and carer communication, multidisciplinary team working and goal-setting in stroke rehabilitation. *Clinical Rehabilitation, 19*(2), 194–199.

Nair, K. P. S., & Wade, D. T. (2003). Changes in life goals of people with neurological disabilities. *Clinical Rehabilitation, 17,* 797–803.

Nijhuis, B. J. G., Reinders-Messelink, H. A., de Blécourt, A. C. E., Boonstra, A. M., Calamé, E. H. M., Groothof, J. W., ... Postema, K. (2008). Goal setting in Dutch paediatric rehabilitation. Are the needs and principal problems of children with cerebral palsy integrated into their rehabilitation goals? *Clinical Rehabilitation, 22,* 348–363.

Parry, R. H. (2004). Communication during goal-setting in physiotherapy treatment sessions. *Clinical Rehabilitation, 18*(6), 668–682.

Parsons, J. G. M., & Parsons, M. J. G. (2012). The effect of a designated tool on person-centred goal identification and service planning among older people receiving homecare in New Zealand. *Health & Social Care in the Community, 20*(6), 653–662.

Pendleton, H. M., & Schultz-Krohn, W. (Eds.). (2005). *Pedretti's occupational therapy practice skills for physical dysfunction* (6th ed.). St. Louis, MO: Mosby/Elsevier.

Phipps, S., & Richardson, P. (2007). Occupational therapy outcomes for clients with traumatic brain injury and stroke using the Canadian Occupational Performance Measure. *American Journal of Occupational Therapy, 61*(3), 328–334.

Playford, E. D., Dawson, L., Limbert, V., Smith, M., Ward, C. D., & Wells, R. (2000). Goal-setting in rehabilitation: Report of a workshop to explore professionals' perceptions of goal-setting. *Clinical Rehabilitation, 14*(5), 491–496.

Playford, E. D., Siegert, R. J., Levack, W., & Freeman, J. (2009). Areas of consensus and disagreement about goal-setting in rehabilitation: A conference report. *Clinical Rehabilitation, 23,* 334–344.

Powell, J., Heslin, J., & Greenwood, R. (2002). Community based rehabilitation after severe traumatic brain injury: A randomised controlled trial. *Journal of Neurology, Neurosurgery & Psychiatry, 72*(2), 193–202.

Randall, K. E., & McEwen, I. R. (2000). Writing patient-centered functional goals. *Physical Therapy, 80*(12), 1197–1203.

Rinpoche, S. (2002). *The Tibetan book of living and dying* (Rev. ed.). Pymble, New South Wales, Australia: HarperCollins Publishers.

Rockwood, K., Joyce, B., & Stolee, P. (1997). Use of goal attainment scaling in measuring clinically important change in cognitive rehabilitation patients. *Journal of Clinical Epidemiology, 50*(5), 581–588.

Rusk, H. A. (1977). *Rehabilitation medicine* (4th ed.). Saint Louis, MO: The C.V. Mosby Company.

Schut, H. A., & Stam, H. J. (1994). Goals in rehabilitation teamwork. *Disability & Rehabilitation, 16*(4), 223–226.

Scobbie, L., Wyke, S., & Dixon, D. (2009). Identifying and applying psychological theory to setting and achieving rehabilitation goals. *Clinical Rehabilitation, 23,* 321–333.

Sewell, L., Singh, S. J., Williams, J. E. A., Collier, R., & Morgan, M. D. L. (2005). Can individualized rehabilitation improve functional independence in elderly patients with COPD? *Chest, 128,* 1194–1200.

Siegert, R. J., McPherson, K. M., & Taylor, W. (2004). Toward a cognitive-affective model of goal-setting in rehabilitation: Is self-regulation theory a key step? *Disability & Rehabilitation, 26*(20), 1175–1183.

Siegert, R. J., & Taylor, W. J. (2004). Theoretical aspects of goal-setting and motivation in rehabilitation. *Disability & Rehabilitation, 26*(1), 1–8.

Sullivan, M. J., Adams, H., Rhodenizer, T., & Stanish, W. D. (2006). A psychosocial risk factor – Targeted intervention for the prevention of chronic pain and disability following whiplash injury. *Physical Therapy, 86*(1), 8–18.

Sutaria, M. C. (1975). Theoretical framework for goal setting and evaluation. *ANPHI Papers, 10*(2–3), 38–41.

Swan, G. S. (1964). The history and development of rehabilitation. *Medical Journal of Australia, 191*, 938–939.

Trieschmann, R. B. (1974). Coping with a disability: A sliding scale of goals. *Archives of Physical Medicine & Rehabilitation, 55*, 556–560.

Trombly, C. A., Radomski, M. V., Trexel, C., & Burnet-Smith, S. E. (2002). Occupational therapy and achievement of self-identified goals by adults with acquired brain injury: Phase II. *American Journal of Occupational Therapy, 56*(5), 489–498.

Turner-Stokes, L. (2008). Goal attainment scaling (GAS) in rehabilitation: A practical guide. *Clinical Rehabilitation, 23*, 362–370.

Turner-Stokes, L., Williams, H., Abraham, R., & Duckett, S. (2000). Clinical standards for inpatient specialist rehabilitation services in the UK. *Clinical Rehabilitation, 14*(5), 468–480.

van Hooren, S. A., Valentijn, S. A., Bosma, H., Ponds, R. W., van Boxtel, M. P., Levine, B., … Jolles, J. (2007). Effect of a structured course involving goal management training in older adults: A randomised controlled trial. *Patient Education and Counseling, 65*(2), 205–213.

Wade, D. T. (1998). Evidence relating to goal planning in rehabilitation. *Clinical Rehabilitation, 12*(4), 273–275.

Wade, D. T. (1999a). Goal planning in stroke rehabilitation: How? *Topics in Stroke Rehabilitation, 6*(2), 16–36.

Wade, D. T. (1999b). Goal planning in stroke rehabilitation: What? *Topics in Stroke Rehabilitation, 6*(2), 8–15.

Wade, D. T. (2009). Goal setting in rehabilitation: An overview of what, why and how. *Clinical Rehabilitation, 23*, 291–295.

Wagner, B. M. (1969). Care plans: Right, reasonable and reachable. *American Journal of Nursing, 69*(5), 986–990.

Wressle, E., Eeg-Olofsson, A. M., Marcusson, J., & Henriksson, C. (2002). Improved client participation in the rehabilitation process using a client-centred goal formulation structure. *Journal of Rehabilitation Medicine, 34*(1), 5–11.

Wressle, E., Lindstrand, J., Neher, M., Marcusson, J., & Henriksson, C. (2003). The Canadian Occupational Performance Measure as an outcome measure and team tool in a day treatment programme. *Disability & Rehabilitation, 25*(10), 497–506.

Zimmerman, D. S., & Gohrka, C. (1970). The goal-directed nursing approach: It does work. *American Journal of Nursing, 70*(2), 306–310.

2

Evidence-Based Goal Setting: Cultivating the Science of Rehabilitation

William M.M. Levack, Sarah G. Dean, Kathryn M. McPherson and Richard J. Siegert

CONTENTS

2.1 Introduction

It is not surprising that goal setting has become so dominant within the practice of clinical rehabilitation. Goal setting is an inherently attractive concept, appearing deceptively simple at first and belying the complex relationships that exist between goals, personality, motivation, mood, self-regulation and other types of cognition. As well as having a long history of influence in psychology and philosophy, the language of goals and goal setting has also become firmly embedded within popular culture and, in particular, within the self-development movement. For instance, one of Covey's (1989) 'seven habits of highly effective people' is to 'begin with the end in mind' (p. 95) – in essence, to start by identifying one's life goals before making decisions about what actions need to be undertaken in order to progress towards them. Thus, goal setting is a concept that will be familiar to all rehabilitation professionals and one that appears, at first blush, to be an inherently credible way to create positive personal change for patients in clinical practice.

In fact, this perspective was espoused in one of the earliest and most widely cited papers on goal setting in rehabilitation (Schut & Stam, 1994). In an article outlining how and why goals should be a central part of the rehabilitation process, Schut and Stam asserted that 'Everyone knows that you have to set goals in order to accomplish anything in life' (p. 223). This statement appears to describe a truism (i.e. a self-evident statement of fact). Implied within it are a number of expectations that all people involved in rehabilitation will be naturally oriented towards explicit goals, will understand the concept of goal setting and will have the capacity and desire to plan ahead and that therefore goal setting should be something of a common currency between health providers and the people who receive their services.

Of course, the chaos and uncertainty of newly acquired chronic disease or disability, coupled with impairments of cognition and disruption of community living that arise from some conditions, can significantly restrict people's ability or willingness to engage with health professionals in goal setting (Brown et al., 2013; Holliday, Ballinger, & Playford, 2007; Laver, Halbert, Stewart, & Crotty, 2010). But, is this necessarily a problem? Is it true that explicit goal setting is *always* required in order to *accomplish anything in life*? Is it possible to be successful in some aspect of one's personal development or in the acquisition of some new ability without having to articulate (to yourself or to other people) what goal, if any, you are specifically working towards? Can a person grow, mature, progress, gain skills or cope with change just by being involved in life in the moment? Indeed, it is arguably a very Western notion that goals are a requirement for personal development. The antithesis of this notion is embodied, for instance, in the practice of *shikantaza* (a form of meditation also known as *just sitting*), which is central to the Soto teaching of Zen Buddhism (Loori, 2004). In shikantaza, all objectives are set aside (even the goal of achieving enlightenment) in order to be in the moment. It is 'an activity completely unconcerned with the benefits or the accomplishment of ulterior goals' (Dallmayr, 1996, p. 179). It is an activity considered beneficial in and of itself.

Is goal setting then always required for good clinical practice in rehabilitation? What would happen if health services were provided without any effort put into the selection and pursuit of specific rehabilitation goals? In a qualitative study investigating clinicians' experiences of goal setting in inpatient rehabilitation, one allied health professional, when pressed to answer this question, ventured to offer the following:

> I don't know if much would happen, yeah – I don't, I mean we probably wouldn't – might not get as far along with clients, yeah – but that's hard to say as well because, you know, I think sometimes we probably just know what to do anyway, we like wouldn't necessarily need a goal to – um, look and think oh we should do this for the client... (Levack, Dean, McPherson, & Siegert, 2006, p. 1442)

Even if the inherent *good* of goal-directed action is undisputed, there remain a number of questions about how goals can be most effectively selected and acted upon, how the goals of individuals can be best incorporated into the goals of a group and about how much clinical time should be invested in goal selection and goal-monitoring activities. Do more elaborate, formal, time-consuming approaches to goal setting produce better clinical outcomes than simpler, more informal methods of incorporating goals into rehabilitation activities? As outlined in Chapter 1, a multitude of approaches to goal setting exist: are some approaches more or less effective than others?

The purpose of this chapter is to discuss the scientific basis of goal setting in clinical rehabilitation. Within it, we will consider the use and misuse of evidence in the promotion and development of goal-setting practice. We will explore the questions of what might count as good evidence of effective goal setting and what might be considered a fair test of different approaches for goal setting in clinical practice. We will also examine a number of difficulties with designing the perfect clinical trial of goal setting in rehabilitation.

In this regard, a number of questions are posed about the best way to conduct such clinical trials. These include questions such as the following: How explicit should the description of the approach to goal setting in a clinical trial be, and what should be included in these descriptions? What is the most appropriate control intervention to use in an experimental trial of the clinical effects of one or more approaches to goal setting? What is the best way to manage cross-group contamination in a clinical trial of goal-setting effects? How can researchers know whether therapists are actually delivering the goal setting intervention as intended or whether patients are actually engaging with goal setting in the way that it is hypothesized? What consideration should be given to the team context in clinical trials on goal setting, and are there variables here that we need to consider when designing clinical trials?

Finally, we end this chapter by outlining a number of principles of good science in this area of inquiry and by making some recommendations for future research. Throughout this chapter, however, there is one central tenet that all assumptions and ideologies about goal setting should be questioned – rigorously, philosophically and scientifically.

2.2 Enthusiasm versus Evidence: The Risk of Confirmation Bias

Perhaps because of our desire to embrace goal setting into clinical practice, we (the rehabilitation community) have at times been quick to accept without question studies that have reported positive results associated with goal setting in rehabilitation contexts. This is known as *confirmation bias* (Kahneman, 2011), that is, a tendency for people to favour information that confirms their beliefs and expectations. A good example of this has been in the use of a study by Webb and Glueckauf (1994) to substantiate claims that higher levels of patient involvement in goal setting improve rehabilitation outcomes.

Webb and Glueckauf's (1994) paper is a historically significant publication as it was one of the earliest attempts to use experimental methods to examine the clinical consequences of enhanced approaches to goal setting in neurological rehabilitation. The paper's main value (we would argue) is simply in expressing the hypothesis that patients with a high level of involvement in the goal-setting process would be more successful in achieving their goals than would patients who had a low level of involvement in goal setting – raising this as a possible research question worthy of asking. The paper also provided some ideas about how one might go about designing a study to answer this kind of question. However, the value of Webb and Glueckauf's study as actual evidence (either positive or negative) of the effectiveness of goal setting in rehabilitation is highly questionable. The main problems with this study are the small sample size, the high attrition of participants, the use of parametric statistical methods for the analysis of goal attainment scaling (GAS) data (the only outcome measure used in the study) and the use of goals as both the dependent and independent variables in the study.

When the sample size of Webb and Glueckauf's (1994) study is described, it is frequently reported as being a study that involved 16 participants with neurological disorders (Boelen, Spikman, & Fasotti, 2011; Cullen, Chundamala, Bayley, & Jutai, 2007; Hart & Evans, 2006; Malec, 1999). Indeed, it is true that 16 participants were randomized at the beginning of this study into one of the two treatment groups (one receiving a high level of involvement in goal setting and goal monitoring; the other having little involvement in the selection or discussion of goals for their rehabilitation). However, 5 of these 16 participants (i.e. over 30%) were lost to follow up at the 2-month data collection period, meaning that the main findings from this study are based on data from just 11 people (5 in the high involvement in goal-setting group and 6 in the low involvement in goal-setting group). Usually this would mean that a clinical trial is considered a *pilot study* at best, with the low sample size producing much less certainty and precision regarding the results. Couple this with the known problems of treating GAS scores as parametric data (Tennant, 2007), the lack of reporting on the process of randomization and concealment of group allocation, and the fact that the only outcome measure used (goal attainment) was directly linked to the study intervention (goal setting), with study participants and therapists being aware of both the study aims and the intended outcome measures, and it is fair to say that this paper provides, at best, only weak evidence that higher levels of patient involvement in goal setting result in better rehabilitation outcomes.

The purpose of this critique is not to belittle Webb and Glueckauf, however, who, as stated earlier, made a significant contribution in terms of breaking new ground in the experimental investigation of goal setting in clinical rehabilitation (and who themselves acknowledge a number of the study's limitations in the discussion of their findings). Rather, our intent is to show how even one study can be highly influential in creating an impression of a strong empirical basis for goal setting in clinical practice, despite the significant limitations inherent in its design. To illustrate this, one needs to only look at how the results from this single study have been reported by other authors and used to substantiate claims regarding goal setting best practice.

According to Thomson Reuters' *Web of Knowledge*, between 1994 (when it was published) and July 2013, Webb and Glueckauf's (1994) study was cited in over 40 peer-reviewed articles. Some of the authors of these articles have been circumspect in their reporting of Webb and Glueckauf, mentioning the sample size involved in the study (Boelen et al., 2011; Cullen et al., 2007; Hart & Evans, 2006; Malec, 1999), identifying that the study has yet to be replicated (Hart & Evans, 2006) or just by using words like *may* to indicate the provisional nature of the study findings (Preminger & Lind, 2012). Others, however, have enthusiastically embraced Webb and Glueckauf's reported findings – using this one paper as the sole source of evidence to substantiate some fairly hefty claims regarding the value of goal setting in rehabilitation. The following is a list of examples of such claims, which have been made in published health science literature, *based entirely on this one study*:

- 'Previous research indicates that goal attainment is optimally realized when consumers are actively involved in the goal-setting process and when goals are defined in concrete terms'. (Balcazar, Keys, Davis, Lardon, & Jones, 2005, p. 41)

- 'Involvement in goal setting has been found... to contribute to greater physical gains'. (Duff, Evans, & Kennedy, 2004, p. 276)

- 'Webb and Glueckauf (1994) found that high patient involvement in setting rehabilitation goals was associated with more optimal outcomes for individuals with a traumatic brain injury'. (Elliott, Uswatte, Lewis, & Palmatier, 2000, p. 263)

- 'Rehabilitation outcomes are better when the patient is involved in setting his/her goals'. (Krasny-Pacini, Hiebel, Pauly, Godon, & Chevignard, 2013)
- '...Webb and Glueckauf found that involving persons with traumatic brain injuries in treatment goal setting and using progress data led to higher ratings of goal attainment'. (Schlund & Pace, 1999, p. 895)
- '...evidence suggests involving patients in setting rehabilitation goals... can effectively improve adaptive functioning in some individuals by increasing the discriminability of relevant behaviour-environment relations'. (Schlund, Pace, & McGready, 2001, p. 1069)
- 'There is moderate evidence that direct patient involvement in neurorehabilitation goal setting results in a significant improvement in obtaining goals from pre-test to post-test that are then maintained at a follow-up of two months'. (Cullen et al., 2007, p. 125)
- '...when compared to individuals with traumatic brain injury (TBI) who were not actively involved in the goal-setting process in their outpatient brain rehabilitation programme, those individuals with greater involvement in collaborative goal-setting were more likely to maintain their treatment gains over time... small adaptations to the process of treatment planning translate to rather striking improvements in the maintenance of treatment gains over time'. (Bergquist et al., 2012, p. 1308)

The point here is that the repeated (and positive) reference to this one study across dozens of publications creates the illusion to the casual reader that there is a higher degree of certainty regarding the scientific evidence underpinning the belief that greater patient involvement in goal setting improves clinical outcomes than actually exists.

Of course, management of bias is one of the key reasons for employing systematic review methods. Systematic reviews involve structured, predetermined and reproducible processes for the identification, selection, critical appraisal, interpretation and synthesis of findings from (ideally) all research on a given topic (Higgins & Green, 2011). To our knowledge, there have been three systematic reviews that have looked at the therapeutic effect of goal setting on clinical outcomes in rehabilitation contexts: two specifically examining the evidence underpinning goal setting in stroke rehabilitation (Rosewilliam, Roskell, & Pandyan, 2011; Sugavanam, Mead, Bulley, Donaghy, & Van Wijck, 2013) and one that has examined goal setting in all rehabilitation literature (Levack, Taylor, Siegert, et al., 2006). The conclusions from these three systematic reviews, however, have been somewhat underwhelming.

The two systematic reviews on goal setting in stroke rehabilitation indicated that there was a modicum of evidence (based on observational and qualitative studies) that active patient participation in goal setting appears to be something that patients value and that structured methods of goal setting seem to increase patients' perceptions of their level of involvement in clinical decision making (i.e. enhancing a sense of self-determination) (Rosewilliam et al., 2011; Sugavanam et al., 2013). In addition, some experimental studies have provided evidence (albeit limited evidence) that goal-setting techniques may increase patient adherence to treatment regimens (Levack, Taylor, Siegert, et al., 2006). However, overall, all three systematic reviews have concluded that at present, there is insufficient experimental research of adequate quality to allow any firm conclusions to be drawn regarding what effect, if any, specific goal-setting practices have on health outcomes (such as recovery rates, improved functional abilities, social participation and quality of life) following rehabilitation.

The main reasons why firmer conclusions could not be reached in these systematic reviews are threefold: (1) in general, most of the research contributing data to these systematic reviews has employed methods with moderate-to-high risk of bias; (2) the research is highly varied in terms of methods used, populations studied and outcomes measured, making it difficult to pool results from two or more studies; and (3) the conclusion of the studies that have been conducted to date are inconsistent at best, with as many studies reporting statistically significant differences as those reporting no significant effects (Levack, Taylor, Siegert, et al., 2006; Rosewilliam et al., 2011; Sugavanam et al., 2013). In other words, while goal theory has an extensive empirical foundation in psychology and some associated disciplines (see Chapters 3, 6, 11 and 14 for more information about this), the evidence base supporting its application to rehabilitation is still in its infancy.

2.3 Conducting a Fair Test of the Effectiveness of Goal Setting in Rehabilitation Contexts

Systematic reviews on questions to do with *treatment effectiveness* rightly place greater emphasis on well-designed randomized controlled trials (RCTs) than on other forms of research. Qualitative research can be extremely valuable for exploring people's perceptions and lived experiences, for challenging the status quo, for generating new ideas and new ways of understanding certain phenomena and for helping us to understand why a particular study result might have occurred (e.g. poor engagement with the intervention, high research burden on participants). Non-randomized clinical trials and observational studies (such as cohort studies and case–control studies) can produce information on associations between variables (and thus can contribute to the development of new hypotheses), but only RCTs can provide strong evidence of whether or not there is a *causal* relationship between one particular intervention (such as an enhanced approach to goal setting) and an outcome of interest (such as improved functional gains following rehabilitation).

The aim of any RCT is to conduct a *fair test* of a particular intervention. In a fair test, two or more types of treatment (e.g. an intervention and a control or two or more different approaches to an intervention) are delivered under identical conditions to similar groups of people. For all participants in any RCT, there ought to be an entirely equal chance that they would receive one treatment or another, and once the participants have been allocated to treatment groups, they should continue to be treated identically except for the intervention under investigation. Studies where patients are not randomly allocated to treatment groups can produce compelling results, but these results can be misleading and are often difficult to interpret from the perspective of their application to clinical practice.

To illustrate this, consider, for instance, Ponte-Allan and Giles' (1999) cohort study examining the relationship between activity-oriented goal setting and functional outcomes after stroke rehabilitation. Ponte-Allan and Giles began with an interesting research question: is it important whether or not stroke patients have rehabilitation goals that focus on topics related to independent performance of functional abilities? To study this question, Ponte-Allan and Giles retrospectively analyzed clinical notes from 46 people with stroke who had completed rehabilitation. They divided these people into two groups: those who were reported to have made functional, independence-focused goal statements on admission and those who had not. They then compared the outcomes achieved by these people on discharge and found that the functional goal cohort achieved significantly better outcomes (as measured by items from the Functional Independence Measure) than did the non-functional goal (or no goal) cohort.

One of the many difficulties with interpreting Ponte-Allan and Giles' (1999) study is that we cannot be sure that the two groups of patients were identical in all ways except for the issue of interest (the types of goals they set). Ponte-Allan and Giles reported that there were no statistically significant differences between their two groups in terms of age, gender, side of brain affected and Functional Independence Measure scores on admission. However, we cannot tell from the information gathered whether or not the groups were also similar in terms of depression, motivation, self-efficacy, communicative ability, cognitive ability and so on because this information was not gathered or reported. In other words, it cannot be concluded from this study that encouraging patients to make more functional, independence-oriented goal statements would result in them being more likely to achieve better outcomes, only that those who *happen* to make such statements are possibly more likely to do better than those that do not.

Development of goal theory in rehabilitation therefore needs to include some well-conducted experimental studies, employing RCT methods. In these studies, it is very important that researchers are clear about which approach, or approaches, to goal setting they are investigating and what the objectives are for using this approach. The manner in which the study is conducted, and the outcome measures used, needs to closely align with the intended function of goal setting under investigation.

There are many published guides to conducting RCTs (e.g. Machin & Fayers, 2010; Matthews, 2006; Solomon, Cavanaugh, & Draine, 2009), and the full extent of possible considerations when attempting to undertake a robust clinical trial is outside the scope of this chapter. However, it is important to note that there are a number of basic methodological principles that have been frequently ignored in RCTs on goal setting in rehabilitation but that are relatively easy to address (Levack, Taylor, Siegert, et al., 2006). These include the need for generating a truly random sequence for use when allocating study participants to treatment groups, the concealment of group allocation during the process of randomization and placement of participants in study groups, the blinding of outcome assessors to group allocation and the application of intention-to-treat analysis when interpreting study results (Higgins & Green, 2011).

However, conducting RCTs is not without its challenges. RCTs can be expensive and complicated to run. Furthermore, goal setting raises some particular challenges that make designing the perfect RCT difficult. These challenges are the subject of the following section.

2.4 Difficulties with Designing the Perfect Experimental Study of Goal Setting in Rehabilitation

There are a number of commonly acknowledged challenges associated with conducting RCTs in rehabilitation. Compared with most drug trials, rehabilitation interventions are often complex in nature, involving multiple people, multiple therapies and with multiple variables present that modify individual patient responses to courses of action (Johnston, 2003; Whyte, 2003). Complex interventions have been described by the UK Medical

Research Council as interventions that contain several interacting components (potentially in both the experimental and control arms of a study), which may also involve management of behaviour of the people delivering and/or receiving the interventions, activities at an organizational as well as an individual level, the tailoring of individual treatments and the use of multiple outcomes to measure change (Craig et al., 2008). Most, if not all, of these characteristics are usually present in any clinical trial of rehabilitation interventions.

Because of this complexity, when rehabilitation interventions are successful, it can be difficult to identify what the active elements of the treatment are. For this reason, rehabilitation has often been described as a *black box* (e.g. Ballinger, Ashburn, Low, & Roderick, 1999; DeJong, Horn, Gassaway, Slavin, & Dijkers, 2004; Grotle et al., 2013; Wade, 2001; Whyte & Hart, 2003). We might broadly know what we *put into* the black box (e.g. a 4-week period of intensive inpatient stroke rehabilitation), and we can measure variables that *come out* of the black box (e.g. functional outcomes, mortality, discharge destination), but we might not be able to say which parts of the intervention contributed to the positive (or negative) outcomes, that is, which were the active ingredients of intervention. These types of issues are common to many clinical trials of rehabilitation interventions. However, there are some nuances to such challenges that are specific to research into goal theory in rehabilitation contexts. The following is a discussion of some of these issues.

2.4.1 Problems with Operationalizing the Treatment Approach

One of the first challenges in designing a clinical trial of goal setting in rehabilitation is the complete and accurate description of what the *intervention* involves. It is important to be able to fully articulate what approach to goal setting was used in a clinical trial so that the study is reproducible in other contexts, so that the results of two or more similar clinical trials can be compared (if reasonable to do so) and so that readers of the trial can be clearly informed of the exact nature of the intervention that achieved the positive (or negative) results, if these occur.

Goal setting, as an intervention, can be altered in a wide range of ways. The process of *goal selection* alone can differ in terms of the number and type of people involved, the restrictions placed on topics deemed to be eligible as the subject of rehabilitation goals, the level of difficulty at which a goal target is set, the way goal statements are formulated for documentation in treatment plans and the degree of influence that patients (or their families) have over the final selection of goals. Goal selection is also usually preceded by a period of clinical assessment. This may be conducted as a multidisciplinary activity, with each member of the clinical team undertaking their own assessment individually, or it may be an activity that is undertaken primarily by a nominated key worker (such as a senior member of the medical, nursing or allied health team). This clinical assessment often includes some evaluation of not only a patient's medical presentation (i.e. their biological, physical and cognitive status) but also evaluation of his or her usual life context and personal values.

Beyond goal selection are variables associated with how goals are used in routine practice. Goals may or may not be subject to review and modification over time. The extent and type of feedback (verbal or written) on progress towards goals may differ from one approach to the next. Goals (and goal progress) may be discussed only in private with the person receiving the rehabilitation in question or may be shared in group settings with peers. Goals may feature in team meetings where rehabilitation plans are reviewed and discussed or be used primarily to motivate the patients and hardly influence clinical decision making at all. If any of these elements is essential to the particular approach to goal setting under investigation, they need to be clearly and accurately described in the method of the study in question.

Currently, published studies investigating the effects of goal setting on rehabilitation outcomes range widely in terms of the amount of information provided regarding the approach to goal setting used. Two good examples of explicit descriptions of goal setting approaches, however, include Åsenlöf, Denison, and Lindberg's (2005) RCT investigating the clinical effect of individually tailored treatments based on the use of the Patient Goal Priority Questionnaire for 122 people receiving therapy for musculoskeletal pain and Holliday, Cano, Freeman, and Playford's (2007) clinical trial of their intervention to increase patient and family participation in goal setting in the context of inpatient neurological rehabilitation. Both these studies clearly outlined what was involved in the process of selection of goals and how the goals were subsequently used by the teams in the planning and delivery of rehabilitation. For the record, Åsenlöf et al. (2005) reported finding that their approach to goal setting (as a behavioural intervention for pain management) resulted in significantly lower levels of pain-related disability, lower maximum pain intensity, higher levels of pain control and lower fear of movement 3 months after enrolment into the study. Holliday, Cano, et al. reported no statistically significant differences in outcomes achieved by their enhanced goal-setting group and outcomes achieved by their control group (as measured by the Functional Independence Measure, London Handicap Scale and General Health Questionnaire). However, the patients in their goal-setting group reported feeling significantly more satisfied with the goal-setting process, having more personal control over the goal selected and that the goals were significantly more personally relevant to individual patients than was reported by people in the control group (Holliday, Cano, et al., 2007).

Of course, some variables associated with goal setting may be much easier to operationalize for the purposes of research than others. It may be relatively easy, for instance, to outline criteria relating to when goal-setting meetings are to occur (e.g. within 2 weeks of admission to a service) and who needs to be at these meetings. It is, in comparison, harder to pre-specify criteria related to the level of difficulty expected of goals set for individual patients. If, for instance, it is considered essential for rehabilitation goals to be achievable or (conversely) highly ambitious and challenging, then some criteria are required to determine when goals do or do not meet these expectations. Furthermore, it must be possible to apply these criteria *before* any therapy has been undertaken if they are to be used for the purposes of distinguishing between two intervention arms in an experimental study. It is not meaningful in a study to classify a goal as being achievable or unrealistic/too difficult *retrospectively* (i.e. because a patient did or did not achieve it) as this completely undermines the entire intent of using experimental methods to study such things.

In this regard, some experimental studies have attempted to standardize the degree of goal difficulty in order to study its effect on patient engagement in therapy or self-management interventions. Researchers have done this either by giving all participants in each study group the exact same goal, with one group having a more challenging target to reach than the other (Miller, Headings, Peyrot, & Nagaraja, 2012), or by using goals that reflect a set percentage increment from baseline levels of functioning for a prescribed task, for example, a 5% improvement on baseline performance for the *easily achievable goal group* versus a 20% improvement for the *challenging/difficult goal group* (Gauggel & Billino, 2002; Gauggel, Leinberger, & Richardt, 2001). Of course, these standardized approaches remove the individualized, person-centred aspect of goal selection that is typically recommended in most rehabilitation practice, so produce results that are limited in other ways (e.g. it may be the set goals were not meaningful or relevant to the people participating in the study).

In addition to the aforementioned discussion, when describing the goal-setting approach under investigation, researchers need to begin with a clearly articulated theory about how their approach to goal setting might result in changes in the outcomes they intend to measure. The UK Medical Research Council guidelines for research into complex interventions state that identifying and developing theory on the hypothesized mechanism of action for the intervention under investigation is an integral first step in any such clinical trial (Craig et al., 2008). As outlined in Chapter 3, there are a number of theories related to goals and human behaviour that rehabilitation researchers could draw upon. Sometimes, however, before launching into a full RCT, it is best to begin with smaller feasibility or pilot studies to examine the assumptions of the theory under investigation. An example of this has been in the development and preliminary testing of theory for using goal setting to address problems with self-regulation after traumatic brain injury before the implementation of a fully powered clinical trial (McPherson, Kayes, & Weatherall, 2009; Siegert, McPherson, & Taylor, 2004; Ylvisaker, McPherson, Kayes, & Pellett, 2008) (see Chapter 6 for more information about the potential application of self-regulation theory to goal-setting practice).

It should be clear from this discussion that providing a complete description of any one goal-setting intervention in rehabilitation is far from a simple matter. In other areas of health research, similar issues have resulted in increased emphasis on *intervention mapping* as a strategy for the development and documentation of complex interventions (Bartholomew, Parcel, & Kok, 1998; Kok, Schaalma, Ruiter, Van Empelen, & Brug, 2004). Intervention mapping provides a framework for the systematic development of interventions from theory, empirical data and information gathered from the target population of interest. It involves a series of six steps, which include (1) identification of the need to be addressed by the intervention, (2) establishment of what is to be achieved by the intervention (known as proximal programme objectives), (3) development of theory-based methods and practical strategies, (4) operationalization of the practical interventions and strategies into a deliverable programme and documentation of this programme, (5) development of a strategy to implement this programme (i.e. pilot the programme) and (6) development of ways to evaluate the effectiveness of the programme (Ammendolia et al., 2009; Bartholomew et al., 1998). While intervention mapping has been primarily implemented in the area of health promotion research, the principles of this technique hold significant potential for research on goal setting in rehabilitation, particularly when it comes to aligning practical and reproducible approaches to goal setting with theories regarding how goal setting is believed to work.

One further advance in contemporary behavioural science research worthy of note is the recent development of the Behaviour Change Technique (BCT) Taxonomy (v1) (Michie et al., 2013). The BCT Taxonomy is a cross-disciplinary classification of 93 distinct BCTs – the first taxonomy of its kind to be developed by expert consensus and empirically tested for reliability (Michie et al., 2013). This taxonomy provides a method for classifying BCTs in clinical practice and in research. Just as the World Health Organization's (2001) *International Classification of Functioning, Disability and Health* has provided a common language for sharing concepts related to human function and disability, so too does the BCT Taxonomy provide a standardized lexicon for discussing concepts related to BCTs. Of particular note, the BCT Taxonomy includes nine behavioural change interventions gathered together under the group label of *goals and planning* (Michie et al., 2013).

The BCT Taxonomy only provides a method for categorization of the *content* of BCTs, however. The authors note that further development of taxonomies of behavioural change interventions could also usefully include ways of categorizing the modes and context of delivery of BCTs (which, for goal setting in rehabilitation, would include some of the issues described earlier) as well as methods for categorization of the competencies required of people who deliver such interventions (Michie et al., 2013). Nonetheless, the BCT Taxonomy, while only in its first iteration, may well provide a useful tool for categorizing various aspects of goal-setting interventions in rehabilitation research.

2.4.2 Problems with Defining a Control Group

As well as being able to clearly describe what was received by the intervention group (or groups) in a goal-setting study, it is also important to be able to outline how this intervention differs from what was provided to the control group. This issue is particularly problematic for research on goal setting because, as has been highlighted in Chapter 1, goal setting is so commonplace in rehabilitation practice that it can be difficult to determine what rehabilitation without goal setting might look like.

One strategy is to compare a newly enhanced method of goal setting (perhaps one that involves a more regulated approach to goal selection or one that encourages greater participation from patients) against what might be considered *usual care*. Indeed, this type of method was employed by both Åsenlöf et al. (2005) and Holliday, Cano, et al. (2007) in the examples described previously. However, if this strategy is to be applied, researchers ought to assiduously describe what *usual care* involves (Craig et al., 2008).

A good example of where this has occurred is in an RCT by Ostelo and colleagues investigating an enhanced approach to goal setting as an adjunct to usual physiotherapy care for 105 people after first-time lumbar disc surgery (Ostelo, de Vet, et al., 2003; Ostelo, Goossens, de Vet, & van den Brandt, 2004; Ostelo, Koke, et al., 2000). Prior to undertaking their full study, Ostelo, Koke, et al. published a report on their intended research methods including, among other things, a complete description of both the intervention and control arms of their study. In their description of the control group, who were to receive *usual care* after surgery, Ostelo, Koke, et al. included not only information about the number and duration of treatment sessions but also information on the treatment philosophy underlying the usual care approach and specifically what types of interventions this did and did not involve. They also included a separate section in their method in which they contrasted the new goal-setting approach with the *usual care* approach, providing criteria that could be used to confirm that the two treatments were indeed fundamentally different from one another.

In the case of this study, Ostelo, de Vet, et al. (2003) reported no statistically significant differences were found between their treatment and control groups at 6 and 12 months on any of their measures of health outcome including measures of functional status, pain intensity, pain catastrophizing, fear of movement, range of motion, general health, social functioning or return to work. They also reported their enhanced goal-setting approach was significantly more costly to deliver, so concluded that it was best to not use this method of behavioural intervention in their particular clinical context (Ostelo, Goossens, et al., 2004).

Other approaches to clinical trials avoid the challenges of having to describe *usual care* by investigating only one aspect of goal setting. For instance, Culley and Evans (2010) and Hart, Hawkey, and Whyte (2002) each investigated the use of electronic media to improve the ability of people with traumatic brain injury to recall their rehabilitation goals (using text messaging and portable voice organizers, respectively). In both these cases, goals were randomly allocated to being included in regular electronic reminders or not. Both groups of authors found that people with traumatic brain injury were significantly better at recalling their rehabilitation goals 1–2 weeks later if they had received electronic reminders. While such studies do not answer the big questions surrounding goal setting in rehabilitation (such as whether or not time invested in goal setting produces better rehabilitation outcomes), these types of clean and relatively simple RCTs are attractive because of their utility in providing data to support (or refute) less dramatic, but nonetheless relevant, hypotheses about aspects of goal-setting practice.

2.4.3 Problems with Blinding

Blinding of study participants, treatment providers and outcome evaluators to treatment group allocation is a commonly recommended strategy to reduce experimenter and observer bias in clinical trials (Schulz & Grimes, 2002). In drug trials, this often involves using two identical sets of pills that are alike in all ways (size, colour, taste, etc.) except for the active ingredient in the pill (i.e. the medicine versus a placebo). If conducted properly, none of the people involved in the delivery of an RCT (the people giving the pills, the people taking the pills, the people measuring the outcomes) should know which participants got which type of pill until the conclusion of the trial. Of course, the blinding of study participants and treatment providers to group allocation is next to impossible in many clinical trials involving rehabilitation interventions (Johnston, 2003; Whyte, 2003). This is because most rehabilitation interventions require active involvement from both therapists and patients in order to be effective. Patients need to know what they are expected to do and why they are doing it in order to adhere to a treatment regime. For this reason, rehabilitation trials are most frequently single-blinded studies at best – with blinding just being applied to the outcome evaluation component of the RCT.

The blinding of outcome evaluation is particularly challenging, however, when RCTs into goal setting involve goal attainment as one of the outcomes of interest. Attempts at blinding study participants to outcome scores based on goal attainment have resulted in some rather convoluted study methods. Howell (1986), for instance, employed the use of *theoretical* goals and *actual* goals in her RCT of GAS in community-based occupational therapy for people with mental health conditions. The *theoretical* GAS goals were set by Howell in discussion with the treating occupational therapist for all 24 participants in the study but were, however, never discussed with the participants themselves. The *actual* GAS goals, by contrast, were set by the treating occupational therapists in discussion with the 13 participants allocated to the intervention condition (with the 11 participants in the control group having no such involvement in any goal setting). For the participants in the intervention condition, these *actual* goals were used to structure therapy sessions over an 8-week period but were not used to evaluate outcomes from the RCT.

At the end of the study period, GAS scores from the *theoretical* goals were collected by Howell (1986) in discussion once more with the treating occupational therapists. The argument here would be that the blinding of participants to the method used for evaluating goal attainment improves the overall validity of study findings. However, it is entirely plausible that the treating occupational therapists, who knew of each participant's allocation to treatment or control groups and who were involved in the delivery of that intervention, may well have been biased in their evaluation of the goal attainment outcomes, skewing the study findings in favour of the GAS intervention.

The best solution to such problems is really just to avoid goal attainment as an outcome in these kinds of studies altogether and to use other forms of standardized outcome measurement instead. Using goal setting as both the independent and dependent variables in experimental studies immediately creates problems with bias. In a clinical trial, the evaluation of whether or not an approach to goal setting in rehabilitation was effective should not be based primarily (if at all) on appraisal of the achievement or non-achievement of those same goals.

Attempts have also been made to conduct studies where the treating therapists have been blinded to goal-setting group allocation. One example of this has been provided by Evans and Hardy (2002). Using a pseudo-RCT method, Evans and Hardy allocated 39 people with sports injuries to one of the three groups: a goal-setting group, a social support group and a control group. In this study, clinical interventions for all participants were provided by a group of physiotherapists who were blinded to group allocation. The goal-setting and social support group interventions were provided separately, but concurrently, by a sport psychologist who was not otherwise involved in the provision of physiotherapy. The findings from this study indicated that treatment adherence and self-efficacy (both based on self-report by the participants, who were of course not blinded to study group allocation) were significantly higher in the group who participated in the goal setting intervention. No data, however, were collected on whether clinical outcomes (such as recovery of functional abilities) were influenced by group allocation.

One slightly odd consequence of Evans and Hardy's (2002) method, however, was that this study involved physiotherapy patients setting goals that the physiotherapists themselves were not informed about. Examples of the types of goals set by the patient and sport psychologist in this study included 'achieving a specified range of muscular tension in muscle groups targeted in rehabilitation activities' and 'completing a specified number of rehabilitation exercises or activity sessions' (Evans & Hardy, 2002, p. 314). What the treating physiotherapists would have made of these goals is something of an open question.

2.4.4 Problems with Cross-Group Contamination

For any RCT to achieve its objective (its objective being to conduct a fair test on one or more hypotheses), it is extremely important that only the intervention group receives the intervention under investigation and that all people in the control group do not. When some people in a control group receive the intervention group protocol by accident or intent (or vice versa, when the intervention groups receive the control protocol), *cross-group contamination* has occurred, and the results of study become difficult, if not impossible, to interpret. The study is no longer a fair test of the intervention in question.

While this statement may seem blindingly obvious, underpinning it are a number of challenges facing all researchers who conduct studies on goal setting in rehabilitation. Imagine, for instance, an RCT where individual patients in an inpatient stroke ward are randomly allocated to either an intervention group, who receive an enhanced approach to patient participation in goal setting, or to a control group, who do not. Maybe this new approach draws on some specific theory of how goal setting influences self-regulation of behaviour or motivation and involves health professionals asking different kinds of questions and interacting in a different kind of way with patients than they usually would. Such an approach would require the health professionals involved to receive training in the new method. Theory-driven approaches to goal setting are often as much about teaching health professionals different ways of thinking about their work and about their patients as it is about actually learning new techniques for doing certain clinical activities. The problem that occurs, however, is that once this new approach is taught and learnt, health professionals then have to actively avoid thinking the same thoughts and using the same strategies when dealing with the people in the control group.

Furthermore, if two patients in one cubicle on the ward have been assigned to different groups in the study, it is possible for the patients in the control group to start behaving differently after observing interactions between fellow patients in the cubicle (who may be in the experimental group) and the ward staff or after informal conversations with their peers in between therapy sessions. Again, this would result in cross-group contamination.

The recommended approach to dealing with cross-group contamination is to keep the groups separate – but this often produces new problems that also have to be addressed. Typically, the problem here is that the act of separating participants results in the study groups no longer being treated identically in all ways except the one related to the study hypothesis. Other factors come into play to contaminate the study findings.

Holliday, Cano, et al.'s (2007) approach to dealing with such cross-group contamination was to implement a non-randomized controlled clinical trial instead of an RCT design. They ran a series of 3-month blocks of intervention, involving 201 people with stroke, over an 18-month period, alternating between their *usual care* approach to goal setting and an approach that increased patient understanding of and involvement in the goal-planning process. (The results of this study are described earlier in this chapter.) Although this study is a considerable addition to the research on goal setting in rehabilitation, non-randomized clinical trials introduce a significant degree of uncertainty to interpretation of study data that can never be fully addressed by any statistical wizardry. This is because we can never completely eliminate the possibility of biases arising from other factors not controlled for in the study – factors that we may be unaware of and that may change over time (Altman & Bland, 1999). For instance, seasonal changes may have an effect on rehabilitation delivery and outcome, or staffing levels may change, with more skilled clinicians being present during some parts of a study than during others.

Another approach to dealing with cross-group contamination in RCTs is to use a cluster RCT design rather than a parallel-group design. In parallel-group RCTs, each individual patient is randomly allocated to a treatment or control group. In cluster RCTs, clusters of patients are randomly allocated to treatment or control groups. For instance, if a study involved randomly assigning a number of different rehabilitation services to either an intervention group or a control group (with the patients in those service receiving whichever protocol had been assigned to that group), this would then be an example of a cluster RCT design.

The limitation of cluster RCTs, however, is that, in general, people within groups tend to be more similar to one another than people between groups. Within a rehabilitation context, this might occur simply because different rehabilitation teams have different levels of resourcing and staff expertise and achieve different levels of success with their patients. For this reason, it is a mistake to conduct randomization at the level of the cluster then analyse at the level of the individual patient, without first accounting for variability in outcomes that occur between the groups (Campbell, Mollison, Steen, Grimshaw, & Eccles, 2000). In order to address this problem, a statistical measure of intracluster dependence (also known as the intracluster coefficient) needs to be incorporated into the analysis.

This approach was attempted in the development of one particular cluster RCT investigating the impact of enhanced interdisciplinary goal setting (based on the use of the Canadian Occupational Performance Measure) on quality of life after inpatient stroke rehabilitation (Taylor et al., 2012). The intent of this study was to randomize rehabilitation services (rather than individual stroke patients) to either the intervention or control condition. However, an initial feasibility study found that there was such a high degree of variability *between* inpatient stroke services in terms of the main outcome measure in question (the Schedule for the Evaluation of Individual Quality of Life) that the fully powered study was effectively impossible to conduct. In this case, it was calculated that if a parallel RCT design were used (ignoring the problems of cross-group contamination), 230 participants would need to be recruited in order to achieve sufficient statistical power to detect a large difference in quality of life between the treatment and control groups. In comparison, a cluster RCT design with 10 clusters, investigating the same hypothesis, would have required a sample size of 923 participants to achieve the same degree of statistical power to detect a significant difference (Taylor et al., 2012). This meant that, while retaining the benefits of randomization and while addressing issues of cross-group contamination, a fully powered cluster RCT would have become too costly to conduct, requiring an impractically large sample size. Dealing with cross-group contamination in RCTs of goal setting in rehabilitation is thus not easy, but it is nevertheless an important issue that needs to be considered when designing such trials.

2.4.5 Problems with Intervention Fidelity

Related to issues with defining the treatment and control group in a goal-setting study, and with the risk of cross-group contamination, are issues to do with intervention fidelity. Ideally, during the delivery of a clinical trial, some attention is directed at evaluating the degree to which the interventions for the treatment and control groups stayed true to the intended protocols for each group – a characteristic known as *intervention fidelity*.

Evaluating intervention fidelity is much easier to do (and report on) when objective criteria have been established in the first place to test whether or not the specific intervention protocols in a study have been followed. Manuals explicitly describing the delivery of the goal setting and control interventions (perhaps based on processes of intervention mapping as described earlier in this chapter) can go a long way towards outlining such criteria. Full reports on the conclusion of RCTs involving complex interventions should include information on these matters. A good example of a study where this has occurred is in the RCT mentioned previously conducted by Åsenlöf et al. (2005). Åsenlöf and colleagues included within their research report extensive information on the compliance of the therapists and participants with the intervention and control protocol, including information on the number and duration of treatment session, as well as information on the exact content of such sessions. They were thus able to confirm that the interventions in the RCT had indeed been delivered in the manner intended.

2.4.6 Problems Arising from Goal Setting Being Primarily Used to Augment Therapy

One slightly unusual aspect of goal setting as a topic for clinical trials is that it is often used only as an add-on to an existing therapy rather than an intervention separate from other clinical activities. Goal setting is not a panacea that makes ineffective rehabilitation suddenly effective. Thus, RCTs that investigate goal setting as an adjunct to particular therapies are not going to produce evidence in favour of goal setting if the underlying therapies are ineffective.

Similarly, goal setting is unlikely to be effective in situations where individualization of treatment is not essential or where patients are already maximally motivated to engage in the rehabilitation in question (i.e. where the therapy in question is already considerably effective). One potential example of this is a study investigating the additive effect of goal setting on pulmonary rehabilitation for 180 people with chronic lung disease (Sewell, Singh, Williams, Collier, & Morgan, 2005). Pulmonary rehabilitation is already known to be an effective form of treatment for lung disease, impacting positively on functional outcomes and quality of life (Lacasse, Goldstein, Lasserson, & Martin, 2006) as well as reducing re-hospitalization and mortality rates after exacerbations (Puhan et al., 2009). Sewell et al. sought to undertake an RCT to investigate whether individualized exercise programmes based on person-centred goal setting enhanced the benefits achieved from pulmonary rehabilitation when compared to the standard approaches based on generic exercises and no goal setting at all. They found that while both approaches to pulmonary rehabilitation (goal-directed versus generic) significantly improved participants' physical activity levels (measured by an accelerometer) and occupational performance (measured by the Canadian Occupational Performance Measure) over the course of the programme, the addition of goal setting and individualization of treatment provided no further benefit.

One possible explanation for Sewell et al.'s (2005) findings is that the treatment in question (generic pulmonary rehabilitation) was already maximally effective – so the addition of goal setting did little to further improve on these clinical results. Another perspective, however, might be that this finding only applies to this particular form of goal setting in the context of pulmonary rehabilitation. Sewell et al.'s approach to goal setting emphasized enhancing the individual meaningfulness of interventions and the specificity of training based on personal goals. While perhaps people with chronic lung disease did not benefit from these mechanisms of goal effect, other approaches to using goals to enhance patient effort and attention during therapy could perhaps have been more advantageous. In particular, perhaps the use of prescribed, specific, difficult goals might have resulted in different conclusions from Sewell et al.'s study, as would be hypothesized by application of Locke and Latham's goal theory (Locke & Latham, 2002) (see Chapter 3 for further details on this theory). Another RCT would of course be required, however, to test whether this new hypothesis could be supported or not.

A caveat to all of this discussion, however, is that while, as argued earlier, goal setting is frequently used to supplement or enhance an existing therapy, in some clinical situations it appears reasonable to speculate that goal setting could have effects independent of other interventions. One thought-provoking example of this can be found in a study by Harwood et al. (2011) on self-management after stroke. In this study, Harwood et al. randomly allocated 172 New Zealand Māori and Pacific Island people with stroke to one of the four research groups. Forty-six of these people participated in a single 80 min, community-based, goal-planning intervention (called a *Take Charge* session), which was designed to facilitate self-directed rehabilitation after stroke. Harwood et al. reported that at a 12-month follow-up assessment, the people who received this intervention scored significantly higher compared to the control group on the Physical Component Summary score of the Short Form 36, were less likely to be physically dependent on others for help with daily activities and had caregivers who scored significantly lower on the Carer Strain Index as a result.

2.4.7 Problems Arising from Not Evaluating Goal Commitment

It is frequently assumed in clinical trials of goal setting (and in clinical practice for that matter) that all patients are equally committed to pursuing and achieving their rehabilitation goals. It also appears to be assumed that simply having patients involved in the goal planning process results in the selection of goals to which they will be immediately and enduringly committed. An important distinction can even be made between the meaningfulness of specific goals to specific people and the degree to which these people are actually committed to achieving their goals. It is entirely conceivable for a rehabilitation patient to contribute to a high level in the selection of subjects and targets for specific rehabilitation goals but to then be relatively equivocal about how important those goals are to achieve.

We also should not assume that all people share our understanding of the concept of goal setting or that all people have the same ability to plan ahead. Problems with engagement in rehabilitation goal setting can occur through lack of prior knowledge and skills in this area (with social and cultural factors having an influence here), through impairments in cognitive capacity or simply as a result of lack of opportunity. The chaos of everyday life, the profound uncertainty that arises from newly acquired disability and daily challenges of the here and now can impede attempts that people make to forward plan (Holliday, Ballinger, et al., 2007; Laver et al., 2010). Furthermore, some people just do not desire to engage in goal planning with health professionals or do not value doing so very highly. Emerging evidence from qualitative research suggests that patients are not always completely forthright with health professionals regarding their own objectives of rehabilitation, particularly when such objectives are deeply personal to them (Brown et al., 2013; Young et al., 2008).

Locke and Latham (2002) have identified goal commitment as an important moderator of the effect of goal setting on human performance and go so far as to state that failure to achieve goal commitment from participants is one of the key reasons why study findings might not match what is predicted by their goal theory on occasions. Any RCT of goal setting in rehabilitation should really therefore include some evaluation of goal commitment to test these assumptions. Currently, few published RCTs on goal setting in health science literature have included evaluation of goal commitment, and indeed, little research has been conducted to examine the best way to evaluate goal commitment in clinical settings. One notable exception to this is Miller et al.'s (2012) RCT on the application of Locke and Latham's goal theory to increase the uptake of lower glycemic index diets among people with type 2 diabetes. Miller et al. were primarily interested in knowing whether difficult dietary goals versus more achievable dietary goals resulted in greater uptake of desirable dietary behaviours by people with diabetes. They found that while both types of goals resulted in increased consumption of lower glycemic index foods, goal difficulty did not appear to facilitate any greater uptake of desirable dietary behaviour. However, because they had measured goal commitment in their study, Miller et al. also discovered that people who had higher levels of goal commitment perceived goals to be easier, and higher levels of self-efficacy appear to be related to higher goal commitment in this context. In general, however, there is a need for far greater attention to evaluating goal commitment in both rehabilitation research and clinical practice.

2.4.8 Consideration of the Group Context of Goal Setting in Interprofessional Rehabilitation

It is acknowledged that goal setting in rehabilitation most often occurs within a team environment and that the process of goal setting can influence factors such as team communication and interprofessional collaboration (Levack, Dean, Siegert, & McPherson, 2006; Levack, Dean, McPherson, et al., 2006). Much of the literature on goal setting in rehabilitation, however, emphasizes the potential for goals to influence patient behaviour rather than team behaviour, examining issues such as the impact of goals on patient adherence to treatment regimens (e.g. Bassett & Petrie, 1999; Cross & Parsons, 1971; Duncan & Pozehl, 2003; Evans & Hardy, 2002; Howell, 1986; LaFerriere & Calsyn, 1978; Miller et al., 2012; Ostelo, de Vet, et al., 2003) rather than, say, on the motivation of health professionals to provide it.

Literature from psychology on goal setting within team environments paints a more complex picture than is typically presented in rehabilitation research. For example, there is experimental evidence from psychological research to suggest that goal effects on group performance are influenced by factors such as group leadership (De Souza & Klein, 1995;

Whittington, Goodwin, & Murray, 2004) and the way in which an individual team member's goals are integrated into the goals of their group (Crown & Rosse, 1995; Kleingeld, van Mierlo, & Arends, 2011). There is also, within psychology, a fascinating and substantial body of research on the phenomena of *social loafing*, a term used to describe the situation where people (e.g. health professionals) deliberately exert less effort to achieve a goal when working in a team environment than when working alone (e.g. Alnuaimi, Robert, & Maruping, 2010; Price, Harrison, & Gavin, 2006; van Dick, Tissington, & Hertel, 2009). Social loafing involves taking work easy because one is in the position of being able to rely on the efforts of others.

These kinds of factors associated with goal setting in a team environment have, to our knowledge, yet to be investigated within a rehabilitation context. It may not be appropriate to simply assume that goal-planning processes designed to enhance patient motivation or patient performance would necessarily provide the best mechanism for maximizing the function of interdisciplinary teams. This is an area for further development in future research.

2.5 Some Principles for Future Research on Goal Setting in Rehabilitation

To summarize the aforementioned discussion, a number of recommendations can be made regarding experimental research into rehabilitation goal setting. These recommendations are as follows:

- Goal setting should be considered as a complex health intervention, and so experimental research on goal setting in rehabilitation should follow established guidelines for complex interventions such as that provided by the UK Medical Research Council (Craig et al., 2008) or similar.

- Experimental studies on goal setting in rehabilitation contexts should include a comprehensive description of what the goal-setting process involved, including (but not limited to) what activities were conducted prior to goal selection, the complete process of goal selection, what restrictions are placed around the content and format of rehabilitation goals and information on how goals are then used to influence patient behaviour, professional behaviour or clinical practice.

- The primary purpose of using goals in clinical practice needs to be carefully considered and documented, and there needs to be alignment between this purpose and the clinical measures used to evaluate patient outcomes.

- The approach taken to goal setting in any one study needs to have a clear theoretical position regarding how the goals (or process of goal setting) are thought to achieve their desired effects. The methods used to set and pursue rehabilitation goals need to align closely with this theoretical foundation, and this alignment ought to be described in detail in the report on the study method.

- The use of established tools such as intervention mapping (Bartholomew et al., 1998; Kok et al., 2004) and the BCT Taxonomy (Michie et al., 2013) may assist with the development and documentation of goal-setting approaches in training manuals for the health professionals who are taking part in the research, to facilitate higher treatment fidelity, to permit replication of the study and to ultimately assist with the wider rollout of service implementation should the approach to goal setting prove effective.

- Careful consideration needs to be given to the comparison intervention (i.e. control group) with which the goal-setting approach is to be compared. This comparison intervention (which may be *usual care* or another modified approach to goal setting) needs to be equally well described in the study method as the primary goal-setting intervention of interest.

- While it is highly likely to be unrealistic to blind study participants and treatment providers to which intervention each participant in an RCT is receiving, all such studies should include blinded evaluation of standardized health outcomes. The use of goal attainment to evaluate the effectiveness of goal setting as an intervention is highly questionable.

- For an RCT, the initial allocation of participants to treatment or control groups, after their enrolment into an RCT, ought to always be blinded, with the sequence of randomization being concealed from those people involved in the recruitment of participants into the study.

- Potential for cross-group contamination needs to be carefully considered in any experimental study of goal setting in clinical rehabilitation. In situations where strategies are used to keep study groups separate to address cross-group contamination, the potential biases resulting from separating treatment groups need to be accounted for (e.g. intracluster dependence needs to be considered whenever cluster RCT designs are to be used).

- Treatment fidelity needs to be evaluated and accounted for in any experimental study of goal setting in rehabilitation to ensure that, first, the right treatment was delivered by the clinicians (fidelity to the protocol) and, second, that the participants truly received and engaged with the approach to goal setting or the control intervention that they were allocated. Both these problems (treatment fidelity and cross contamination) can to some extent be mitigated by using the appropriate intention to treat analysis approach.

- In situations where goal setting is to be used to enhance the treatment effect of an existing rehabilitation intervention, researchers first need to firmly establish that the rehabilitation intervention in question is capable of producing sufficient, but not maximal, effect such that the goal-setting approach can have a measureable influence on it.

- Goal commitment should be measured in all experimental studies of goal setting in rehabilitation, and not simply assumed.

- It would be beneficial if future research on goal-setting interventions in interprofessional rehabilitation takes into consideration the effects of goals on health professional behaviour and interprofessional teamwork.

2.6 Conclusions

There has been substantial interest in the development of research evidence on which to base goal-setting practice in rehabilitation. Research on rehabilitation goal setting needs to be interpreted cautiously, however, as it is easy to begin with an expectation that any form of goal setting is a universal good and thus biases the way we view studies on its application to clinical practice. While various types of research offer considerable potential for furthering our understanding of goal setting in rehabilitation, experimental studies (and in particular RCT methods) are essential for us to develop a strong evidence base about the best way to use goal setting as an intervention to maximize the health benefits that people gain from receiving rehabilitation services.

Goal setting in rehabilitation should be considered a complex intervention. As such, the methods for experimental studies that examine its impact on health outcomes need to be carefully thought-out. RCTs on goal setting in rehabilitation can be challenging to design, but if goal theory in rehabilitation is to progress, more of these types of studies need to be undertaken. Indeed, the future for rehabilitation research is very promising. There has been considerable growth in the development and refinement of methods for conducting clinical trials in rehabilitation in recent years. The introduction of standards for conducting studies on complex interventions, the rise of interest in intervention mapping and the increasing uptake of fidelity checking in rehabilitation trials are just some of the examples of such developments. As these new approaches filter through to applied research, we can expect to see new understandings of goal theory in rehabilitation emerging. The more we approach goal setting from a scientific perspective – critically and objectively – the more sophisticated our understanding of goal setting in rehabilitation will become. The more we understand goal setting, the better we can serve our patients.

References

Alnuaimi, O. A., Robert, L. P., & Maruping, L. M. (2010). Team size, dispersion, and social loafing in technology-supported teams: A perspective on the theory of moral disengagement. *Journal of Management Information Systems*, 27(1), 203–230.

Altman, D. G., & Bland, J. M. (1999). Statistics notes: Treatment allocation in controlled trials: Why randomise? *British Medical Journal*, 318(7192), 1209.

Ammendolia, C., Cassidy, D., Steenstra, I., Soklaridis, S., Boyle, E., Eng, S., ... Côté, P. (2009). Designing a workplace return-to-work program for occupational low back pain: An intervention mapping approach. *BMC Musculoskeletal Disorders*, 10(1), 65.

Åsenlöf, P., Denison, E., & Lindberg, P. (2005). Individually tailored treatment targeting activity, motor behavior, and cognition reduces pain-related disability: A randomized controlled trial in patients with musculoskeletal pain. *The Journal of Pain*, 6(9), 588–603.

Balcazar, F. E., Keys, C. B., Davis, M., Lardon, C., & Jones, C. (2005). Strengths and challenges of intervention research in vocational rehabilitation: An illustration of agency-university collaboration. *Journal of Rehabilitation*, 71(2), 40–48.

Ballinger, C., Ashburn, A., Low, J., & Roderick, P. (1999). Unpacking the black box of therapy – A pilot study to describe occupational therapy and physiotherapy interventions for people with stroke. *Clinical Rehabilitation*, 13(4), 301–309.

Bartholomew, L. K., Parcel, G. S., & Kok, G. (1998). Intervention mapping: A process for developing theory and evidence-based health education programs. *Health Education & Behavior*, 25(5), 545–563.

Bassett, S. F., & Petrie, K. J. (1999). The effect of treatment goals on patient compliance with physiotherapy exercise programmes. *Physiotherapy*, 85(3), 130–137.

Bergquist, T. F., Micklewright, J. L., Yutsis, M., Smigielski, J. S., Gehl, C., & Brown, A. W. (2012). Achievement of client-centred goals by persons with acquired brain injury in comprehensive day treatment is associated with improved functional outcomes. *Brain Injury*, 26(11), 1307–1314. doi:10.3109/02699052.2012.706355

Boelen, D. H. E., Spikman, J. M., & Fasotti, L. (2011). Rehabilitation of executive disorders after brain injury: Are interventions effective? *Journal of Neuropsychology*, *5*, 73–113. doi:10.1348/174866410x516434

Brown, M., Levack, W., McPherson, K. M., Dean, S. G., Reed, K., Weatherall, M., & Taylor, W. J. (2013). Survival, momentum, and things that make me 'me': Patients' perceptions of goal setting after stroke. *Disability and Rehabilitation*, [Early Online], 1–7.

Campbell, M. K., Mollison, J., Steen, N., Grimshaw, J. M., & Eccles, M. (2000). Analysis of cluster randomized trials in primary care: A practical approach. *Family Practice*, *17*(2), 192–196.

Covey, S. R. (1989). *The 7 habits of highly effective people*. New York, NY: Simon & Schuster.

Craig, P., Dieppe, P., Macintyre, S., Michie, S., Nazareth, I., & Petticrew, M. (2008). Developing and evaluating complex interventions: The new Medical Research Council guidance. *British Medical Journal*, *337*, 979–983.

Cross, J. E., & Parsons, C. R. (1971). Nurse-teaching and goal-directed nurse-teaching to motivate change in food selection behavior of hospitalized patients. *Nursing Research*, *20*(5), 454–458.

Crown, D. F., & Rosse, J. G. (1995). Yours, mine, and ours: Facilitating group productivity through the integration of individual and group goals. *Organizational Behavior and Human Decision Processes*, *64*(2), 138–150.

Cullen, N., Chundamala, J., Bayley, M., & Jutai, J. (2007). The efficacy of acquired brain injury rehabilitation. *Brain Injury*, *21*(2), 113–132.

Culley, C., & Evans, J. J. (2010). SMS text messaging as a means of increasing recall of therapy goals in brain injury rehabilitation: A single-blind within-subjects trial. *Neuropsychological Rehabilitation*, *20*(1), 103–119.

Dallmayr, F. R. (1996). *Beyond orientalism: Essays on cross-cultural encounter*. Albany, NY: State University of New York Press.

De Souza, G., & Klein, H. J. (1995). Emergent leadership in the group goal-setting process. *Small Group Research*, *26*(4), 475–496.

DeJong, G., Horn, S. D., Gassaway, J. A., Slavin, M. D., & Dijkers, M. P. (2004). Toward a taxonomy of rehabilitation interventions: Using an inductive approach to examine the "black box" of rehabilitation. *Archives of Physical Medicine and Rehabilitation*, *85*(4), 678–686.

Duff, J., Evans, M. J., & Kennedy, P. (2004). Goal planning: A retrospective audit of rehabilitation process and outcome. *Clinical Rehabilitation*, *18*(3), 275–286. doi:10.1191/0269215504cr720oa

Duncan, K., & Pozehl, B. (2003). Effects of an exercise adherence intervention on outcomes in patients with heart failure. *Rehabilitation Nursing*, *28*(4), 117–122.

Elliott, T. R., Uswatte, G., Lewis, L., & Palmatier, A. (2000). Goal instability and adjustment to physical disability. *Journal of Counseling Psychology*, *47*(2), 251–265. doi:10.1037//0022-0167.47.2.251

Evans, L., & Hardy, L. (2002). Injury rehabilitation: A goal-setting intervention study. *Research Quarterly for Exercise and Sport*, *73*(3), 310–319.

Gauggel, S., & Billino, J. (2002). The effects of goal setting on the arithmetic performance of brain-damaged patients. *Archives of Clinical Neuropsychology*, *17*(3), 283–294.

Gauggel, S., Leinberger, R., & Richardt, M. (2001). Goal setting and reaction time performance in brain-damaged patients. *Journal of Clinical and Experimental Neuropsychology*, *23*(3), 351–361.

Grotle, M., Klokkerud, M., Kjeken, I., Bremander, A., Hagel, S., Strombeck, B., … Hagen, K. B. (2013). What's in the black box of arthritis rehabilitation? A comparison of rehabilitation practice for patients with inflammatory arthritis in Northern Europe. *Journal of Rehabilitation Medicine*, *45*(5), 458–466.

Hart, T., & Evans, J. (2006). Self-regulation and goal theories in brain injury rehabilitation. *Journal of Head Trauma Rehabilitation*, *21*(2), 142–155.

Hart, T., Hawkey, K., & Whyte, J. (2002). Use of a portable voice organizer to remember therapy goals in traumatic brain injury rehabilitation: A within-subjects trial. *Journal of Head Trauma Rehabilitation*, *17*(6), 556–570.

Harwood, M., Weatherall, M., Talemaitoga, A., Barlier, P.A., Gommans, J., Taylor, W., & McNaughton, H. (2011). Taking charge after stroke: Promoting self-directed rehabilitation to improve quality of life–a randomized controlled trial. *Clinical Rehabilitation, 26*(6), 493–501. doi:10.1177/0269215511426017.

Higgins, J. P. T., & Green, S. (Eds.). (2011). *Cochrane handbook for systematic reviews of interventions – Version 5.1.0.* Oxford, U.K.: The Cochrane Collaboration.

Holliday, R. C., Ballinger, C., & Playford, E. D. (2007). Goal setting in neurological rehabilitation: Patients' perspectives. *Disability and Rehabilitation, 29*(5), 389–394.

Holliday, R. C., Cano, S., Freeman, J. A., & Playford, E. D. (2007). Should patients participate in clinical decision making? An optimised balance block design controlled study of goal setting in a rehabilitation unit. *Journal of Neurology, Neurosurgery and Psychiatry, 78*(6), 576–580.

Howell, C. (1986). A controlled trial of goal setting for long-term community psychiatric patients. *British Journal of Occupational Therapy, 49*, 264–268.

Johnston, M. V. (2003). Desiderata for clinical trials in medical rehabilitation. *American Journal of Physical Medicine and Rehabilitation, 82*(Suppl.), S3–S7.

Kahneman, D. (2011). *Thinking: Fast and slow.* London, U.K.: Penguin Books.

Kleingeld, A., van Mierlo, H., & Arends, L. (2011). The effect of goal setting on group performance: A meta-analysis. *Journal of Applied Psychology, 96*(6), 1289–1304.

Kok, G., Schaalma, H., Ruiter, R. A., Van Empelen, P., & Brug, J. (2004). Intervention mapping: Protocol for applying health psychology theory to prevention programmes. *Journal of Health Psychology, 9*(1), 85–98.

Krasny-Pacini, A., Hiebel, J., Pauly, F., Godon, S., & Chevignard, M. (2013). Goal Attainment Scaling in rehabilitation: A literature-based update. *Annals of Physical and Rehabilitation Medicine, 56*(3), 212–230.

Lacasse, Y., Goldstein, R., Lasserson, T. J., & Martin, S. (2006). Pulmonary rehabilitation for chronic obstructive pulmonary disease. *Cochrane Database of Systematic Reviews, 4*, CD003793. doi:10.1002/14651858

LaFerriere, L., & Calsyn, R. (1978). Goal attainment scaling: An effective treatment technique in short-term therapy. *American Journal of Community Psychology, 6*(3), 271–282.

Laver, K., Halbert, J., Stewart, M., & Crotty, M. (2010). Patient readiness and ability to set recovery goals during the first 6 months after stroke. *Journal of Allied Health, 39*(4), e149–e154.

Levack, W. M. M., Dean, S., Siegert, R. J., & McPherson, K. M. (2006). Purposes and mechanisms of goal planning in rehabilitation: The need for a critical distinction. *Disability and Rehabilitation, 28*(12), 741–749.

Levack, W. M. M., Dean, S. G., McPherson, K. M., & Siegert, R. J. (2006). How clinicians talk about the application of goal planning to rehabilitation for people with brain injury –Variable interpretations of value and purpose. *Brain Injury, 20*(13–14), 1439–1449.

Levack, W. M. M., Taylor, K., Siegert, R. J., Dean, S. G., McPherson, K. M., & Weatherall, M. (2006). Is goal planning in rehabilitation effective? A systematic review. *Clinical Rehabilitation, 20*(9), 739–755.

Locke, E. A., & Latham, G. P. (2002). Building a practically useful theory of goal setting and task motivation: A 35-year odyssey. *American Psychologist, 57*(9), 705–717.

Loori, J. D. (Ed.). (2004). *The art of just sitting: Essential writings on the Zen practice of Shikantaza* (2nd ed.). Somerville, MA: Wisdom Publications.

Machin, D., & Fayers, P. (2010). *Randomized clinical trials: Design, practice and reporting.* West Sussex, U.K.: Wiley-Blackwell.

Malec, J. F. (1999). Goal attainment scaling in rehabilitation. *Neuropsychological Rehabilitation, 9*(3/4), 253–275.

Matthews, J. N. S. (2006). *An introduction to randomized controlled clinical trials* (2nd ed.). Boca Raton, FL: Chapman & Hall/CRC.

McPherson, K. M., Kayes, N., & Weatherall, M. (2009). A pilot study of self-regulation informed goal setting in people with traumatic brain injury. *Clinical Rehabilitation, 23*, 296–309.

Michie, S., Richardson, M., Johnston, M., Abraham, C., Francis, J., Hardeman, W., ... Wood, C. E. (2013). The behavior change technique taxonomy (v1) of 93 hierarchically clustered techniques: Building an international consensus for the reporting of behavior change interventions. *Annals of Behavioral Medicine, 46*, 81–95.

Miller, C. K., Headings, A., Peyrot, M., & Nagaraja, H. (2012). Goal difficulty and goal commitment affect adoption of a lower glycemic index diet in adults with type 2 diabetes. *Patient Education and Counseling, 86*(1), 84–90.

Ostelo, R. W. J. G., de Vet, H. C. W., Vlaeyen, J. W., Kerckhoffs, M. R., Berfelo, M. W., Wolters, P. M. J. C., & van den Brandt, P. A. (2003). Behavioral graded activity following first-time lumbar disc surgery. *Spine, 28*(16), 1757–1765.

Ostelo, R. W. J. G., Goossens, M. E. J. B., de Vet, H. C. W., & van den Brandt, P. A. (2004). Economic evaluation of a behavioral-graded activity program compared to physical therapy for patients following lumbar disc surgery. *Spine, 29*(6), 615–622.

Ostelo, R. W. J. G., Koke, A. J. A., Beurskens, A. J. H. M., de Vet, H. C. W., Kerckhoffs, M. R., Vlaeyen, J. W., ... van den Brandt, P. A. (2000). Behavioral-graded activity compared with usual care after first-time disk surgery: Considerations of the design of a randomized clinical trial. *Journal of Manipulative and Physiological Therapeutics, 23*(5), 312–319.

Ponte-Allan, M., & Giles, G. (1999). Goal-setting and functional outcomes in rehabilitation. *American Journal of Occupational Therapy, 53*, 646–649.

Preminger, J. E., & Lind, C. (2012). Assisting communication partners in the setting of treatment goals: The development of the goal sharing for partners strategy. *Seminars in Hearing, 33*(1), 53–64. doi:10.1055/s-0032-1304728

Price, K. H., Harrison, D. A., & Gavin, J. H. (2006). Withholding inputs in team contexts: Member composition, interaction processes, evaluation structure, and social loafing. *Journal of Applied Psychology, 91*(6), 1375.

Puhan, M. A., Gimeno-Santos, E., Scharplatz, M., Troosters, T., Walters, E., & Steurer, J. (2009). Pulmonary rehabilitation following exacerbations of chronic obstructive pulmonary disease. *Cochrane Database of Systematic Reviews*, Issue 1. Art No.: CD005305. doi: 10.1002/14651858. CD005305.pub2.

Rosewilliam, S., Roskell, C. A., & Pandyan, A. D. (2011). A systematic review and synthesis of the quantitative and qualitative evidence behind patient-centred goal setting in stroke rehabilitation. *Clinical Rehabilitation, 25*(6), 501–514.

Schlund, M. W., & Pace, G. (1999). Relations between traumatic brain injury and the environment: Feedback reduces maladaptive behaviour exhibited by three persons with traumatic brain injury. *Brain Injury, 13*(11), 889–897.

Schlund, M. W., Pace, G. M., & McGready, J. (2001). Relations between decision-making deficits and discriminating contingencies following brain injury. *Brain Injury, 15*(12), 1061–1071. doi:10.1080/02699050110086887

Schulz, K. F., & Grimes, D. A. (2002). Blinding in randomised trials: Hiding who got what. *The Lancet, 359*(9307), 696–700.

Schut, H. A., & Stam, H. J. (1994). Goals in rehabilitation teamwork. *Disability and Rehabilitation, 16*(4), 223–226.

Sewell, L., Singh, S. J., Williams, J. E., Collier, R., & Morgan, M. D. (2005). Can individualized rehabilitation improve functional independence in elderly patients with COPD? *Chest, 128*(3), 1194–1200.

Siegert, R. J., McPherson, K. M., & Taylor, W. (2004). Toward a cognitive-affective model of goal-setting in rehabilitation: Is self-regulation theory a key step? *Disability and Rehabilitation, 26*(20), 1175–1183.

Solomon, P., Cavanaugh, M. M., & Draine, J. (2009). *Randomized controlled trials: Design and implementation for community-based psychosocial interventions.* Oxford, U.K.: Oxford University Press.

Sugavanam, T., Mead, G., Bulley, C., Donaghy, M., & Van Wijck, F. (2013). The effects and experiences of goal setting in stroke rehabilitation – A systematic review. *Disability and Rehabilitation, 35*(5), 177–190.

Taylor, W. J., Brown, M., Levack, W., McPherson, K. M., Reed, K., Dean, S.G., & Weatherall, M. (2012). A pilot cluster randomised controlled trial of structured goal-setting following stroke. *Clinical Rehabilitation, 26*(4), 327–338.

Tennant, A. (2007). Goal attainment scaling: Current methodological challenges. *Disability and Rehabilitation, 29,* 1583–1588.

van Dick, R., Tissington, P. A., & Hertel, G. (2009). Do many hands make light work? How to overcome social loafing and gain motivation in work teams. *European Business Review, 21*(3), 233–245.

Wade, D. T. (2001). Research into the black box of rehabilitation: The risks of a Type III error. *Clinical Rehabilitation, 15*(1), 1–4.

Webb, P. M., & Glueckauf, R. L. (1994). The effects of direct involvement in goal setting on rehabilitation outcome for persons with traumatic brain injuries. *Rehabilitation Psychology, 39*(3), 179–188.

Whittington, J. L., Goodwin, V. L., & Murray, B. (2004). Transformational leadership, goal difficulty, and job design: Independent and interactive effects on employee outcomes. *The Leadership Quarterly, 15*(5), 593–606.

Whyte, J. (2003). Clinical trials in rehabilitation: What are the obstacles? *American Journal of Physical Medicine and Rehabilitation, 82*(Suppl.), S16–S21.

Whyte, J., & Hart, T. (2003). It's more than a black box; it's a Russian doll: Defining rehabilitation treatments. *American Journal of Physical Medicine & Rehabilitation, 82*(8), 639–652.

World Health Organization. (2001). *International Classification of Functioning, Disability and Health.* Geneva, Switzerland: WHO.

Ylvisaker, M., McPherson, K., Kayes, N., & Pellett, E. (2008). Metaphoric identity mapping: Facilitating goal setting and engagement in rehabilitation after traumatic brain injury. *Neuropsychological Rehabilitation, 18*(5–6), 713–741.

Young, C. A., Manmathan, G. P., Ward, J. C., Young, C. A., Manmathan, G. P., & Ward, J. C. R. (2008). Perceptions of goal setting in a neurological rehabilitation unit: A qualitative study of patients, carers and staff. *Journal of Rehabilitation Medicine, 40*(3), 190–194.

3

Psychology, Goals and Rehabilitation: Providing a Theoretical Foundation

Richard J. Siegert, Christine O'Connell and William M.M. Levack

CONTENTS

3.1 Introduction

> We define goals as internal representations of desired states, where states are broadly construed as outcomes, events, or processes. Internally represented desired states range from biological set points for internal processes (e.g. body temperature) to complex cognitive depictions of desired outcomes (e.g. career success). Likewise, goals span from the moment to a life span and from the neurological to the interpersonal.

Austin and Vancouver (1996, p. 338)

There is growing acknowledgement that scientific progress in rehabilitation requires development of theories in addition to empirical research (Dunn & Elliot, 2008; Siegert, McPherson, & Dean, 2005; Siegert & Taylor, 2004). While a *grand unified theory* of rehabilitation seems highly unlikely to emerge, there is increasing acceptance that sophisticated theoretical accounts of important phenomena in rehabilitation are necessary to understand complex processes and predict outcomes (Scobbie, Wyke, & Dixon, 2009; Siegert, McPherson, & Taylor, 2004; Whyte, 2007). This awareness of the important role of theory building and theory testing in a scientific rehabilitation is a recent development. Rehabilitation theory of goal setting still lags well behind goal-setting research in fields such as industrial–organizational psychology, education and sport psychology. This imbalance between theory development and empirical research limits the scientific credibility of rehabilitation (Siegert et al., 2005). More importantly, it does our clients or patients a disservice. It assumes that all we need is evidence about which interventions are effective – without a comprehensive understanding of *how* an intervention works for an individual client with a particular set of problems in a unique psychosocial context.

Goal setting provides a prime example of the relative neglect of theory development in rehabilitation when compared to the time and resources spent on gathering quantitative evidence – this neglect of theory building has led to some conceptual confusion. For example, one of the theories most frequently cited as a basis for using goal setting in rehabilitation is Locke and Latham's goal-setting theory (GST) (Latham & Locke, 2007; Locke & Latham, 1990, 2002; Scobbie et al., 2009). This is perhaps not surprising since GST is a well-established and clearly formulated theory with a formidable amount of support from quantitative studies. However, Locke and Latham are industrial–organizational psychologists whose original research focused on enhancing performance in work settings where the goals are most often dictated by the organization, not the individual. Indeed, the most consistent finding from numerous studies of GST has been that individuals perform at a higher level when they are set specific, difficult goals – a finding in direct conflict with the conventional wisdom in rehabilitation that a patient's goal must be achievable or attainable (Barnes & Ward, 2000; Playford, Siegert, Levack, & Freeman, 2009; Schut & Stam, 1994). Moreover, it is axiomatic in rehabilitation that the client or patient should actively participate in determining what their goals are. In contrast, in GST, the importance of goal commitment is acknowledged only as one of many possible *moderators* of goal-directed performance, and it is not considered essential to involve employees in goal setting to achieve goal commitment (Locke & Latham, 2007). Thus, one of the theories most frequently cited to justify the use of goal setting in rehabilitation actually conflicts with some important aspects of how goal setting is typically practised in rehabilitation. Moreover, we are not aware of any research study that has actually tested GST directly in the context of a rehabilitation programme (such as that provided by a multidisciplinary team over a period of several weeks).

The point at issue is that rehabilitation needs robust scientific theories and nowhere is this more evident than in rehabilitation goal setting. Borrowing existing theories from psychology to develop stronger theoretical frameworks within rehabilitation seems a reasonable and productive strategy. At the same time, science proceeds by two related activities – theory building and theory testing (Dubin, 1969). Thus, when a well-known theory is borrowed from psychology, to justify an intervention such as goal setting in a rehabilitation context, it is essential that the theory is tested in the new context and modified in the light of empirical findings.

Evidence to support this perspective can be found in the literature on the development of goal theory in sport psychology. Following the development of their GST in industrial–organizational psychology, Locke and Latham (1985) proposed that their findings (regarding a linear relationship between specific, difficult goals and human performance) would be even more pronounced in sport settings. They based this argument on an assumption that the measurement of individual performance tended to be more objective in sports compared to industrial and organizational contexts and therefore would provide a better basis for goal selection and evaluation (Locke & Latham, 2007). As it turned out however, scores of experimental studies into goal theory in sport psychology failed to provide the evidence to support this assertion (Burton & Naylor, 2002; Hall & Kerr, 2001). Although goal setting does appear to have a desirable effect on sport performance, the overall effect of specific, difficult goals has been found to be lower in sport contexts than that reported in industrial–organizational settings (Burton & Naylor, 2002; Hall & Kerr, 2001). The reason behind this difference appeared to relate, at least partly, to the differences in human cognition and behaviour that occur in sport versus work contexts. To give just one example, many athletes are already driven by their own superordinate goals (such as to win a competition or achieve a personal best). The addition of specific, difficult goals on top of these superordinate goals therefore does not have the same effect as it might do in a work setting, where employees are not internally driven to the same extent (Hall & Kerr, 2001). Thus, Hall and Kerr have stated that 'while there is little doubt that goal setting is an effective performance-enhancing technique, claims for its effectiveness as a motivational technique must also consider the context in which participants are being asked to set goals' (p. 194).

The aim of this chapter is to highlight some psychological theories, a number of which have previously been drawn upon in the rehabilitation literature, and to consider their respective merits for developing rehabilitation GST. One challenge here is the large and diverse body of knowledge regarding goals and human performance that exists outside of rehabilitation. Goal setting has been extensively researched in education (Boekaerts & Niemivirta, 2000; Pintrich, 2000), organizational psychology (Latham & Locke, 2007; Locke & Latham, 1990, 2002), social cognition and personality (Austin & Vancouver, 1996; Custers & Aarts, 2010; Grant & Gelety, 2009) and sport psychology (Burton, Pickering, Weinberg, Yukelson, & Weigand, 2010; Wilson, Hardy, & Harwood, 2006). Therefore, the present discussion will constitute at best a rather selective, narrative review of a limited number of potentially useful theories that have already received some attention in the rehabilitation literature. In particular, we will consider the following approaches:

- Neuropsychological and neurophysiological perspectives on goals
- Carver and Scheier's self-regulation theory
- Bandura's self-efficacy theory
- Locke and Latham's GST
- Social cognitive research on implicit goals

3.2 Neuropsychological and Neurophysiological Perspectives on Goals and Goal Setting

Contemporary neuropsychology views goals as important elements in the organization of human behaviour and the prefrontal cortex of the brain as playing an important role in goal-directed behaviour (Berkman & Lieberman, 2009). Indeed, the prefrontal cortex is widely considered to be the *executive centre* of the brain, responsible for functions that include '...goal formation, planning, carrying out goal-directed plans, and effective performance' (Jurado & Rosselli, 2007, p. 213). Badre, Hoffman, Cooney, and D'Esposito (2009) noted that 'the function of the prefrontal cortex... is closely associated with cognitive control or the ability of humans and other primates to internally guide behaviour in accordance with goals, plans and broader contextual knowledge' (p. 515). Much of the evidence for the role of the prefrontal cortex in regulating goal-directed behaviour has come from case studies and group studies of people who have suffered lesions to the prefrontal cortex stemming back as far as the famous case of Phineas Gage* in the mid-nineteenth century (Macmillan, 2008). The epidemic of prefrontal lobotomy in the treatment of schizophrenia which occurred in the United States and parts of Europe in the 1950s also demonstrated rather dramatically the importance of the frontal cortex for goal-directed behaviour and motivation – resulting as it frequently did in listless, apathetic individuals (Lerner, 2005; Valenstein, 1986). More recently, advances in neuroimaging techniques have also further supported the notion of the prefrontal cortex as critical in goal-directed behaviour (Berkman & Lieberman, 2009).

In reviewing the literature on neuroscience and goal pursuit, Berkman and Lieberman (2009) commented that neuroscience has traditionally not been concerned with goal pursuit per se but rather with the cognitive components or sub-components that contribute to it. For example, they cite the role of the dorsolateral prefrontal cortex in maintaining rules and planning rule-based action. They also observed that neuroscience has largely been concerned with short-term, concrete goals, whereas social psychology has tended to study more abstract, life goals. This suggests that neuropsychological perspectives on goal setting in rehabilitation will be most relevant at the micro level – perhaps in relation to achieving short-term goals, completing specific tasks and motor skill learning. One neuropsychological theory that has been proposed to account for the problems that people with frontal lobe injuries sometimes experience in goal-directed behaviour is that of Norman and Shallice (1980).

3.2.1 Norman and Shallice Model of Action Control

Norman and Shallice developed this theory partly to explain the behaviour of certain patients with frontal lesions who coped perfectly well with routine behaviour but struggled when faced with unexpected or novel problems. Norman and Shallice (1980) described a model of hierarchical information processing which distinguished between *willed* and *automatic* behaviours. Shallice (1982) proposed that routine actions and cognitions (known as *schema*) are activated by an input, such as a perception or another schema, and result in an *automatic* output, such as a behavioural response or thought process. This practice involves a mechanism referred to as *contention scheduling*, an automatic process which is said to mediate schema selection by opting for compatible schemas and, depending on the specific environment or situation, ensuring the highest priority schema is activated (Cooper & Shallice, 2006).

However, the model holds that for situations involving decision making, planning and goal-directed behaviour, this automatic response is not sufficient. For the execution of tasks requiring such processes, a non-habitual schema selection is necessary. This involves a supervisory attentional system, a planning system thought to be located in the prefrontal cortex (Shallice, 2002), which is invoked in order to bias the operation of contention scheduling and override automatic behaviours (Cooper & Shallice, 2006). According to Shallice (1982), support for the existence of the supervisory attentional system comes from

---

* Phineas Gage was a foreman who worked on railroads in Virginia in the United States in the nineteenth century. An explosion accidentally fired a metal rod through his skull, and although he made an excellent physical recovery, his social behaviour was severely affected. Phineas had been a model citizen before the accident and afterwards displayed the disorganization and disinhibition that are now known to characterize serious damage to the frontal lobes.

the concept of *action lapses*. For example, a routine task, such as driving home from work, which does not require the supervisory attentional system, can be carried out by using contention scheduling alone, while the supervisory attentional system is focused on a non-competing action or thought process, such as planning a shopping list. Stopping at the supermarket, however, may not be part of the routine of driving home, and the routine behaviour may be completed without fulfilling this task. In this case, the supervisory attentional system, being engaged with planning the shopping list, has not overridden the automatic behaviour so one has an action lapse (Norman, 1981). The model therefore assumes that while the two processes (i.e. automatic/habitual and planned/non-habitual schema selection) interact, performance on a novel task can be impeded independently of performance on a practised task, which is consistent with the problems experienced by people with frontal lobe injuries.

3.2.2 Goal Management Training

Goal management training (GMT) was originally developed by Ian Robertson in 1996 for patients with traumatic brain injury. GMT is a self-regulation approach to goal-directed behaviour aimed at training individuals to structure intentions and manage goal-planning activities (Levine et al., 2000; Robertson, 1996). This intervention has its grounding in various executive theories of goal neglect, sustained attention and disorganization of behaviour and in the Norman and Shallice model of action control (Cooper & Shallice, 2006; Duncan, 1986; Duncan, Emslie, Williams, Johnson, & Freer, 1996; Robertson & Garavan, 2000). GMT, which centres on attention control and awareness, has also recently been linked to *mindfulness*, a therapeutic intervention which has its origins in eastern contemplative traditions. Kabat-Zinn (2003), who pioneered the introduction of mindfulness in health and clinical settings, described this concept as 'the awareness that emerges through paying attention on purpose, in the present moment' (p. 145). The development of a metacognitive awareness through the ability to view one's thoughts from a different perspective is fundamental to both mindfulness and GMT.

According to GMT, goal-directed behaviour is a structured process managed in the prefrontal cortex of the brain. It is controlled by a set of hierarchical task requirements (or steps) derived from environmental or internal information. Specifically, when the current situation is at variance with the desired situation, a number of actions may be considered to resolve the discrepancy. Each action represents a step towards goal execution. These actions are subsequently activated in an ordered process. However, interfering internal or external cues can disrupt this step-by-step process resulting in the individual neglecting to maintain their original goals. For example, John is at work but needs to leave early to post an important parcel before 5 o'clock, when the post office closes. Just as he is about to switch off his computer, he spots an e-mail from a friend he has not seen since university days. John quickly scans the e-mail and becomes nostalgic reminiscing about his college days. He then hits the *reply* button and begins to write, forgetting about time and the parcel beside him on the desk. When he has finished his reply, he glances at his watch. It is quarter past five and he has missed the deadline to post his package. This unconscious disregard of a task requirement (leaving before 5 o'clock), in spite of the fact that it has been encoded and comprehended, is known as *goal neglect*. This is instigated by internal and external distractions along with poor construction and use of goal-planning procedures, which, according to the Norman and Shallice model of action control, occurs commonly among healthy individuals and is often a significant impairment in people with frontal lobe dysfunction (Cooper & Shallice, 2006; Duncan, 1986; Levine et al., 2000).

GMT comprises five stages, each of which relates to a central element of goal focused behaviour. Stage 1 refers to the *stop strategy* which encourages individuals to stop and think about what they are doing. Defining the main goal or task at hand comprises Stage 2 of GMT. During Stage 3, clients are required to list the necessary steps involved in executing their goal. Stage 4 involves carrying out each step in turn. Finally, Stage 5 involves the individual using the *stop strategy* once more and *checking* if their current behaviour is still advancing them towards the original main goal.

In several clinical and non-clinical randomized controlled trials, GMT's efficacy in improving goal management has been illustrated in groups including individuals who have suffered TBI, patients characterized by frontal lobe damage (although this study was only partially randomized) and older adults (Levine et al., 2000, 2011; van Hooren et al., 2007). Specifically, the value of GMT has been illustrated in relation to goal neglect and attention (Levine et al., 2000, 2011). In addition, its usefulness in improving the management of executive failures has been identified (van Hooren et al., 2007). The effectiveness of this intervention combined with mindfulness meditation in reducing executive and decision-making deficits has also been demonstrated in a non-randomized controlled study (Alfonso, Caracuel, Delgado-Pastor, & Verdejo-Garcia, 2011). Thus, GMT may be described as an experimentally validated clinical intervention with firm theoretical underpinnings for neurological rehabilitation.

3.2.3 Summary and Comments

Neuropsychology and related neurosciences have enhanced our current understanding of goal setting by identifying the specific brain regions associated with goal-directed behaviour and through the detailed examination of the behavioural deficits of people with damage to the prefrontal cortex. This has already led to the development of specific neuropsychological models of executive behaviour and executive dysfunction and of at least one therapeutic intervention specifically targeted at goal management for people with executive dysfunction. Although the neuropsychological perspective is not a theory of goal setting per se, it is an important body of knowledge that informs and enhances our understanding of goal setting in rehabilitation. With the rapid emergence of the new discipline of social neuroscience, we expect to see exciting theoretical developments in the next few years that will have substantial relevance for clinical rehabilitation.

3.3 Carver and Scheier's Self-Regulation Theory

There has been an upsurge of interest in the relevance of self-regulation models for rehabilitation in the past decade (Hart & Evans, 2006; Jones & Riazi, 2011; Siegert et al., 2004). Self-regulation has in part gained prominence in health sciences because of its association with self-responsibility in increasingly overburdened health economies worldwide (Maes & Karoly, 2005). Self-regulation, as a theory from applied psychology, is not just about health behaviour however. In fact, self-regulation is rather difficult to define as a concept because of the multitude of ideas that have been associated with it. Self-regulation has been variously described as self-determination, self-control, self-management and self-direction (Ylvisaker & Feeney, 2002) and has been related to the concepts of self-monitoring and self-care (Wilde & Garvin, 2007). It is considered a 'multi-component, multi-level, iterative, self-steering process' (Boekaerts, Maes, & Karoly, 2005, p. 150). In other words, self-regulation results from complex and repeating interactions between many factors, both personal (i.e. traits, beliefs, expectancies, values and abilities) and environmental (i.e. the social, cultural, political, organizational and societal context in which one lives and operates).

Self-regulation is however explicitly linked to goal setting. While there are a large number of theories about or related to self-regulation, Siegert et al. (2004) have suggested that all major self-regulation approaches share some, or all, of the following assumptions:

1. Most human behaviour is goal directed.
2. People strive towards multiple goals simultaneously.
3. Progress or failure in achieving desired goals has emotional consequences.
4. Goal attainment, motivation and affect are inextricably linked and interact.
5. Success at achieving important personal goals will often be determined by the individual's ability to regulate their own thoughts, emotions and behaviour.

It has been stated that the more explicitly aware people are of their goals and how their goal systems (in its broadest sense) works, the more successful they will be in directing their own behaviour (Boekaerts et al., 2005). Furthermore, the more conscious individuals are about the influence of environmental factors on their choices, persistence and ability to complete personal objectives, the more successful they will be with achieving their goals (Boekaerts et al., 2005). Thus, what might be considered *metacognition* (i.e. thinking about how you think) and being *streetwise* (i.e. knowing how the environment one is in works and how to successfully work within it) are fundamentally important attributes for successful self-regulation.

Favouring a process-oriented definition rather than a personality-oriented one, Maes and Karoly (2005) have offered the following as a definition of self-regulation for a health science context:

> Self-regulation can be more specifically defined as a goal-guidance process, occurring in iterative phases, that requires the self-reflective implementation of various change and maintenance mechanisms that are aimed at task- and time-specific outcomes. (p. 269)

One approach to thinking about self-regulation that is potentially very valuable in a rehabilitation context is Carver and Scheier's control-process model of self-regulation (Carver & Scheier, 1990, 1998). Within this model, human behaviour is viewed from a cybernetic perspective, whereby cognition is presented as a system of inputs, outputs and feedback loops much like a computer programme within a machine. Central to Carver and Scheier's self-regulation theory is the notion of a negative feedback system. In this system, a person has a goal and seeks to moderate their behaviour to achieve that goal. They do this by (explicitly or implicitly) evaluating the discrepancy between their current situation and their desired state and then acting to reduce this discrepancy (hence the reference to *negative* feedback).

In Carver and Scheier's self-regulation theory, the *goal* (or desired state) is called a *reference value* because it is the set point towards which all action is directed. The individual's perception of their current situation is referred to as an *input function* – providing information about the environment and the individual's current state in the self-regulation system. Also required within this system is something Carver and

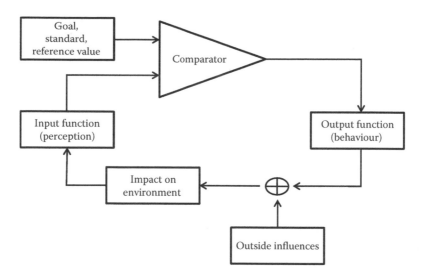

FIGURE 3.1
Schematic depiction of a feedback loop, the basic unit of cybernetic control. (Reproduced from Carver, C.S. and Scheier, M.F., *On the Self-Regulation of Behavior*, Cambridge University Press, Cambridge, U.K. With permission.)

Scheier refer to as a *comparator* – a component of the system (i.e. part of the brain) that allows for a comparison to be made between the input and the reference value. The *output function* from this system is the behaviour implemented to correct the discrepancy between the input and reference values, in response to an *error signal* from the comparator. The output function feeds forwards into the system, to adjust behaviour with the intention of changing the current situation to be more in line with the desired one. Figure 3.1 provides an overview of these processes.

Another central part of Carver and Scheier's self-regulation model is the idea that individuals are never pursuing only one goal at a time. In fact, Carver and Scheier have proposed that there is a hierarchy of goals which influence our behaviour, ranging from high-level abstract goals to very concrete goals related to specific actions, through to physiological goals our bodies respond to in order to achieve certain outcomes (Carver & Scheier, 1998). This hierarchy is presented as comprised of four levels: (1) system concept, (2) principles, (3) programmes and (4) sequences. At the top of this hierarchy is a person's *system concept*: the mental image they hold of their idealized self and the person they ultimately want to be in life. The *principles* are the values and philosophies that a person chooses to adhere to or pursue (e.g. to be a good person, to become a productive researcher, to be seen as a wise clinician or to create an environmentally sustainable world). The *programmes* are the specific activities that they endeavour to engage in (e.g. reading, shopping, washing, driving, studying, recycling, gardening, caregiving), and *sequences* are the highly routine or automatic behaviours that people undertake in their daily life (e.g. motor sequences are involved in walking).

The idea here is that people are motivated to pursue lower-order goals and behaviours that will contribute to their higher-order life goals. For instance, after a spinal cord injury resulting in paraplegia, a 39-year-old man might hold as his *system concept* the idea of once again returning to his role as the primary income earner for his family, loving partner to his wife and father to his children. Evaluation of his current situation would highlight a discrepancy between where he is at now (unable to walk and being in hospital) to this

TABLE 3.1

Comparison of Terminology and Concepts Related to Life Goals Used by Nair and Carver and Scheier

Nair's Representation of a Hierarchy of Life Goals	Carver and Scheier's Hierarchy of Behaviour and Goals	Examples
1. Idealized self-image	1. System concept	The person one wants to be
2. Abstract motivations	2. Principles	Power, fame, fortune
3. Personal goals		Career, family, relationships
4. Contextual goals		Striving for better grades at school
5. Immediate actions	3. Programmes	Specific activities like reading, writing, playing
n/a	4. Sequences	Highly practised, automatic routines such as motor sequences

desired state. This man then may seek information from his current environment (such as from books, from fellow patients within the hospital and from the health professionals he interacts with) to determine not only what might be possible to achieve in the future but also what types of personal attributes (principles) and activities (programmes) would most help him with ways of returning to his idealized self. His evolving beliefs regarding his idealized self, personal attributes and activities he believes he needs to pursue all become reference values which guide his behaviour over the coming weeks and months of rehabilitation.

Building on the work of Carver and Scheier (1990) and others (Austin & Vancouver, 1996; McGrath & Adams, 1999; Roberts & Roins, 2000), Nair (2003) further developed this hierarchy in his work on life goals in rehabilitation. Instead of a *system concept*, Nair referred to an *idealized self-image*, but the concept is essentially the same. Nair's hierarchy has a few more subcategories of goals which seem closely related to Carver and Scheier's concept of *principles*, and he has one less category of goals related to the notion of *sequences*, but overall, Nair argued for a very similar structure linking lower-order activities to higher-order abstract objectives. Table 3.1 presents a comparison of Nair and Carver and Scheier's hierarchies of behaviours and goals.

Of course modifying one's behaviour to better improve chances of achieving a particular goal is not the only possible response to a discrepancy between a current state (or at least one's perception of a current state) and a desired end point. Another approach would be to adjust the reference value or to give up on it altogether. This is also something that Carver and Scheier's model accommodates. Indeed, Carver and Scheier have proposed that at times it may be healthiest to know when to *quit* pursuing an unattainable goal or perhaps when to quit pursuing a goal where the end point does not justify the personal resources expended (Wrosch, Scheier, Miller, Schulz, & Carver, 2003). This concept is known as *goal disengagement*.

The concept of goal disengagement has bearing on goal setting for rehabilitation in two ways. First, a planned process for goal disengagement may be useful during therapy when it becomes apparent that current clinical goals are not going to be achieved. Second, people entering into rehabilitation services often have had substantial changes to their capacity to pursue goals they held prior to acquiring a disability. In this context, providing patients and family members with support and guidance through the process of life goal disengagement and re-engagement could potentially be an important part of the rehabilitation process. In fact, it has been suggested that the emphasis in goal setting for rehabilitation should be on being 'opportunistic and discriminative in goal pursuit' (Neter, Litvak, & Miller, 2009, p. 175).

In one of the few studies on goal disengagement in rehabilitation, Neter et al. (2009) investigated the influence of continuing to pursue or ceasing pursuit of life goals on emotional well-being, among people with multiple sclerosis. One of the key findings in Neter et al. research was that problems with depression following increasing disability are not so much associated with failure to achieve a life goal per se, but rather from a failure to reengage with new, meaningful goals when older goals become untenable. In particular, they found that the study participants who had high levels of disengagement but low levels of re-engagement (i.e. who gave up previously held goals but did not replace these with new goals to pursue) were significantly more depressed than other participants. Surprisingly, participants who had low levels of disengagement with previous life goals and low levels of re-engagement with new goals were the least depressed. These findings suggested that health professionals, when working with people facing life changes as a result of a degenerative condition such as multiple sclerosis, need to be cautious about counselling patients to give up on what might be considered, from the health professional's perspective, unrealistic life goals. Furthermore, if such a person overtly needs to give up on a previously held goal, their general well-being will be influenced by the degree to which they successfully re-engage with a new goal. This is clearly an area where health professionals could provide advice and support.

Carver and Scheier's model of self-regulation is not without its detractors, however. It has been criticized for being too mechanistic and for avoiding consideration of the significant capacity humans have for actively deciding which goals are important to pursue and which to avoid (Locke & Latham, 1990). It has also been highlighted that Carver and Scheier's model is primarily about the *how* of goals and behaviour (i.e. how people stay engaged with goals) but little about the *what* and *why* of goal setting (i.e. how people decide which goals are most important to them and why they choose certain goals over others) (Deci & Ryan, 2000). Nevertheless, Carver and Scheier's model contains a number of important ideas for rehabilitation providers to consider and is certainly worthy of further examination in future research.

3.3.1 Summary and Comments

While little research has been conducted examining the application of Carver and Scheier's model of self-regulation to rehabilitation settings, the model appears to provide a promising framework for better understanding how patients in rehabilitation respond to goal setting. Carver and Scheier's model also highlights that as well as the clinical goals which health professionals identify or negotiate with their patients, people within rehabilitation services will also have a number of other *reference values* against which they will be evaluating their current situation and consequently modifying their behaviour. These people may be consciously aware of their most influential reference values and may tell their health professionals about them or choose not to disclose them at all, or they may hold some reference values that they are not entirely able to articulate (to themselves or to others) but which nevertheless have a profound influence over their decisions and behaviour.

The concept of goal disengagement is also one which rehabilitation researchers need to pay considerably more attention to. How well people navigate through their life after disability will in part relate to how they respond to decisions regarding giving up on, or sticking with, previously held goals and to their ability to set new priorities. At present, we have very little data on the effect of goal engagement and disengagement on rehabilitation outcomes, and yet this is an area of patients' lives in which health professionals potentially have a significant influence.

3.4 Bandura's Self-Efficacy Theory

Self-efficacy is an essential component in Albert Bandura's social cognitive theory of human behaviour (Bandura, 2001). Put simply, self-efficacy is the confidence one has in one's own ability to succeed at a particular task or to achieve a certain goal and a belief in possessing the ability necessary to cope with any challenges that arise. Moreover, self-efficacy in relation to any specific task or goal facilitates or promotes success at completing that task or achieving the goal (Bandura, 1977). Self-efficacy is one of the most frequently applied psychological theories within rehabilitation research and goal-setting research in particular. Scobbie and colleagues (2009) completed a systematic search of the rehabilitation literature to identify those articles which had used a specific theory of behaviour change in reviewing or reporting original research on goal setting in a rehabilitation context and noted that 13 out of the 24 articles they retrieved used social cognitive theory and self-efficacy as their theoretical underpinning. Scobbie et al. included social cognitive theory among the three theoretical approaches that they considered had the greatest potential to inform clinical practice based upon clinical utility and empirical support. They noted: 'Self-efficacy is theorized to exert its influence on health outcomes by improving motivation to set and pursue goals and to increase resilience in the face of setbacks during goal pursuit' (Scobbie et al., 2009, p. 323). Self-efficacy is also an influential construct within the broader field of rehabilitation research as well as the specific domain of goal setting. It has been extensively studied in relation to the management or rehabilitation of chronic conditions including arthritis, diabetes, respiratory disease, coronary heart disease and stroke (Bentsen, Wentzel-Larsen, Henriksen, Rokne, & Wahl, 2010; Jones & Riazi, 2011; Marks, Allegrante, & Lorig, 2005; Woodgate & Brawley, 2008). A specific example of its application to self-management after stroke can be found in Chapter 14 of this book.

Research on self-efficacy in rehabilitation is likely to develop quickly with the increasing availability of self-efficacy scales that are specific to rehabilitation settings and for conditions that frequently require rehabilitation such as spinal cord injury, chronic obstructive pulmonary disease and multiple sclerosis (Davis, Figueredo, Fahy, & Rawiworrakul, 2007; Fliess-Douer, Van Der Woude, & Vanlandewijck, 2011; Rigby, Domenech, Thornton, Tedman, & Young, 2003; Stevens, van den Akker-Scheek, & van Horn, 2005). While the idea that a person is more likely to be successful at a task that they feel confident about hardly seems surprising or even informative, this is just one important implication of social cognitive theory, and to understand self-efficacy and its implications for rehabilitation, it is necessary to first examine social cognitive theory, self-efficacy and the image of human functioning that they assume.

3.4.1 Social Cognitive Theory, Self-Efficacy and Human Agency

Bandura argues that social cognitive theory is based on a conception of human beings as agents who act consciously and deliberately to mould the course of their daily lives (Bandura, 2001). Social cognitive theory was developed as an alternative to the two dominant paradigms in psychology in the late twentieth century, namely, behaviourism and information-processing approaches. Behaviourism viewed human behaviour as the product of learned associations between stimuli and responses acquired through Pavlovian and operant conditioning and placed little emphasis on unobservable thought processes. Information-processing approaches sought to replace the rat and pigeon with the modern high-speed computer as the best paradigm for understanding human beings while focusing on cognition rather than observable behaviour (Hunt, 1993). Social cognitive theory, while drawing substantially from both these schools of thought, maintained at the same time that 'the capacity to exercise control over the nature and quality of one's life is the essence of humanness' (Bandura, 2001, p. 1).

Bandura has argued that this quality of human agency entails four essential features which he labels (1) intentionality, (2) forethought, (3) self-reactiveness and (4) self-reflectiveness. *Intentionality* means the ability to plan for a specific outcome and to commit to a course of action to achieve the desired outcome. For this intentionality to succeed however requires *forethought* or forward planning. Bandura (2001) framed forethought in the language of goal setting commenting that 'People set goals for themselves, anticipate the likely consequences of prospective actions, and select and create courses of action likely to produce desired outcomes and avoid detrimental ones' (p. 7). *Self-reactiveness* describes the ability of people to motivate themselves and to monitor their own behaviour and progress towards a desired end or goal. Most importantly, it also involves the capacity to modify or self-regulate one's own thoughts, feelings and behaviour in response to perceived progress or failure. Finally, *self-reflectiveness* refers to the ability to self-examine or reflect on who one is and where one is going in life at a high level. Linking these four characteristics of human agency is the concept of perceived self-efficacy which is posited as a mechanism that determines our coping ability, effort expended and endurance when faced with a challenge.

According to the social cognitive theory, the information that people use to judge or calibrate their self-efficacy in relation to a particular task, challenge or goal is gleaned from four sources (Bandura, 1982):

1. *Mastery experience* (i.e. direct experience of the activity concerned and perceived success or failure). In Bandura's (1982) words, 'Successes heighten perceived self-efficacy; repeated failures lower it' (p. 126).

2. *Vicarious experience* (i.e. observing other people's successful or unsuccessful performance and modelling of specific behaviours).

3. *Verbal persuasion* (i.e. direct encouragement and inducement by others, such as peers, family members or health professionals).

4. *Physiological feedback* (i.e. interpretation of physical or emotional feelings, such as elevated heart rate, tiredness or a heightened sense of anxiety).

Bandura gives examples of each of these four sources of information using the example of a person recovering from a heart attack and their sense of self-efficacy in regard to resuming physical activity (Bandura, 1982). First, he suggests the rehabilitation process might involve carefully graduated treadmill exercises designed to provide direct experience of strenuous physical exertion in a controlled setting. Second is modelling which is typically achieved in cardiac rehabilitation programmes by involving former patients in education and support groups for current patients. Third is verbal persuasion which is provided by physicians and nurses directly and also through the use of pamphlets and video and Internet resources. The fourth source of information is physiological cues or sensations. For example, physiological feedback might relate to how the person interprets bodily sensations such as breathlessness. If perceived as signs of heart failure, breathlessness might undermine self-efficacy, but if perceived positively as an indication that one is working at an appropriate level of effort to make positive gains, self-efficacy could be enhanced.

3.4.2 Summary and Comments

Self-efficacy is a construct that has been extensively researched by social and clinical psychologists, and so far, the evidence has indicated that it is an important influence on successful coping and effective performance in a range of situations. Self-efficacy has also become increasingly popular with researchers attempting to explain rehabilitation outcomes, and it is probably the most frequently studied explanatory variable in rehabilitation goal-setting research (Scobbie et al., 2009). However, some researchers have challenged the notion that high self-efficacy always results in better performance or coping with a difficult task or in a stressful situation. Vancouver and colleagues have argued that a positive correlation between self-efficacy and motivation or performance does not demonstrate cause and effect and their own research has suggested a more complex relationship whereby performance can effect self-efficacy as well as self-efficacy effecting performance (Vancouver, More, & Yoder, 2008; Vancouver, Thompson, & Williams, 2001). However, much of the research by Vancouver and colleagues has had an organizational psychology focus and has used undergraduate psychology student participants. What are now needed are methodologically sound studies of self-efficacy in relation to the application of goal setting in rehabilitation contexts.

3.5 Locke and Latham's GST

One theory that has been frequently cited to support the use of goal setting in rehabilitation is GST, developed by the organizational psychologists Edwin Locke and Gary Latham (Locke & Latham, 1990, 2002). GST is probably the most well-researched theory of goal setting and human motivation in psychology. At the heart of GST is the finding (from numerous studies of human performance involving an extensive range of different tasks) that people perform at a higher level when given specific, difficult or challenging goals compared to if they are given a specific, easy goal or if they are simply told to *do your best* (representative of a non-specific goal). Moreover, Locke and Latham proposed that there is a linear relationship between goal difficulty and behaviour so that as goals become more difficult, so too does an individual's effort – and achievement tends to rise to match the stated expectation. This does not mean that people necessarily always achieve stated goals that are difficult, but just that their performance is better overall when striving towards difficult goals. For example, if someone is set the goal of peeling 30 potatoes in an hour, they might meet this goal, but not peel as many potatoes as someone who is set a goal of peeling 50 potatoes. Whether this second person peels 35 potatoes or 50 potatoes is not the point – the issue of interest is whether they achieved more overall than the person who was set the goal of peeling only 30 potatoes. To extend this example further, according to Locke and Latham's research, if people are instructed to just *do their best* at peeling as many potatoes as they can in 1 h (a non-specific goal), on average, they tend to do worse than if set a specific goal. The way Locke and Latham (2002) have explained this response is by saying that 'when people are asked to do their best, they do not do so' (p.706). Moreover, this is not just speculation or opinion. Locke and Latham (2002) have noted that research supporting their theory has involved 'over 100 different tasks involving more than 40,000 participants in at least eight countries working in laboratory, simulation and field settings' (p. 714).

According to Locke and Latham, goals affect performance on a task through four mechanisms:

1. Goals can serve to enhance performance through a directive function – which means they help people to focus their attention and skills on information and activities that are relevant to the particular task and to ignore distractions or competing demands.

2. Goals can have an energizing role – in other words, we put more conscious effort into performing well as a result of having specific goals.

3. Goals can also affect performance through raising persistence. This means we strive for longer and are less likely to give up in the face of obstacles or setbacks.

4. Goals can also function indirectly by assisting in the use of task-relevant knowledge and strategies and in discovering new and more effective strategies.

In addition to these four mechanisms through which goals influence performance, Locke and Latham (2002) also posit a number of variables which can moderate the relationship between a goal and related performance, in what they call the *high-performance cycle* (see Figure 3.2). Three of the most important moderators of performance are (1) goal commitment, (2) feedback and (3) task complexity. Goal commitment means simply that a person

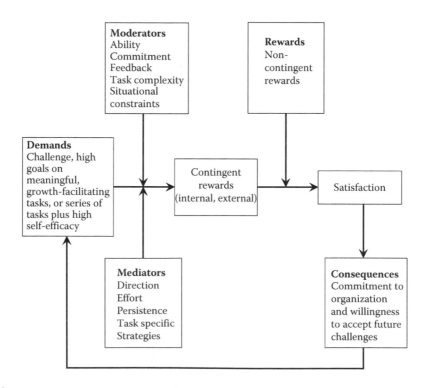

FIGURE 3.2
The high-performance cycle from Locke and Latham's GST. (Reproduced from Latham, G.P. and Locke, E.A., *Eur. Psychol.*, 12(4), 290, 2007. With permission. Copyright 2007 Hogrefe and Huber Publisher, www.hogrefe.com.)

will perform at a higher level on a goal that seems important to them and one that they regard as relevant and important.

Interestingly from a rehabilitation perspective, Locke and Latham do not consider involvement in defining or setting goals as very important in determining commitment to a goal, perhaps reflecting the origins of GST in industrial–organizational psychology. Indeed, they comment that 'meta-analyses of the effect of participation in decision making on performance, for those studies that measured performance objectively, yielded an effect size of only. 0.11' (Locke & Latham, 2002, p. 708). The two variables they consider that are both important in determining a person's level of goal commitment are the importance of the goal and self-efficacy. In other words, people are likely to work harder to achieve a goal that they perceive as important and one that they are confident they can succeed at. In this regard, it is possible for a health professional, who is well regarded as a clinician by their patients, to have an influence over what is potentially considered an important goal for an individual's rehabilitation and over what patients believe they could be capable of achieving.

Feedback is also important for goal commitment, and GST suggests that people need regular objective feedback on their performance level so that they can adjust their effort and behaviour accordingly. The third factor that can influence goal commitment is the complexity of the task. Here, Locke and Latham (2002) have noted that more complex tasks demand the ability to develop new strategies and individuals vary widely in this ability; hence, the linear relationship between task difficulty and performance is not as strong here. This is particularly relevant to consider in rehabilitation, as some tasks (such as retraining of physical function) can be relatively simple, whereas others (such as return to work) can involve multiple variables, complex social relationships and difficult decisions regarding investment of attention and energy. Thus, Locke and Latham's goal theory might be more appropriate for some aspects of rehabilitation than others.

Some of the best evidence for GST in rehabilitation comes from a series of elegant studies by Siegfried Gauggel, who examined performance on reaction time, motor speed and mental arithmetic tasks in people with an acquired brain injury (Gauggel & Billino, 2002; Gauggel & Fischer, 2001; Gauggel, Hoop, & Werner, 2002; Gauggel, Leinberger, & Richard, 2001). Gauggel's group found participants who were set specific, challenging goals performed better than a group instructed to *do your best*. This relationship was not moderated by clinical variables (e.g. mood or executive function). Gauggel's group has replicated these results and shown that assigning specific, challenging goals results in better performance than when people with a brain injury are told to set their own goals – supporting Locke and Latham's GST (Gauggel & Billino, 2002; Gauggel & Fischer, 2001; Gauggel et al., 2001, 2002). Similarly, controlled trials have demonstrated that specific goals may enhance physical performance when compared to no goals or non-specific goals for people undertaking a quadriceps strengthening programme after knee arthroscopy (Theodorakis, Beneca, Malliou, & Goudas, 1997) and that goal planning can result in higher levels of treatment adherence and patient self-efficacy in a population of injured athletes (Evans & Hardy, 2002).

3.5.1 Summary and Comments

While GST has often been cited in the rehabilitation literature as part of the theoretical rationale underpinning the practice of goal setting, there are some elements of GST which seem to conflict with widely accepted beliefs concerning the way in which rehabilitation should be practised. In particular, the idea that goals should be difficult or challenging contradicts the conventional wisdom that patient's or client's rehabilitation goals should be realistic, achievable or attainable (Playford et al., 2009; Wade, 2009). Similarly, it is an axiom in rehabilitation that the patient or client should be actively involved in developing their own goals and indeed the entire process of setting goals needs to be *client centred* (McGrath & Adams, 1999; McPherson & Siegert, 2007). However, Locke and Latham might dispute this notion – at least in terms of the effect of goals on motivation and performance in the workplace (Locke & Latham, 2002). Once again, this highlights the limitations in borrowing a theory from one branch of psychology without (1) a careful theoretical analysis of how the theory might transfer to clinical rehabilitation and (2) a rigorous empirical evaluation of how well it works in the new setting. In our opinion, GST is one of the most promising theories to help us to better understand goal setting in rehabilitation. However, there remain a number of issues yet to be explored. For example, in the context of a newly acquired disability where prognostic uncertainty can exist, how can one predetermine how *difficult* a goal needs to be to achieve desired motivational effects? Does failure to meet a goal carry with it any real psychological risks that health professionals ought to be concerned about, or are patients less concerned about goal failure than health professionals realize? The time (and resources) for some serious quantitative studies of GST in clinical rehabilitation is long overdue.

3.6 Social Cognitive Research on Implicit Goals: The Cutting Edge of Goal-Setting and Psychological Theory

Wade (2009) has suggested that rehabilitation goals have two essential characteristics. First, they involve an 'intended future state' (Wade, 2009, p. 291), and second, this state must be the deliberate or intended outcome of an intervention by a rehabilitation professional or team. Wade also specifies that this goal must be explicitly developed through the rehabilitation professionals collaborating with the client to develop explicit goals. Compare this with the definition of a goal from two psychologists, Austin and Vancouver (1996), at the start of this chapter. For Austin and Vancouver, a goal is an internal representation of a desired state – in other words, a goal is first and foremost a cognitive or psychological phenomenon. It is important to acknowledge then that while rehabilitation has profitably drawn from psychological theories of goals and goal setting, there are some important differences in the general approach each discipline takes to goal setting. Most importantly, rehabilitation tends to view goals as observable outcomes that are negotiated or agreed upon by a client and the rehabilitation team, whereas psychology typically regards the goal as a part of an individual's cognitive or mental world.

This difference between the concept of a goal in psychology and in rehabilitation is especially evident when we consider research within psychology on implicit or unconscious goals (Custers & Aarts, 2010). For not only are goals in psychology typically viewed as mental representations but goals and goal-related behaviour are both considered to be influenced by environmental stimuli in the absence of conscious awareness (Bargh & Chartrand, 1999; Custers & Aarts, 2010). This reflects an extensive body of research in contemporary cognitive psychology that attests to the impact of implicit or non-conscious influences upon human behaviour. Consider just a few recent examples of this line of research. In a series of studies, Holland, Hendriks and Aarts were able to show that simply exposing research participants to the citrus-like odour of a household cleaner resulted in better performance on a word task in which some of the correct answers were synonymous with hygiene or tidiness and also resulted in participants leaving less mess after eating

(Holland, Hendriks, & Aarts, 2005). Importantly, participants seemed totally unaware of any influence of the odour upon their own behaviour. A series of studies by Kay, Wheeler, Bargh and Ross (2004) showed that simply exposing participants to objects connected with the business world, such as a briefcase or boardroom table, increased the cognitive accessibility of the idea of competition. For example, their participants were more likely to interpret an ambiguous social scenario as reflecting competition or to award themselves a larger monetary reward relative to co-participants on a game.

A key concept in both of the two series of studies just described (and in modern cognitive psychology generally) is the notion of *priming*. Priming is a phenomenon whereby the presence of a stimulus in a person's environment facilitates or makes a certain related response more probable. The important point about priming is that it can occur without conscious awareness on the part of the person whose behaviour is being influenced.

In a review of the psychological literature on goals, attention and consciousness, Dijksterhuis and Aarts (2010) argued that 'goals guide attention and thereby often behaviour, and both goals and attention are largely independent from consciousness' (p. 469) and, moreover, that 'goals can be activated unconsciously by features of the environment' (p. 470). Perhaps what is most striking about this quote from a rehabilitation perspective is the gap it highlights between current psychological thinking on goals and current thinking in rehabilitation about goal setting. To our knowledge, there has been no discussion of the concept of implicit goals and their relationship to motivation and no discussion of phenomena such as priming in the rehabilitation literature. Indeed, the hottest topic in current psychological research on goals is not mentioned in the rehabilitation goal-setting literature. This probably reflects the fact that rehabilitation is an applied field concerned with assisting people with major physical and cognitive impairments, and consequently, the focus is a pragmatic one. Nevertheless, rehabilitation professionals may be missing an important element of goal setting if they are unaware of or choose to ignore the implications of implicit goals.

The problem with the literature on implicit or unconscious goals, fascinating though it seems, is quite what it means in practice. After all, how does a clinician determine if a patient has an implicit goal, if the goal itself is outside the patient's conscious awareness? This is a difficult question and there is no simple answer. However, we believe that research on goal setting in rehabilitation might well benefit from a closer examination of the burgeoning research on implicit goals and motivation. Most clinicians have encountered clients whose behaviour seemed to work against attaining the very goals they stated verbally as important to achieve. For example, failing to care for oneself adequately might satisfy an implicit goal to be cared for, which the person either will not reveal or is not consciously aware of. Similarly, many patients will have experience of rehabilitation services where subtle non-verbal cues served to discourage striving towards challenging goals regardless of what explicit goals were stated verbally. It is important to note that rehabilitation would not be the only field to benefit were this research synergy to occur. Psychological research on goals and motivation might have more influence and prestige in the public domain if there were less reliance on studies using psychology undergraduates as participants and more evidence from clinical participants.

3.6.1 Summary and Comments

There has been extensive research in psychology in the past few decades on the role of unconscious or implicit influences on human goals and on people's motivation and behaviour towards achieving such goals. To date, this research has been largely ignored by rehabilitation clinicians and researchers, possibly because they are simply unaware of it or perhaps because it seems somewhat esoteric and impractical. For example, much of the evidence for implicit goals comes from experiments in which subtle environmental cues have been shown to influence the behaviour of university students working on artificial laboratory tasks. Given the evidence that effective motor rehabilitation techniques involve extensive repetition of monotonous and fatiguing tasks (e.g. constraint therapy, treadmill training and robotics), there seems potential scope for similar studies examining implicit influences (e.g. wall posters, music) on motivation and performance in the rehabilitation gym or clinic.

3.7 Conclusion

The field of clinical rehabilitation is increasingly characterized by more sophisticated theories and models underpinning both clinical practice and research. Goal setting in rehabilitation has used psychology as a rich source of relevant theories for understanding and planning the application of goal setting with patients. This chapter has reviewed some of the most frequently used psychological theories and also suggested some new directions. Most importantly, it has been argued here that each theory must be critically evaluated conceptually and empirically tested in the rehabilitation context and not simply *transplanted* from the psychology laboratory to the clinic. However, with this caveat in mind, we believe that closer integration between GST in psychology and rehabilitation has much to offer both disciplines and the consumers of rehabilitation services.

References

Alfonso, J. P., Caracuel, A., Delgado-Pastor, L. C., & Verdejo-Garcia, A. (2011). Combined goal management training and mindfulness meditation improve executive functions and decision-making performance in abstinent polysubstance abusers. *Drug and Alcohol Dependency, 117*(1), 78–81.

Austin, J. T., & Vancouver, J. B. (1996). Goal constructs in psychology: Structure, process and content. *Psychological Bulletin, 120*(3), 338–375.

Badre, D., Hoffman, J., Cooney, J. W., & D'Esposito, M. (2009). Hierarchical cognitive control deficits following damage to the human frontal lobe. *Nature Neuroscience, 12*(4), 515–522.

Bandura, A. (1977). Self-efficacy: Toward a unifying theory of behavioral change. *Psychological Review, 84*(2), 191–215.

Bandura, A. (1982). Self-efficacy mechanism in human agency. *American Psychologist, 37*(2), 122–147.

Bandura, A. (2001). Social cognitive theory: An agentic perspective. *Annual Review of Psychology, 52*, 1–26.

Bargh, J. A., & Chartrand, T. K. (1999). The unbearable automaticity of being. *American Psychologist, 54*(7), 462–479.

Barnes, M. P., & Ward, A. B. (2000). *Textbook of rehabilitation medicine*. Oxford, U.K.: Oxford University Press.

Bentsen, S. B., Wentzel-Larsen, T., Henriksen, A. H., Rokne, B., & Wahl, A. K. (2010). Self-efficacy as a predictor of improvement in health status and overall quality of life in pulmonary rehabilitation – An exploratory study. *Patient Education and Counseling, 81*(1), 5–13.

Berkman, E. T., & Lieberman, M. D. (2009). The neuroscience of goal pursuit. In G. B. Moskowitz & H. Grant (Eds.), *The psychology of goals* (pp. 98–126). New York, NY: The Guilford Press.

Boekaerts, M., Maes, S., & Karoly, P. (2005). Self-regulation across domains of applied psychology: Is there an emerging consensus? *Applied Psychology, 54*(2), 149–154.

Boekaerts, M., & Niemivirta, M. (2000). Self-regulated learning: Finding a balance between learning goals and ego-protective goals. In M. Boekaerts, P. R. Pintrich, & M. Zeidner (Eds.), *Handbook of self-regulation* (pp. 417–451). San Diego, CA: Academic Press.

Burton, D., & Naylor, S. (2002). The Jekyll/Hyde nature of goals: Revisiting and updating goal-setting in sport. In T. Horn (Ed.), *Advances in sport psychology* (pp. 459–499). Champaign, IL: Human Kinetics.

Burton, D., Pickering, M., Weinberg, R., Yukelson, D., & Weigand, D. (2010). The competitive goal effectiveness paradox revisited: Examining the goal practices of prospective olympic athletes. *Journal of Applied Sports Psychology, 22*, 72–86.

Carver, C. S., & Scheier, M. F. (1990). Origins and functions of positive and negative affect: A control-process view. *Psychological Review, 1990*(97), 19–35.

Carver, C. S., & Scheier, M. F. (1998). *On the self-regulation of behavior*. Cambridge, U.K.: Cambridge University Press.

Cooper, R. P., & Shallice, T. (2006). Hierarchical schemas and goals in the control of sequential behavior. *Psychological Review, 113*(4), 887–916.

Custers, R., & Aarts, H. (2010). The unconscious will: How the pursuit of goals operates outside of conscious awareness. *Science, 329*, 47–50.

Davis, A. H. T., Figueredo, A. J., Fahy, B. F., & Rawiworrakul, T. (2007). Reliability and validity of the exercise self-regulation efficacy scale for individuals with chronic obstructive pulmonary disease. *Heart & Lung, 36*, 205–216.

Deci, E. L., & Ryan, R. M. (2000). The 'what' and 'why' of goal pursuits: Human needs and the self-determination of behavior. *Psychological Inquiry, 11*, 227–268.

Dijksterhuis, A., & Aarts, H. (2010). Goals, attention and (un)consciousness. *Annual Review of Psychology, 61*, 467–490.

Dubin, R. (1969). *Theory building*. New York, NY: The Free Press.

Duncan, J. (1986). Disorganization of behavior after frontal-lobe damage. *Cognitive Neuropsychology, 3*(3), 271–290.

Duncan, J., Emslie, H., Williams, P., Johnson, R., & Freer, C. (1996). Intelligence and the frontal lobe: The organization of goal-directed behavior. *Cognitive Psychology, 30*(3), 257–303.

Dunn, D., & Elliot, T. (2008). The place of theory in rehabilitation psychology research. *Rehabilitation Psychology, 53*, 254–267.

Evans, L., & Hardy, L. (2002). Injury rehabilitation: A goal-setting intervention study. *Research Quarterly for Exercise and Sport, 73*(3), 310–319.

Fliess-Douer, O., Van Der Woude, L. H. V., & Vanlandewijck, Y. C. (2011). Development of a new scale for perceived self-efficacy in manual wheeled mobility: A pilot study. *Journal of Rehabilitation Medicine, 43*, 602–608.

Gauggel, S., & Billino, J. (2002). The effects of goal setting on the arithmetic performance of brain-damaged patients. *Archives of Clinical Neuropsychology, 17*, 283–294.

Gauggel, S., & Fischer, S. (2001). The effect of goal setting on motor performance and motor learning in brain-damaged patients. *Neuropsychological Rehabilitation, 11*, 33–44.

Gauggel, S., Hoop, M., & Werner, K. (2002). Assigned versus self-set goals and their impact on the performance of brain-damaged patients. *Journal of Clinical and Experimental Neuropsychology, 24*(8), 1070–1080.

Gauggel, S., Leinberger, R., & Richard, M. (2001). Goal setting and reaction time performance in brain-damaged patients. *Journal of Clinical and Experimental Neuropsychology, 23*(3), 351–361.

Grant, H., & Gelety, L. (2009). Goal content theories: Why differences in what we are striving for matter. In G. B. Moskowitz & H. Grant (Eds.), *The psychology of goals* (pp.77–97). New York, NY: The Guilford Press.

Hall, H. K., & Kerr, A. W. (2001). Goal setting in sport and physical activity: Tracing empirical developments and establishing conceptual direction. In G. C. Roberts (Ed.), *Advances in motivation in sport and exercise* (pp. 183–233). Champaign, IL: Human Kinetic.

Hart, T., & Evans, J. (2006). Self-regulation and goal theories in brain injury rehabilitation. *Journal of Head Trauma Rehabilitation, 21*(2), 142–155.

Holland, R. W., Hendriks, M., & Aarts, H. (2005). Smells like clean spirit: Nonconscious effects of scent on cognition and behavior. *Psychological Science, 16*, 689–693.

Hunt, M. (1993). *The story of psychology*. New York, NY: Doubleday.

Jones, F., & Riazi, A. (2011). Self-efficacy and self-management after stroke: A systematic review. *Disability and Rehabilitation, 33*(10), 797–810.

Jurado, M. B., & Rosselli, M. (2007). The elusive nature of executive functions: A review of our current understanding. *Neuropsychological Review, 17*, 213–233.

Kabat-Zinn, J. (2003). Mindfulness-based interventions in context: Past, present, and future. *Clinical Psychology: Science and Practice, 10*(2), 144–156.

Kay, A. C., Wheeler, S. C., Bargh, J. A., & Ross, L. (2004). Material priming: The influence of mundane physical objects on situational construal and competitive behavioral choice. *Organizational Behavior and Human Decision Processes, 95*, 83–96.

Latham, G. P., & Locke, E. A. (2007). New developments in and directions for goal-setting research. *European Psychologist, 12*(4), 290–300. doi:10.1027/1016-9040.12.4.290

Lerner, B. H. (2005). Last-ditch medical therapy – Revisiting lobotomy. *New England Journal of Medicine, 353*(2), 119–121.

Levine, B., Robertson, I. H., Clare, L., Carter, G., Hong, J., Wilson, B. A., … Stuss, D. T. (2000). Rehabilitation of executive functioning: An experimental–clinical validation of goal management training. *Journal of the International Neuropsychological Society, 6*(3), 299–312.

Levine, B., Schweizer, T. A., O'Connor, C., Turner, G., Gillingham, S., Stuss, D. T., … Robertson, I. H. (2011). Rehabilitation of executive functioning in patients with frontal lobe brain damage with goal management training. *Frontiers of Human Neuroscience, 5*, 9.

Locke, E. A., & Latham, G. P. (1985). The application of goal setting to sports psychology. *Journal of Sports Psychology, 7*, 205–222.

Locke, E. A., & Latham, G. P. (1990). *A theory of goal setting and human performance*. Englewood Cliffs, NJ: Prentice Hall.

Locke, E. A., & Latham, G. P. (2002). Building a practically useful theory of goal setting and task motivation: A 35-year odyssey. *American Psychologist, 57*(9), 705–717.

Macmillan, M. (2008). Phineas Gage – Unravelling the myth. *The Psychologist, 21*(9), 828–831.

Maes, S., & Karoly, P. (2005). Self-regulation assessment and intervention in physical health and illness: A review. *Applied Psychology, 54*(2), 267–299.

Marks, R., Allegrante, J. P., & Lorig, K. (2005). A review and synthesis of research evidence for self-efficacy-enhancing interventions for reducing chronic disability: Implications for health education practice (Part II). *Health Promotion Practice, 6*(2), 148–156.

McGrath, J. R., & Adams, L. (1999). Patient-centered goal planning: A systematic psychological therapy? *Topics in Stroke Rehabilitation, 6*, 43–50.

McPherson, K. M., & Siegert, R. J. (2007). Person-centred rehabilitation: Rhetoric or reality? *Disability and Rehabilitation, 29*, 1551–1554.

Nair, K. P. S. (2003). Life goals: The concept and its relevance to rehabilitation. *Clinical Rehabilitation, 17*, 192–202.

Neter, E., Litvak, A., & Miller, A. (2009). Goal disengagement and goal re-engagement among multiple sclerosis patients: Relationship to well-being and illness representation. *Psychology and Health, 24*(2), 175–186.

Norman, D. A. (1981). Categorization of action slips. *Physiological Review, 88*(1), 1–15.

Norman, D. A., & Shallice, T. (1980). *Attention to action: Willed and automatic control of behavior* (Tech. Rep. 99). La Jolla, CA: Centre for Human Information Processing, University of California.

Pintrich, P. R. (2000). The role of goal orientation in self-regulated learning. In M. Boekaerts, P. R. Pintrich, & M. Zeidner (Eds.), *Handbook of self-regulation* (pp. 451–502). San Diego, CA: Academic Press.

Playford, E. D., Siegert, R. J., Levack, W. M. M., & Freeman, J. (2009). Areas of consensus and controversy about goal-setting in rehabilitation: A conference report. *Clinical Rehabilitation, 23*, 334–344.

Rigby, S. A., Domenech, C., Thornton, E. W., Tedman, S., & Young, C. A. (2003). Development and validation of a self-efficacy measure for people with multiple sclerosis: The Multiple Sclerosis Self-efficacy Scale. *Multiple Sclerosis, 9,* 73–81.

Roberts, B. W., & Roins, R. W. (2000). Broad dispositions, broad aspirations: The intersection of personality traits and major life goals. *Personality and Social Psychology Bulletin, 26,* 1284–1296.

Robertson, I. H. (1996). *Goal management training: A clinical manual.* Cambridge, U.K.: PsyConsult.

Robertson, I. H., & Garavan, H. (2000). Vigilant attention. In M. Gazzaniga (Ed.), *New cognitive neurosciences* (pp. 563–578). Cambridge, MA: MIT Press.

Schut, H. A., & Stam, H. J. (1994). Goals in rehabilitation teamwork. *Disability and Rehabilitation, 16*(4), 223–226.

Scobbie, L., Wyke, S., & Dixon, D. (2009). Identifying and applying psychological theory to setting and achieving rehabilitation goals. *Clinical Rehabilitation, 23,* 321–323.

Shallice, T. (1982). Specific impairments of planning. *Philosophical Transactions of the Royal Society of London B: Biological Sciences, 298*(1089), 199–209.

Shallice, T. (2002). Fractionation of the supervisory system. In D. T. Stuss & R. T. Knight (Eds.), *Principles of frontal lobe function* (pp. 261–277). New York, NY: Oxford University Press.

Siegert, R. J., McPherson, K. M., & Dean, S. J. (2005). Theory development and a science of rehabilitation. *Disability and Rehabilitation, 27,* 1493–1501.

Siegert, R. J., McPherson, K. M., & Taylor, W. (2004). Toward a cognitive-affective model of goal-setting in rehabilitation: Is self-regulation theory a key step? *Disability and Rehabilitation, 26*(20), 1175–1183.

Siegert, R. J., & Taylor, W. J. (2004). Theoretical aspects of goal-setting and motivation in rehabilitation. *Disability and Rehabilitation, 26*(1), 1–8.

Stevens, M., van den Akker-Scheek, I., & van Horn, J. R. (2005). A Dutch translation of the Self-Efficacy for Rehabilitation Outcome Scale (SER): A first impression on reliability and validity. *Patient Education and Counselling, 58,* 121–126.

Theodorakis, Y., Beneca, A., Malliou, P., & Goudas, M. (1997). Examining psychological factors during injury rehabilitation. *Journal of Sport Rehabilitation, 6,* 355–363.

Valenstein, E. S. (1986). *Great and desperate cures: The rise and decline of psychosurgery and other radical treatments for mental illness.* New York, NY: Basic Books.

van Hooren, S. A., Valentijn, S. A., Bosma, H., Ponds, R. W., van Boxtel, M. P., Levine, B., … Jolles, J. (2007). Effect of a structured course involving goal management training in older adults: A randomised controlled trial. *Patient Education and Counseling, 65*(2), 205–213.

Vancouver, J. B., More, K. M., & Yoder, R. J. (2008). Self-efficacy and resource allocation: Support for a nonmonotonic, discontinuous model. *Journal of Applied Psychology, 93*(1), 35–47.

Vancouver, J. B., Thompson, C. M., & Williams, A. A. (2001). The changing signs in the relationships among self-efficacy, personal goals, and performance. *Journal of Applied Psychology, 86*(4), 605–620.

Wade, D. T. (2009). Goal setting in rehabilitation: An overview of what, why and how. *Clinical Rehabilitation, 23,* 291–295.

Whyte, J. (2007). A grand unified theory of rehabilitation (we wish!). The 57th John Stanley Coulter Memorial Lecture. *Archives of Physical Medicine and Rehabilitation, 89,* 203–209.

Wilde, M. H., & Garvin, S. (2007). A concept analysis of self-monitoring. *Journal of Advanced Nursing, 57*(3), 339–350.

Wilson, K. M., Hardy, L., & Harwood, C. G. (2006). Investigating the relationship between achievement goals and process goals in rugby union players. *Journal of Applied Sports Psychology, 18,* 297–311.

Woodgate, J., & Brawley, L. R. (2008). Self-efficacy for exercise in cardiac rehabilitation: Review and recommendations. *Journal of Health Psychology, 13*(3), 366–387.

Wrosch, C., Scheier, M. F., Miller, G. E., Schulz, R., & Carver, C. S. (2003). Adaptive self-regulation of unattainable goals: Goal disengagement, goal reengagement, and subjective well-being. *Personality and Social Psychology Bulletin, 29,* 1494–1608.

Ylvisaker, M., & Feeney, T. (2002). Executive functions, self-regulation, and learned optimism in paediatric rehabilitation: A review and implications for intervention. *Pediatric Rehabilitation, 5*(2), 51–70.

4

Ethics and Goal Setting

William M.M. Levack, Richard J. Siegert and Neil Pickering

CONTENTS

4.1 Introduction

In rehabilitation, the value that patients place on particular goals is considered a central concern. Patients often are in positions of disempowerment, and one of the objectives of intervention is usually to maximize their level of control over their lives. Patient involvement in goal setting is viewed as one of the main ways that health professionals can share control over clinical decision making with their clients, thus beginning their journey towards greater independence (Baird, Tempest, & Warland, 2010; Blackmer, 2000). However, a number of factors can complicate the process of involving patients in goal setting, and it is not always easy to determine the most ethical approach for individual people. It would be comforting if we, as health professionals, could simply decide that the goals of rehabilitation should be whatever patients wished to work towards, regardless of the context of the clinical situation, but such a perspective greatly oversimplifies the complexities of work in the *real world* of rehabilitation. Furthermore, challenges around maximizing patient autonomy are not the only ethical issues relevant to goal setting in rehabilitation – far from it. Consider the following:

> Mr Roberts is an 84-year-old man with a below-knee amputation subsequent to peripheral vascular disease, diabetes and smoking. His goal for rehabilitation is to return home where he says his wife, Mrs Roberts, will take care of him, helping him with showering, toileting and dressing. The rehabilitation team is concerned about the impact of this

goal on Mrs Roberts' health, who is similarly aged and frail, but who does not appear to be the dominant partner in the relationship. Furthermore, Mrs Roberts would need to give up many of her social roles and activities in the community if she is to become Mr Roberts' primary carer in the home.

This is only one of many possible scenarios where aspects of goal setting ideology (in this case, that of setting objectives for rehabilitation which are meaningful and valued by the patient) can conflict with other apparent moral responsibilities. In this chapter, goal setting is considered from the perspective of bioethics. As will emerge, in common with nearly all other areas of health-care provision, rehabilitation is rife with such ethical challenges. But we had better say from the outset that this chapter will not provide you with any algorithm for resolving these ethical difficulties. Its aim is more modest, but also more realistic: to provide the reader with a richer way of appreciating, discussing and perhaps finding a way through the ethical issues that the practice of goal setting in rehabilitation throws up.

In this chapter, we will promote one approach to ethics in rehabilitation, that of *principlism*. We will argue that principlism, while a commonly recommended approach to medical ethics, has at times been oversimplified in rehabilitation literature. In addition to arguing in favour of principlism, we will introduce an important associated concept: *value pluralism*. We will examine in more detail the four main principles associated with this approach to bioethics – beneficence, non-maleficence, autonomy and justice – and will discuss how a pluralist approach to these principles requires each individual clinical scenario to be considered within its own particular set of circumstances and moral considerations. These principles in themselves will not be new to many readers of this chapter, but we aim to provide a fresh perspective on understanding them and applying them to clinical practice. This chapter will also address common criticisms of principlism, and lastly, a discussion will be provided regarding the ethics *of* goal setting in rehabilitation, as opposed to ethics *in* goal setting, and an argument will be presented in favour of explicit goal setting as a moral responsibility of rehabilitation providers.

4.2 What Is Ethics?

Ethics is a branch of philosophy that explores the concepts of right and wrong, and as such, ethics is also sometimes known as *moral philosophy* (Thompson, 1994). *Applied ethics* involves the use of ethical theory or an agreed set of moral values to examine appropriateness of actions, events or beliefs in *real-world* settings, such as, in the case of this chapter, health-care or disability support services. From an ethical perspective, actions can be considered one of three things: moral, immoral or amoral. *Moral actions* are those which are considered *good* or *right* to the extent that they match a person's values or those of their community. *Immoral actions* are those which conflict with a person's values or their community's values, while *amoral actions* are those which are unrelated to personal or social values. As an example of the latter, while it is usually considered immoral for one human to take another's life, a cat killing a bird is considered an amoral act rather than an immoral one because the cat is only acting according to its nature and does not have the capacity for ethical reflection on that action. Of course, decisions regarding what actions in which circumstances might be moral, immoral or amoral for humans are frequently and hotly debated. This debate is central to the study of ethics.

4.3 Why No Ethical Algorithm?

It may be asked why, as we have suggested, some sort of ethical calculation or problem-solving algorithm cannot be provided in this chapter on ethics and goal setting. After all, there are ethical theories (several, in fact) that could be used as the basis of such a calculation. In most areas of study, a theory will provide everyone with an agreed way of understanding what is going on and hopefully some way forward. Chemists work with theories about the chemical properties of molecules, and this helps them frame problems in chemistry and find solutions (no pun intended). Why should it be any different in ethics?

Unfortunately, in ethics, this hope is highly likely to be disappointed. For a start, there are a number of ethical theories to choose from: consequentialist theories of various kinds (e.g. utilitarianism), deontological theories (e.g. duty-based theories) and theories focusing on virtues, rights and so on (Levack, 2009; Siegert & Ward, 2010; Siegert, Ward, & Playford, 2010). Each of these approaches has been subject to significant scrutiny and debate, and no theory is without its critics. This criticism applies just as much to the ethical approach promoted in this chapter, principlism, which has, for example, been criticized by feminist theorists for being too prescriptive and for ignoring the role of human relationships and sociopolitical contexts in practice (but more on this later). In place of principlism, theories such as *the ethics of care* (Held, 2005) and *narrative ethics* (Adams, 2008) have been advanced (Box 4.1).

Nevertheless, even supposing we all shared a favourite ethical theory, it is far from clear that this would resolve all or indeed many of our ethical problems. As an example of this from outside of rehabilitation literature, rights theorists may be deeply divided by the issue of abortion; does the foetus have a right to life or not? Is any right it has of greater significance than that of the mother to control what happens to her body? A less divisive but more relevant example to rehabilitation might be the sexual rights of people with disability. The vast majority of people in Western countries are likely to agree that all people with disabilities should have access to resources and services related to sexual health at an equal level compared to those received by non-disabled people. However, opinion is more likely to be divided regarding the extent of rights that people with disabilities should have to additional resources and services to compensate for impairments of sexual function arising from their health condition. If a person with spinal cord injury needs to have a medical intervention (e.g. medication, an implant to facilitate erection or in vitro fertilization) in order to conceive a child, is this a human right? If so, is there a limit on the amount of publicly funded health-care resources that should be invested if these individuals continue to be unsuccessful in conceiving a child? What about if they need a medical intervention in order to have sexual intercourse purely for pleasure? Is this a luxury or a right? Such arguments quickly reduce to an almost farcical level. If a person is considered to have a right to a pill that compensates for erectile dysfunction, how many pills a week do they have a right to receive, and who decides? To view this problem from a completely different perspective, is the way these very questions are framed misguided and potentially immoral in itself, given that such questions reduce a socially constructed phenomenon (intimate sexual relationships) to the status of a biomedical *problem*? If we take up an alternative approach to ethics, say a narrative approach, such problems of interpretation remain. In the case of narrative theory, for instance, there remains an open ethical question as to what narrative we accept: and upon this question, many other ethical questions may turn. The point is that ethics is the sort of area where radical disagreement can exist and persist despite and indeed within theoretical agreement.

BOX 4.1 DESCRIPTIONS OF SOME COMMON THEORIES OF ETHICS

Consequentialism: An approach to ethics that judges that the *consequences* of a particular action form the basis for any valid moral judgement about that action. In other words, the *ends* justify the *means*. How the consequences of certain actions are judged (i.e. which type of *ends* are valued) differs from one type of consequentialism to another. Utilitarianism is one form for consequentialism that values maximizing *utility* as its desired end point.

Deontology: An approach to ethics that judges the morality of an action on the basis of that action's adherence to a rule or rules. From this perspective, actions (such as killing, forgiving, lying) are considered inherently moral or immoral regardless of the consequences of those actions. An example of a deontological belief might be that killing another human being is always wrong, regardless of the consequences of killing that person (e.g. who else might be saved or helped as a result). Some deontologists, however, create exceptions to these rules which can become increasingly complicated or only apply them under certain conditions (e.g. killing is never moral, except for killing in self-defence or killing in defence of others, etc.). Deontologists may emphasize *duties* (such as to one family) with these rules of ethics (McNaughton & Rawling, 2007).

Utilitarianism: A form of ethics that is characterized by evaluating the consequences of actions in terms of the maximization of utility. *Utility* can be considered whatever is useful, profitable or beneficial, but typically utilitarianism is considered in terms of maximizing happiness or pleasure or minimizing harm and suffering, summed among all sentient beings involved, directly or indirectly, in any particular situation. (Thus, a person becoming happy because they steal a sports car is not considered moral due to the unhappiness experienced by the person whom the car originally belongs to!) Utilitarians can differ over their definitions of *utility* and the way they judge *maximization of utility* to be best estimated.

Ethics of care: An approach to ethics based on the premise that men and women view ethical issues in different ways. Gilligan (1982), for instance, has maintained that men tend to intellectualize ethics in a somewhat detached manner, placing an emphasis on universal rights and principles. In comparison, women, argued Gilligan, view ethics more in terms of responsibilities of care within meaningful relationships. The *ethics of care* thus is a moral framework based on focusing on specific relationships within specific situations rather than on general principles (Held, 2005; Roberts, 2004).

Narrative ethics: A relatively new approach to bioethics, which places communication at its core. Narrative ethics is based on the assumption that every moral situation is unique, unable to be reduced to any set of universal rules or principles. Therefore, all moral issues in health-care contexts have to be resolved by considering how subsequent actions and options can be justified in terms of how well they fit with the life story (or *narrative*) of the person in question. This requires the people involved in the situation, actions and options to debate the issues related to their individual and shared meanings around the ethical situation in question. The aim of this debate is not to create a unifying account of the situation but instead to acknowledge the multiplicity of moral perspectives, enriching understanding for all regarding the situation and the possible responses of the various people involved.

Having said that, rational discussion is very much a part of ethics, and this chapter will be a rational discussion. Furthermore, it may be that rational discussion will lead those who originally differed to agree. At the very least, it may begin to develop a basis of specific principles and rules of thumb, which may form a starting point for further discussion. So, though this chapter does not promise answers, we will not simply be throwing up our hands in the face of ethical difficulties either.

4.4 What Is Principlism?

Within bioethics as a discipline, the most common theoretical approach is that of *principlism*, an approach promulgated by Beauchamp and Childress through their book, *Principles of Biomedical Ethics*, originally published in 1979, now in its seventh edition (2013). Beauchamp and Childress argue that all people *who are committed to morality* endeavour to adhere to the same standards, which Beauchamp and Childress call *the common morality*. The common morality comprises a set of *moral norms*, with *principles* being the most general and comprehensive of these norms. In particular, Beauchamp and Childress have promoted four key principles within the field of biomedical ethics:

1. *Respect for autonomy* – recognizing and supporting people's self-determination
2. *Beneficence* – acting to the benefit of others
3. *Non-maleficence* – avoiding causing harm to others
4. *Justice* – treating all people fairly in terms of distributing benefits, risks and costs

These principles, as a tool for dealing with ethical issues in health care, have particularly dominated discussion of ethics in clinical rehabilitation over the last few decades (Blackmer, 2000) and have been used specifically to discuss ethical challenges that arise during goal setting for rehabilitation (Haas, 1993).

The *common morality* promoted by Beauchamp and Childress (2013) is not however limited to just these principles. Several types of other moral norms (rules, obligations, rights and traits) have also been included in this ethical approach. While there is no absolute distinction between *principles* and *rules*, rules have been presented as moral norms which focus more on specific content and restricted circumstances than do principles. Examples of these rules include the following: substantive rules (such as truth telling, privacy, informed consent, confidentiality), authority rules (e.g. about who may or may not make decisions and perform actions) and procedural rules related to specific decisions or circumstances (e.g. procedures for deciding who should be prioritized to go to a post-acute rehabilitation unit after a stroke). Moral character traits, by way of comparison, are described by Beauchamp and Childress to be commonly recognized virtues that people may possess, such as honesty, integrity, trustworthiness, kindness and non-malevolence.

One of the key arguments within principlism is that these *moral norms* are *universal*, that is, 'so widely shared that they form a stable social compact' (Beauchamp and Childress, 2013, p. 3). In other words, these moral norms are said to be relevant to all people who are serious about morality, regardless of place, culture or time. We may debate *which* exact rules, obligations and traits actually fit within a list of moral norms, but regardless of the specifics of this debate, Beauchamp and Childress assert that moral norms do exist and are universal in the manner they propose.

However, Beauchamp and Childress (2013) have also been careful to state that just because they claim that moral norms are *universal* does not mean they are asserting that moral norms are also *absolute*. An absolute moral norm would be one which should always be followed or acted on in all occasions in which it applies. Beauchamp and Childress recognize that moral principles (and other moral norms) can and do conflict in everyday decision making, and so there are some circumstances where pursuing some moral norms may be unethical. For instance, it may sometimes be morally appropriate to prevent a person (such as Mr Roberts at the start of the chapter) from setting or pursuing his own goal for therapy (undermining the principle of autonomy) if in doing so one was to prevent harm occurring to another individual (in this case, Mrs Roberts). The challenge then is to be able to decide when one principle should override another and in which situation, and on this subject, many an ethical debate is to be had.

When it comes to such dilemmas, Beauchamp and Childress (2013) have discussed the options of *specifying* and *balancing*. *Specifying* is a process which involves adding information to assist with understanding and interpreting the circumstances in which an action should be pursued or avoided. It is about providing clarity regarding when, where, why and in what manner the rules or obligations related to one particular principle should be applied. An example of specifying would include a description of when it might be appropriate to have a third party (such as a family member) set goals on behalf of a patient. This may be appropriate where, for example, the patient lacks capacity to decide (Levack, Siegert, Dean, & McPherson, 2009; McClain, 2005; Wade, 1999). In this case, the specification limits the application of the principle of autonomy to cases where people are able to make decisions on their own behalf.

In contrast, *balancing* involves weighing up the relative strength and importance of various considerations arising from different moral norms when deciding or justifying the most appropriate course of action *in any one situation*. As an example of *balancing*, in the case of Mr Roberts, the rehabilitation team may decide to hold a conversation with Mrs Roberts without her husband present regarding his possible goals for therapy. This discussion might include an attempt to uncover what Mrs Roberts' own views are regarding her obligations, her preferences for care arrangements (thus taking her autonomy into account) and the possible risks and benefits to her if she were to become Mr Roberts' primary carer (thus achieving a richer sense of the benefits and harms of different actions). Based on this discussion, and along with other information the rehabilitation team has gleaned, the rehabilitation team may decide on balance that the most moral thing to do would be to support Mr Roberts in the pursuit of his goal to return home with his wife as his main carer *or* they may decide that such an approach would be immoral and that Mr Roberts should be encouraged to modify his goal to reflect an outcome that is less demanding on his wife.

So, when *balancing* and *specifying*, which moral norms are the most important to emphasize? Is the principle of autonomy the most important to champion in general? Or is it the principle of beneficence or the principle of justice? Or are there some other values (perhaps treating people with respect and dignity) that are most important? The answer, at least according to Beauchamp and Childress (2013), is none of the above. All moral norms need to be considered from the perspective of value pluralism.

4.5 What Is Value Pluralism?

It has been noted already that, at least in Beauchamp and Childress's approach, the four main principles of principlism, while universal, are not absolute. In some contexts, a decision may be made in which considerations arising under the broad heading of (say) autonomy would be seen as less important than considerations arising under the broad heading of (say) beneficence or non-maleficence. This reflects a second important point about principlism, namely, that there is *no hierarchy of moral norms*: no one principle is said to be more or less important than another. In this regard, the principles approach encompasses the notion of *value pluralism*. For any clinical decision, the relevant ethical issues associated with each principle need to be considered before an overall perspective on the situation is reached. Value pluralism, as an approach to medical ethics, can be contrasted with *value monism* in which all ethical questions are reduced to a single value. Two examples of value monism are the following: the rights-based approach to medical ethics, where human rights are considered to trump all other ethical considerations (Siegert et al., 2010) and the utilitarian approach, where all ethical decisions are evaluated on the basis of the degree to which they maximize *utility* (Levack, 2009).

As suggested earlier, challenges arise from value pluralism when two or more principles appear to conflict. For example, when a patient with acquired disability refuses to *give up* on goals that their health professionals consider to be increasingly unrealistic, the health professionals may feel that continuing to encourage pursuit of these goals (supporting autonomy) might conflict with helping these patients emotionally and socially adjust to life after disability (reducing the beneficence and non-maleficence of the health professionals' actions). They may also consider that pursuit of unachievable goals would result in money being spent on ineffective interventions resulting in others with rehabilitation needs missing out (an unjust distribution of health-care resources).

The point here is that under value pluralism, all such decisions are context dependent. The ethical principles in themselves do not tell health professionals how to manage complex moral decisions; rather they provide a useful framework for discussing and considering these issues. The benefit of course of working in a rehabilitation team is that no one individual health professional has to make such decisions on their own. They can support one another to consider all the factors involved, challenge each other's assumptions and decide together on the most appropriate course of action for any given situation to the best of their collective ability.

Interestingly, a value pluralist perspective does not always seem to be associated with some authors' representations of principlism. For example, Barnitt (1998), in a survey on ethical dilemmas experienced by UK-based occupational therapists and physical therapists, explicitly asked participating clinicians to rank ethical principles. These principles were then reported in terms of their frequency and importance in the clinicians' work.

It is not uncommon to see some principles being promoted as perhaps more or less important than others. For instance, it sometimes appears as if, at least for health professionals, the principle of autonomy is considered a fundamentally more important *moral norm* to pursue than the principle of beneficence or the principle of justice. From this perspective, the principle of beneficence may be reduced to a gross version of medical paternalism and associated with the image of the arrogant clinician who always thinks he or she *knows best* regardless of the patient's perspectives and preferences, whereas the principle of justice may be equated to cold-hearted clinical decision making based on how best to make maximal health gains from each health-care dollar spent regardless of the *human cost* of such decisions. Blackmer (2000), for instance, while acknowledging that health professionals need to encourage patients to consider the impact of their decisions on their family and society as a whole, still suggested that the physician's first responsibility is to the patient (ahead of, e.g. consideration of resource limitations at a societal level) and concluded that when it comes to selection of goals of therapy, 'If the patient is competent, his or her wishes must prevail' (p. 54). We would argue however that there is no absolute ethical requirement to uphold the principle of autonomy (or any other principles) over other moral norms. Health professionals have multiple moral responsibilities, and each action, decision or interaction needs to be continually considered and re-evaluated in the light of these as part of routine clinical practice.

4.6 Examining the Principles

4.6.1 Autonomy

Consider the following:

> Mrs Jones is a 78-year-old woman with Alzheimer's disease who recently fell and broke her hip. Her occupational therapist wants to involve her in goal setting following internal fixation of her fractured neck of femur but is uncertain how much Mrs Jones actually understands about her current situation.

- To what degree should Mrs Jones be involved in setting her own goals for therapy?
- Are all people capable of acting autonomously, even when free to do so?

Perhaps, at one time, rehabilitation professionals would have set and pursued goals for rehabilitation without much reference to the wishes of the patients. However, since the late 1970s, a powerful social movement began to pass more power into the hands of the patient. We can trace this development to wider social movements which placed oppressed individuals (in some cases) or oppressed groups (in many others) on the road to taking greater control over their own lives. These movements are sometimes referred to in terms of rights: *civil rights*, *human rights* and so on. The jargon terminology in health care is *patient autonomy*.

Philosophers working in the world of bioethics have theorized patient autonomy in various ways. Patient autonomy, as a term and as a concept, has most obviously been taken up by the *four principles* approach but, like all the other principles, has much deeper roots in moral philosophy than just Beauchamp and Childress's (1979) text. For example, the term *autonomy* and a number of important concepts related to this term come from the work of Immanuel Kant. Kant, the eighteenth-century philosopher, argued that all humans had a duty to live life in a moral way and that morality could be determined by reason alone. Kant's expression of this rational vision is his *categorical imperative*, one version of which demands that all people be treated as *ends in themselves* (Kant, 1948). As Thompson (1994) puts it, the requirement is that all people be considered equally as 'autonomous moral agents... free to act on their freely chosen maxims' (p. 98).

However, to more fully understand the concept of autonomy, a number of insights need to be garnered from various theories. There are perhaps three issues of paramount importance. These are the ideas that autonomy consists of (1) *liberty* from outside coercion, (2) *freedom from internal barriers* to realizing one's values and pursuing one's own life and (3) the idea that an individual's autonomy is *relational* – that it is built up and makes sense only in the context of human society.

The concept of liberty from outside coercion has at least some roots in utilitarianism. The nineteenth century utilitarian philosopher John Stuart Mill argued that liberty to pursue one's own idea of the good life for one's self in one's own way was a central value. He saw this as the best way to ensure general happiness; but his notion of liberty has been taken up in modern discussions of autonomy and the right to self-determination. Mill was particularly concerned with people's liberty from the interference of others, including those acting on behalf of the state. Thus, he opposed any attempt to force people into accepting goals for their lives which they did not want. He argued that the coercion of the state could be justified only on the grounds of preventing harm. If a person's goals involved harming others, then this would justify the intervention of the state in order to prevent that harm. Mill's insights have been greatly developed by others – and of course, there have been objections to his approach too, but his concern with liberty is what is relevant to us here.

Freedom from internal barriers to autonomy is a slightly more complex notion. However, consider this question: can a young child be considered autonomous? One's inclination is to answer *no*. The reason would be in part because children have their goals set for them by others – principally their parents, but also the state and its institutions. Children should of course be *involved* in decisions about their lives, and creating opportunities for children to develop skills in self-determination and self-regulation is important, but ultimately, adults are responsible for any important decisions regarding the life, health and well-being of a child.

The reason for this lies in the nature of the child. A child has not yet developed a sufficiently mature approach to either selecting or achieving goals for himself or herself. Children are generally not allowed to be solely responsible for choices about their rehabilitation because, for example, they might not be able to understand the long-term consequences of choices, or appreciate the significance of their choices on their future, or reason about alternatives, or even communicate their choices fully. (Incidentally, whether non-disabled parents are the best people to make decisions for disabled children has also been contested [e.g. For parents only, n.d.], but this is outside the scope of this discussion.) In contrast, the autonomous individual adult is generally considered to have all these capacities: indeed, having them is a requirement of autonomy.

The idea that autonomy is relational is in some ways more recent than these other ideas and, in some ways, very ancient. Aristotle (350 BCE) famously observed that 'man is by nature a political animal' (Book 1, Part II) – meaning that it is of the nature of people to be part of a social group. This insight has been revived in response to the very individualistic turn which a concern with autonomy is sometimes said to have taken over the last few decades (Kenny, Sherwin, & Baylis, 2010). We grow up and learn in nurturing groups such as families; we take up or reject opportunities and roles offered to us by our society; we imbibe values which are communicated to us by others; and we may reflect upon them and judge them with techniques of reflection and judgement available to us in the public domain of language and thought. We are autonomous in a social context. This is a highly significant element of autonomy, for it implies that without some sort of social input, we cannot achieve our goals or even develop any goals to achieve.

To return then to the case of Mrs Jones, the barrier to her achieving full autonomy might not be restrictions placed on her liberty (e.g. by health professionals acting against her will or without due consideration of her wishes) but rather as a result of internal barriers (e.g. her lack of capacity to act as an autonomous individual: fully aware of her surroundings, her health and well-being and the events leading up to her hospitalization and having full capacity to make decisions about her current situation and her future). Yet, if health professionals are to make decisions about Mrs Jones' capacity for acting autonomously, and therefore the degree to which she should be involved in selecting goals for her rehabilitation, by what criteria should her capacity for autonomy be judged?

In fact, the criteria used depend in part on the way capacity for autonomy is conceptualized. In this regard, Macciocchi and Stringer (2001) have proposed that tests of capacity for autonomy can range from very liberal (e.g. able to make a choice) to very strict (e.g. able to 'demonstrate complete understanding of a situation, make decisions based on rational reasons, and fully understand the outcomes', p. S16). In between these extremes are more moderate criteria such as that people will be able to make decisions based on rational reasons. Macciocchi and Stringer have also rightly suggested that capacity for autonomy is contextually determined (i.e. dependent in part on the type of decision being made and the associated conditions). Mrs Jones may be capable of consenting to a goal that has been set on her behalf by a third party, for instance (e.g. a family member or health professional), but not capable of selecting her own goal for rehabilitation without fairly explicit direction and support. Macciocchi and Stringer argued that tests for capacity to act autonomously need to be flexible, including consideration of not only the complexity of the decision but also the risks associated with it. They added the caveat however that the aim of any such capacity testing should always be to maximize autonomy wherever possible.

This perspective highlights one other issue: conceptualization of what the main objectives of rehabilitation should be in general. Often rehabilitation is broadly presented as an intervention to enable people to do various things that they have lost the power or opportunity to do as a result of disability. These *things* might be activities (such as walking, talking or dressing) or social roles (such as being a worker, spouse or parent). Thus, we talk about rehabilitation in terms of maximizing people's ability to function. However, a broader perspective on what *things* should be the desired end point of rehabilitation might include maximization of self-determination and self-regulation, that is, the capacity to be autonomous. One's ability to be autonomous might be impeded by cognitive impairments (e.g. memory loss, communicative problems), but it could also be impeded by physical impairments (e.g. requiring assistance to perform certain tasks and therefore depending on the control, in its physical sense, of others). Thus, the function of goal setting could in itself be to help people with disabilities improve skills in self-regulation and gain greater autonomy in other aspects of their life outside clinical rehabilitation.

4.6.2 Beneficence and Non-Maleficence

Consider the following:

> Trevor is a 20-year-old man who is extremely ataxic following surgical removal of a benign cerebellar tumour. The only goal he will consider for rehabilitation is *to walk again* stating that (in his words) 'I don't want to look like a retard for the rest of my life'. While his parents can pay for almost endless physical therapy, after 6 months of intensive rehabilitation, his clinical team concludes that Trevor is unlikely to ever walk again. They begin to suspect that continued pursuit of an unachievable goal is detrimental to Trevor moving on with his life after disability.

- What constitutes *doing good* in a rehabilitation context?
- Does *doing good* in rehabilitation include challenging belief systems? Challenging personal values or public policies when these seem wrong? Allowing people the opportunity to learn from mistakes and so on?

The *principle of beneficence* is encapsulated by the notion that health professionals should always endeavour to do good by their patients. The *principle of non-maleficence* is the related value that health professionals should never act to cause harm. While it is possible to distinguish between beneficence and non-maleficence on the basis of the specific effects of certain decisions and actions, for the purposes of this chapter, they will be considered in tandem.

These two principles have arguably had a longer association with the provision of health care than has the principle of autonomy as, unlike the principle of autonomy, they can be traced back to the *Hippocratic model* of patient–clinician interactions and thus can be considered values that have been held by medical practitioners for two and a half millennia (Haas, 1993). (*Note*: the principle of autonomy is not the only modern-day common moral that was omitted from the original fifth-century BC version of the Hippocratic Oath – obligations for doctors to tell the truth or to be responsible for fair distribution of health-care resources, for instance, were also not included.)

At first glance, these principles seem fairly straightforward. However, there are a couple of big questions lurking within them when examined more closely. Two particular questions that we will address now are as follows: (1) What might be considered *good* or *harm*, and (2) is there a difference between *good* we are obliged to do and *good* that would be ideal for us to do?

One interpretation of what might constitute *good* is the concept of biomedical good: 'the good that can be achieved by applying expert technical medical knowledge – cure, containment of disease, prevention, amelioration of symptoms, or prolongation of life' (Pellegrino & Thomasma, 1988, p. 78). In fact at times, it seems that in health science literature, this interpretation of *good* is the entirety of the *good* intended by the principle of beneficence. Usually however, this version of *good* is promoted as a way of asserting the primacy of the principle of autonomy over the principles of beneficence. Blackmer (2000), for example, when promoting the need for clinicians to maximize their patients' opportunities for self-determination, has warned that health professionals 'must be very careful to avoid practising persistent beneficence, which will be to the patient's detriment over the long run' (p. 54). Another way of expressing this is doing *good* on behalf of patients for too long eventually results in causing harm. This perspective equates overly enthusiastic beneficence with *medical paternalism*, whereby clinicians take full responsibility for all decisions regarding a patient's health, without any specific consultation with the patient around their views and preferences and without necessarily their consent to treatment even.

However, others have argued that this is a limited version of beneficence. Pellegrino and Thomasma (1988), for instance, have drawn a line between medical paternalism and beneficence by stating that beneficence is essentially about protecting the patient's best interests and that 'the best interests of patients are intimately linked with their preference' (p. 29). This is not to say that supporting patients' right to self-determination is always synonymous with protecting their best interest of course. A patient may enjoy smoking, for instance, but few would consider it *good* for a health professional to condone this behaviour simply because the patient gains enjoyment from it. While we would ultimately disagree with Pellegrino and Thomasma, who take their argument further, arguing in fact for the primacy of beneficence over all other ethical principles in medicine, we would agree with their notion that patient preferences and values need to be a significant part of any decision regarding what is in their best interest.

In the case of Trevor earlier then, it could be argued that regardless of his understandable desire to achieve a goal of walking again and despite his family's ability to pay for treatment to pursue this goal, it would not be moral to consent to this goal if it is truly considered impossible to achieve. It could also be considered immoral to continue to work with him without actively (albeit sensitively) challenging his beliefs regarding the ability of people in wheelchairs to achieve meaningful and valued lives. Indeed, the rehabilitation team could introduce activities that might expose Trevor to different ways of viewing disability: they might engage a mentor who is also in a wheelchair to work with Trevor to redefine his life goals, or they might take him to a game of wheelchair rugby to watch other young, fit men with disabilities participate in competitive sport.

Thinking about what a rehabilitation team *could* do in the case of Trevor raises the second issue for discussion here, namely, what *good* rehabilitation providers are obliged to do versus what *good* could they ideally do? The distinction between obligatory beneficence and ideal beneficence relates to the degree to which particular acts require people to put others' interests ahead of their own and in what contexts (Beauchamp and Childress, 2013). We might all agree, for example, that therapists within a rehabilitation unit have an obligation to provide at least some rehabilitation interventions for all people who enter into their service regardless of who those people are, what they have done in their lives or whether they are likeable or despicable individuals. However, the majority of us are also likely to agree that we have no such obligation to provide rehabilitation for free and in our own time (such as on weekends), although would probably admire the generosity of people who do just that. Pellegrino and Thomasma (1988) argued that 'some degree of effacement of personal self-interest has always been understood as a physician's duty' (p. 27), and this can certainly be extended to include the duty of nurses and allied health professionals. Thus, it can be assumed that some degree of ideal beneficence is often offered to patients alongside obligatory beneficence. Nevertheless, it is important to note that there are limitations regarding the level of beneficence that any one health professional can be expected to achieve in usual daily practice.

A discussion of the principle of beneficence would not be complete without recognition of its potential to conflict with the principle of autonomy. This is a topic that has been discussed by a number of authors (Beauchamp & Childress, 2013; Blackmer, 2000; Haas, 1993; Macciocchi & Stringer, 2001) and is one which resonates strongly with health professionals in clinical practice. Conflicts between beneficence and autonomy can occur when patients wish to pursue goals or activities that health professionals do not believe are in their best interests. The case of Trevor earlier is one example of this. Another example might involve an elderly patient in an inpatient rehabilitation ward who wishes to set a goal for rehabilitation of returning to live at home alone when the health professionals involved believe that any such attempt is very likely to end in a disastrous accident.

Of course, if a person is completely impaired in terms of their ability to regulate their behaviour or express their opinions (i.e. they are entirely unable to control their actions or thought processes, or are unable to express a basic *yes/no* in response to questions), then no such conflict really exists. This is because the person is incapable of acting autonomously even if free to do so, as previously described. However, it is perhaps more common for a patient's ability to act autonomously to be partially rather than completely compromised (e.g. by partial cognitive or communicative impairments).

One suggestion in response to such situations is to employ a *fiduciary* approach to interacting with patients (Blackmer, 2000; Haas, 1993). The word *fiduciary* is more commonly used in legal rather than health-care contexts where it refers to something which is held *in trust* by one person for another. What is being held in trust in the context of a fiduciary model of patient–clinician interaction is the patient's right to self-determination. The fiduciary model stems from an acknowledgement that in the early days of post-acute rehabilitation, particularly after severe injury or illness, patients are often not in the right space or the right mind-set to take full responsibility for decisions about their health and their lives. Indeed, studies have suggested that more paternalistic approaches can be preferred by some patients in certain contexts (Zandbelt, Smets, Oort, Godfried, & deHaes, 2006).

Patients can need time to come to terms with the implications of a newly acquired disability. They need to gather information about their disease or injury and about what degree of recovery they could reasonably hope for or expect. They need to emotionally adjust to the implications of their situation before truly being able to consider their future and their goals with a clear mind. It should not really be surprising then that when health professionals ask for patients (recently admitted to hospital) to provide a perspective on their goals for rehabilitation, they receive the ubiquitous *to go home*, or *to walk again*, or simply *to get better* response. In these contexts, the fiduciary model allows health professionals to adopt a more paternalistic role in clinical decision making during the early days of post-acute rehabilitation, passing increasing control of autonomy back to patients as they gain in confidence, awareness, ability and experience. Yes, clinicians have an obligation to listen to patients, to seek an understanding of their values and perspectives and to respect their liberty to pursue their own idea of a good life (as John Stuart Mill put its), but *equally*, they have a professional obligation to share their clinical experience, to challenge belief systems that might impede a patient's opportunity for a full and rich life and to do what they can to improve the overall well-being and quality of life of the people in their care.

4.6.3 Justice

Consider the following:

> Rebecca is a speech therapist working in a busy outpatient service. Mr Samuel is referred to Rebecca's clinic by the community rehabilitation team as he continues to have problems with severe dysphasia 6 months following a stroke. After reviewing the case and seeing that *extensive periods of therapy have been provided in the past*, Rebecca refuses to work towards this goal. While Rebecca agrees that further intensive rehabilitation *could* result in Mr Samuel improving his ability to make *speech sounds* (i.e. to articulate different noises), she thinks it is highly unlikely that further intervention would result in improved *functional speech* at this stage in the man's recovery (i.e. his ability to communicate with others verbally). Rebecca's clinical manager disagrees with this decision, stating that any improvement in oral production of sound is a step forward for Mr Samuel and so should be pursued. Rebecca argues that there are several other people on her waiting list, who are far more likely to benefit from her input than Mr Samuel. She believes that it would be a better use of resources (and Mr Samuel's needs would be better served) if he were to join a community group for people with stroke, with a goal set for Mr Samuel at the level of social participation rather than bodily function.

- What responsibility do rehabilitation professionals have to fair distribution of their services to the countries and communities that they serve?
- Is any such responsibility to a community more or less important than the health professional's responsibility to the individual patients who come to see them in their clinic?

All health-care resources are rationed. Populations around the world are ageing at an unprecedented rate (United Nations, 2001). People are also surviving injuries and diseases that used to be almost inevitably fatal 50 or so years ago. But people are ageing and surviving with disability. As a consequence, demand for rehabilitation is growing. Add to this the technological and scientific advancements in health care that have created new and wonderful ways of spending money. We now have on the market wheelchairs that climb stairs, robotic exoskeletons to enhance muscle power, designer pharmaceuticals and virtual reality environments for rehabilitation. Health care is an industry where demand inevitably exceeds supply.

In countries like the United Kingdom, Canada, Australia and New Zealand, public health services ration health care through waiting lists and prioritization systems. In the United States, health care is rationed more on the basis of price and the ability to pay. People in the United States with health insurance can receive gold standard services, but for the 45 million US citizens without health insurance, access to this care is limited. Even for those with health insurance, coverage is not limitless. Increasing health-care costs are passed directly back to those paying for insurance in the form of premiums, and thus in the past decade, health insurance premiums in the United States have risen at a rate four times faster than wages (Singer, 2009).

So what relevance does any of this have to goal setting in rehabilitation? Well, if we assume that goal setting is an integral part of the process of rehabilitation planning, then it is an important step along the way to committing health-care resources to certain activities. A large part of these resources are likely to be the amount of professional contact time that individual patients receive from various members of the interdisciplinary team, but it could also include access to costly inpatient or residential facilities, the prescription of equipment or the onward referral to other specialist services. Rehabilitation providers are gatekeepers of health-care resources, whether they want to be or not. Rehabilitation providers therefore have a moral responsibility to encourage, ensure or support the fair distribution of these resources, and this is the subject of the fourth ethical principle to be discussed in this chapter, the *principle of justice*.

Justice is often thought of in connection with legal processes. However, in the context of health care, the principle of justice is almost entirely about *distributive justice*: ensuring fairness to all people when sharing out limited resources. In practice however, deciding what might actually constitute a *fair* distribution of health-care resources is somewhat tricky. Should all people be allocated the exact same amount of health-care resources – say 60 h of physical therapy for all patients, no more, no less – regardless of how injured or unwell they are (a resource egalitarian approach)? Should severely impaired people receive the lion's share of health-care resources, regardless of their ability to benefit from those resources, simply because they are the least well off (a welfare egalitarian approach)? Should decisions regarding the fairness of resource allocation be determined instead by an approach that involves trying to maximize the best outcomes for the most number of people within the resources available (a utilitarian approach)?

In practice (and this is a gross generalization), rehabilitation professionals usually seem to consider a fair distribution of collectively funded resources to be partly determined by the perceived need of individual patients and partly determined by the perceived ability of those individuals to benefit from the resources in question, although this is moderated by the funding structure underpinning the delivery of rehabilitation. For instance, in the United States, access to any intervention covered by an insurance claim can be considered an individual entitlement that has been paid for rather than a resource that is shared with other members of an insurance group.

Nevertheless, some clinicians can be hesitant about embracing a responsibility to watch how the health dollar is spent. Blackmer (2000), for instance, has suggested that asking clinicians to consider resources on a large scale is like asking them to 'put aside their basic commitment and compassion for individual patients' (p. 52), implying that health professionals have greater responsibility to the individual people in their clinic than those in the wider community. Blackmer is also particularly concerned about people with severe disability missing out if a cost-effectiveness approach is followed at all. As we have pointed out elsewhere however (Levack, 2009), even a utilitarian method for the distribution of health-care resource does not necessarily result in arguments to cut services for the most disabled people, provided a full calculation of the benefits and cost of rehabilitation interventions are taken into consideration. For instance, Turner-Stokes, Paul, and Williams (2006) have illustrated that small gains in levels of functional ability can have a substantial impact on reducing the cost of ongoing care for people with severe disability. In fact, based on changes in scores on the Northwick Park Dependency and Care Needs Assessment, which can be used to estimate the cost of care for people with disability, Turner-Stokes et al. (2006) demonstrated that the cost of specialist inpatient rehabilitation for people with the highest levels of disability can be offset far more quickly by the resultant savings in ongoing care, when compared to rehabilitation for people with less severe disability, despite the cost of rehabilitation for those with severe disability being initially higher. This is because small gains in physical independence can result in large cost saving associated with the delivery of attendant care if people have high levels of impairment (and thus high cost-of-care needs) to begin with.

In reality, however, undertaking calculations to determine what might be considered a *fair* distribution of resources is often difficult (although perhaps no more difficult than trying to determine exactly what constitutes *facilitating autonomy* or *acting in the best interests of patients*). The significance of the principle of justice in any particular case may vary depending on the context, and what is considered *just* can be influenced by a range of social, political and cultural factors underlying each situation. Moreover, questions such as how much money should be spent on rehabilitation services as opposed to emergency, intensive care or public health services add further complexities to these discussions.

Nonetheless, we would argue that clinicians do have an ethical responsibility to actively consider justice at a community level when delivering services to individual patients and that this responsibility is not fundamentally less important than that of the other moral considerations outlined in the principles earlier. The principle of justice can also be considered to provide an ethical justification to pursue an evidence-based approach to clinical decision making. This is because it behoves all health professionals to not waste time and money on ineffective treatment modalities or even, in some cases, interventions that required considerable investment of time and money for little clinical gain. Therefore, Rebecca, the speech therapist at the beginning of this section, is correct to question the value of providing an intervention just because she can or just because there is any chance whatsoever of effecting change, no matter how small, in a patient.

One final point regarding the principle of justice, the discussion earlier has centred on the most effective use of limited resources within health services. The principle of justice can also be viewed however at a national or international level. Thus, while rehabilitation professionals have a moral responsibility to make best use of the limited resources at their disposal, they also have a moral responsibility to advocate for a fairer distribution of a country's or the world's resources to people with chronic illness or disability and to perhaps even be politically active when doing so.

4.7 Addressing Criticisms of Principlism

Like all ethical theories, principlism is not without its critics. Walker (2009), for instance, has criticized principlism for being an incomplete ethical framework. While Walker has not challenged the possible existence of *common morals* that are universally shared, he has argued that the four principles of principlism are insufficient for dealing with all ethical issues that arise in clinical practice. To illustrate this, Walker has suggested that desecration of the dead would be considered immoral by most people yet would not contravene any of the principles of autonomy, beneficence, non-maleficence or justice. (The specific example he uses is urinating on a memorial to the dead, but perhaps a more relevant example to clinical practice might be leaving a recently dead body unclothed, uncovered and unattended in a general medical ward cubicle.) Walker also has argued that there are some moral principles that are culturally specific (yet still important) and that therefore it is not possible to encapsulate everything relevant to discussion of ethics within four principles that are universally shared. Principlism misses, according to Walker, important parts of the broader ethical debate.

In response to this, Sokol (2009) has argued that Walker's (2009) perspective is gross oversimplification of principlism. He has stated that an in-depth, sophisticated appreciation of the four principles is required, rather than a superficial interpretation of the principles based on their most basic definitions. Taking Walker's example of desecration of the dead, Sokol has suggested that a broader understanding of autonomy would include the preferences of the living regarding the treatment of their bodies after death and inclusion of harm done to friends and family of the deceased individual is sufficient to justify why urinating on a person's memorial (or disrespectful treatment of dead bodies in hospital wards) is immoral. Additional principles are not required to explain why these acts are unacceptable.

Furthermore, Sokol (2009) has provided clarification regarding the place of *culturally specific* moral norms within a framework of universal moral principles. Sokol stated that the process of *specification*, which is an essential component of principlism (as described at the beginning of this chapter), is about the creation of context-sensitive norms when applying the four universal principles to specific situations. Principlism is indeed impractical (if not meaningless) without the specification and balancing of common morals. Principlism, Sokol argued, thus can be considered to already involve a partial degree of cultural relativism at the level of interpretation of the four principles in specific cases and situations – provided that the belief in a universal set of fundamental moral principles remains at the core of the approach.

This perspective however raises another criticism, which is that with all this discussion about specifying, balancing and interpretation, principlism provides little guidance to health professionals regarding what is actually right or wrong to *do*. The problem here, according to philosophers such as Gert, Culver and Clouser (2000), is that principlism is not linked to any underlying single theory of ethics, that 'morality is a system that includes much more than moral rules and principles' (p. 310). Gert et al. (2000) proposed that a *moral system* includes, in addition to moral principles, moral ideals, morally relevant features and 'a two-step procedure for determining when it is justified to violate a moral rule' (p. 311). This two-step procedure involves firstly describing any particular act in terms of its morally relevant features, then secondly 'estimating the harms resulting from everyone knowing that everyone is allowed to violate that moral rule in this kind of circumstance versus the harms resulting from everyone knowing that no one is allowed to violate the moral rule in these circumstances' allow (Gert et al., 2000, p. 313).

While some, such as Richardson (2000), have argued that this is merely a slightly different version of global balancing – a suggestion which Gert et al. have vehemently opposed – the simplest response to these sort of criticisms is to acknowledge that, yes, this lack of procedural guides is indeed a feature of principlism, but that it is an intended feature, and that perhaps principlism is none the worse for this lack of restriction on its application. Principlism provides a framework for discussion of such procedures for considering ethical issues; it does not restrain them.

Another significant thread of criticism against principlism has come from feminist philosophers, who have argued that *principlism* (along with a number of other traditional approaches to ethics) represents a particularly male view of morality, one which centres on the interests of the individual and which has prioritized 'rational, universal and detached ethical reasoning' (Roberts, 2004, p. 585). What is missing from this worldview, it is argued, is the significance of interpersonal relationships and an overarching emphasis on *care* and *caring* in health-care contexts. In place of individualistically oriented ethics, feminist philosophers have proposed the value of *relational ethics* (Sherwin, 2008) and *the ethics of care* (Gilligan, 1982). These theories place individual relationships back at the centre of the discussion on bioethics.

A similar sort of argument has been raised by those who promote *narrative ethics* – an approach to bioethics which places communication rather than principles at its core (McCarthy, 2003). A key argument within narrative ethics is that all situations begging a bioethical analysis are unique, individual and nuanced depending on the context of the situation and the various factors involved. No list of universal principles or common morals can therefore help with resolving ethical issues in these situations. Instead, communication is required in order to elucidate and understand the various perspectives of all people involved. One counter-argument to this however has been that both principlism and narrative ethics benefit from incorporation of both consideration of principles *and* narrative tendencies (McCarthy, 2003). Principlism is enriched by the inclusion of communication and personal narratives when universal principles are being discussed, specified and balanced, but likewise narrative ethics gains when life stories are discussed and shared using a common language, such as can be provided by principlism. These approaches in other words are not necessarily mutually exclusive.

Lastly, a general comment on Beauchamp and Childress's (2013) approach is that with all the specification and balancing, principlism could be viewed as being open to potentially endless re-interpretation and ad hoc changes. This could lead some to be suspicious of its credibility as a method of addressing ethical dilemmas in health-care settings. However, this at least shows that principlism has a certain flexibility, which may be welcomed by others.

4.8 Ethics of Goal Setting versus Ethics in Goal Setting

So far in this chapter, we have discussed how principlism can provide a useful framework for addressing ethical issues that arise during goal setting in rehabilitation. To extend this discussion further, we propose that undertaking goal setting with patients is in itself an ethical responsibility for all clinicians working in rehabilitation services. This, of course, is a substantive moral claim. How is it to be evaluated and justified? In particular, how can it be justified given the values plural/principlist approach outlined earlier?

One apparent problem for the substantive moral claim we are making is that it is a general claim about the practice of rehabilitation. Our values plural/principlist approach may seem better suited to moral decision making in particular, concrete and richly described cases, such as those we have provided in this chapter. In any such case, specification and balancing seems to provide a way forward, without committing us to making the same decision in another case with any substantive relevant differences. In short, the whole approach may seem better oriented to a case-by-case analysis than to an analysis of practice in general.

However, we hold that the approach we have outlined is just as capable of justifying such general moral claims about a practice as a whole, as it is of justifying specific decisions. There is nothing in the approach which dictates that it cannot handle ethical issues at a general level. Of course, it does dictate that justification of a general rule of approach such as *always undertake goal setting with your rehabilitation patients* will rest upon a multiplicity of considerations rather than just one.

What considerations, then, should go into evaluating this substantive claim, and how does it come out in the light of these considerations? All four principles seem to be pertinent to considering the claim. To undertake discussions with patients about outcomes clearly has implications for patient autonomy, the aim to do the best for patients and avoid harming them, and is clearly an issue in resource allocation, as discussions take time and other resources. Our argument is that when we apply all four principles to this particular claim, we see that the form in which it has been stated is appropriately modest. It states only that goal setting should be undertaken with patients as a part of all rehabilitation practice. It does not state that the goals set through this process should always be followed.

Patient autonomy is clearly a consideration in evaluating the claim and also supports its modest scope. Considerations of patient autonomy do not support the stronger claim that the goals preferred by the patient as a result of discussion should be what determine practice. This is because, as we have already argued in looking at specific cases, doing what the patient wants is not always the right thing to do. Finding what the patient wants and why is however the right thing to do in the vast majority of cases, limited only by instances where the patient is unable to engage in such discussions. This is in part because successful rehabilitation must be individualized to the patient's case, and the individual case cannot be fully described in purely physiological and functional terms. Rehabilitation medicine deals with people, not types of problems. The rehabilitation process is essentially a problem-solving one, where no two patients present with the same problems (Levack & Dean, 2012). Rehabilitation clinicians therefore are required to find out what makes each patient unique. This includes information about their clinical presentation, their life goals, their social context and what makes their life worth living.

Beneficence is also clearly a consideration in evaluating this claim. In general, it might be expected that a practice which includes a discussion of outcomes with patients is likely to contribute to fostering the achievement of outcomes the patient values, avoiding the pursuit of outcomes the patient may consider harmful or not in their best interests and enhancing the patient's knowledge of what outcomes are possible. However, there is no support for the idea that goal setting discussions actually and inevitably improve outcomes for all patients who have engaged with health professionals in clinical rehabilitation. Rather, the evidence is equivocal (Levack et al., 2006); goal setting (by itself) does not always enhance the patient's best interests. However, this evidence has to be evaluated against what may happen if no such discussions takes place, or takes place only haphazardly or randomly.

Our view is that equivocal evidence of benefit is not a sufficient consideration against routine discussion of rehabilitation plans to achieve individualized patient outcomes.

Justice requires that we ask about the resource implications of any proposed action. To require that discussions about expected outcomes take place with all patients is to make a demand upon health professionals' time. It will also require the provision of space in which discussions can proceed with a reasonable degree of privacy and perhaps greater provision of training in communication for health professionals. All these have resource implications. The question, then, is how far investing resources in this process is justified in contrast to some other use of them. It is difficult to answer this question without specifying what other uses are possible. However, we can note the following in favour of using resources to ensure goals of therapy are discussed with all patients. First, it is fair in the sense that these resources are to be distributed equally, at least insofar as every patient who is capable is to be given the opportunity to engage in such discussions. This is better than a system in which some, but not all, patients have outcomes discussed with them, where there is no good reason for the discrimination. Second, what is being distributed is a *good* – that is to say, it represents the opportunity for each patient to enhance that patient's autonomy and serves as a basis for individualized practice. At the same time, considerations of justice also support the modest scope of the proposal. It does not license the pursuit of patient demands irrespective of their implications for resources.

It is our belief that considerations based upon the values plural/principlist approach supports the idea that rehabilitation clinicians need to do more than just pursue this type of activity unconsciously. Goal setting needs to be transparent and explicit process. The ethical approach we have pursued in this chapter supports the idea that goal setting discussions with capable patients should be a part of all rehabilitation practice. Without it, rehabilitation is morally lacking.

4.9 Conclusion

In this chapter, we have reintroduced a familiar moral framework that has been previously used in health-care work – that of Beauchamp and Childress's (2013) principlism approach to ethics. We have expanded on the four core ethical principles underlying the principlism approach and have emphasized the need to retain value pluralism at the centre of any discussion of the application of these principles. This requires all four of the core principles (autonomy, beneficence, non-maleficence and justice) to be held as equally important to one another, using the processes of specification and balancing to determine their application to individual clinical (or indeed non-clinical) situations. We have raised a number of common criticisms of the principlism approach, acknowledging these criticisms as relevant but nevertheless still maintaining that principlism provides a useful foundation for everyday consideration of moral issues in clinical practice. Finally, we have presented an argument that regardless of the current evidence regarding the effectiveness of goal setting to improve outcomes for rehabilitation patients in terms of improvements on standardized outcome measurement, rehabilitation professionals have an ethical obligation to engage in goal setting in rehabilitation contexts, and to not do so, actively and explicitly, results in a moral deficit in clinical practice.

References

Adams, T. E. (2008). A review of narrative ethics. *Qualitative Inquiry, 14*(2), 175–194.

Aristotle. (350 BCE). Politics (B. Jowett, Trans.). Retrieved from http://classics.mit.edu/Aristotle/politics.html. Accessed on 4 December, 2011.

Baird, T., Tempest, S., & Warland, A. (2010). Service users' perceptions and experiences of goal setting theory and practice in an inpatient neurorehabilitation unit. *British Journal of Occupational Therapy, 73*(8), 373–378.

Barnitt, R. (1998). Ethical dilemmas in occupational therapy and physical therapy: A survey of practitioners in the UK National Health Service. *Journal of Medical Ethics, 24,* 193–199.

Beauchamp, T. L., & Childress, J. F. (1979/2013). *Principles of biomedical ethics* (1st/7th edn). New York, NY: Oxford University Press.

Blackmer, J. (2000). Ethical issues in rehabilitation medicine. *Scandinavian Journal of Rehabilitation Medicine, 32*(2), 51–55.

For parents only. (n.d.). Retrieved 12 October 2011, from http://www.cochlearwar.com/for_parents_only.html.

Gert, B., Culver, C. M., & Clouser, K. D. (2000). Common morality versus specified principlism: Reply to Richardson. *Journal of Medicine and Philosophy, 25*(3), 308–322.

Gilligan, C. (1982). *In a different voice: Psychological theory and women's development.* London, U.K.: Harvard University Press.

Haas, J. (1993). Ethical considerations of goal setting for patient care in rehabilitation medicine. *American Journal of Physical Medicine & Rehabilitation, 72,* 228–232.

Held, V. (2005). *The ethics of care.* Oxford, U.K.: Oxford University Press.

Kant, I. (1948). *The moral law: Kant's Groundwork of the metaphysic of morals* (H. J. Paton, Trans.). London, U.K.: Hutchinson University Library.

Kenny, N. P., Sherwin, S. B., & Baylis, F. E. (2010). Re-visioning public health ethics: A relational perspective. *Ethics in Public Health, 101*(1), 9–11.

Levack, W., & Dean, S. (2012). Processes in rehabilitation. In S. Dean, R. Siegert, & W. Taylor (Eds.), *Interprofessional Rehabilitation: A Person-Centred Approach.* (pp. 79–108). Chichester, U.K.: John Wiley & Sons.

Levack, W. M. M. (2009). Ethics in goal planning for rehabilitation: A utilitarian perspective. *Clinical Rehabilitation, 23*(4), 345–351.

Levack, W. M. M., Siegert, R. J., Dean, S. G., & McPherson, K. M. (2009). Goal planning for adults with acquired brain injury: How clinicians talk about involving family. *Brain Injury, 23*(3), 192–202.

Levack, W. M. M., Taylor, K., Siegert, R. J., Dean, S. G., McPherson, K. M., & Weatherall, M. (2006). Is goal planning in rehabilitation effective? A systematic review. *Clinical Rehabilitation, 20*(9), 739–755.

Macciocchi, S., & Stringer, A. (2001). Assessing risk and harm: The convergence of ethical and empirical considerations. *Archives of Physical Medicine and Rehabilitation, 82*(Suppl. 2), S15–S19.

McCarthy, J. (2003). Principlism or narrative ethics: Must we choose between them? *Medical Humanities, 29*(2), 65–71.

McClain, C. (2005). Collaborative rehabilitation goal setting. *Topics in Stroke Rehabilitation, 12*(4), 56–60.

McNaughton, D. A., & Rawling, J. P. (2007). Deontology. In R. E. Ashcroft, A. Dawson, H. Draper, & J. R. McMillan (Eds.), *Principles of health care ethics* (2nd ed.), (pp. 65–72). Chichester, U.K.: John Wiley & Sons.

Pellegrino, E., & Thomasma, D. C. (1988). *For the patient's good: The restoration of beneficence in health care.* New York, NY: Oxford University Press.

Richardson, H. S. (2000). Specifying, balancing and interpreting bioethical principles. *Journal of Medicine and Philosophy, 25*(3), 285–307.

Roberts, M. (2004). Psychiatric ethics; a critical introduction for mental health nurses. *Journal of Psychiatric and Mental Health Nursing, 11,* 583–588.

Sherwin, S. (2008). Whither bioethics? How feminism can help reorient bioethics. *International Journal of Feminist Approaches to Bioethics, 1*(1), 7–27.

Siegert, R. J., & Ward, A. B. (2010). Dignity, rights and capabilities in clinical rehabilitation. *Disability and Rehabilitation, 32*(25), 2138–2146.

Siegert, R. J., Ward, T., & Playford, E. D. (2010). Human rights and rehabilitation outcomes. *Disability and Rehabilitation, 32*(12), 965–971.

Singer, P. (2009, July 15). Why we must ration health care. *The New York Times.* Retrieved from http://www.nytimes.com/2009/07/19/magazine/19healthcare-t.html.

Sokol, D. K. (2009). Sweetening the scent: Commentary on "What principlism misses". *Journal of Medical Ethics, 35,* 232–233.

Thompson, M. (1994). *Understanding ethics.* London, U.K.: Hodder Education.

Turner-Stokes, L., Paul, S., & Williams, H. (2006). Efficiency of specialist rehabilitation in reducing dependency and costs of continuing care for adults with complex acquired brain injuries. *Journal of Neurology, Neurosurgery and Psychiatry, 77,* 634–639.

United Nations. (2001). *World population ageing: 1950–2050.* Retrieved from http://www.un.org/esa/population/publications/worldageing19502050/.

Wade, D. T. (1999). Goal planning in stroke rehabilitation: How? *Topics in Stroke Rehabilitation, 6*(2), 16–36.

Walker, T. (2009). What principlism misses. *Journal of Medical Ethics, 35,* 229–231.

Zandbelt, L. C., Smets, E. M. A., Oort, F. J., Godfried, M. H., & de Haes, H. C. J. M. (2006). Determinants of physicians' patient-centred behaviour in the medical specialist encounter. *Social Science & Medicine, 63,* 899–910.

5

Goal Setting as Shared Decision Making

E. Diane Playford

CONTENTS

5.1 Introduction

The aim of this chapter is to consider goal setting in the context of the growing literature on shared decision making and patient decision aids. Goal setting in rehabilitation will be compared with shared decision making in the management of chronic disease. The nature of preference-sensitive decisions and the importance of understanding an individual's personal values, beliefs and preferences in making such decisions will be discussed. The barriers to shared decision making and goal setting will be considered, with attention paid to situations often considered as difficult, including how to involve patients with cognitive impairment and sudden disabling diagnoses. The criteria for judging shared decision-making processes will be described, with each of the steps in supporting shared decision making explained.

5.2 Goal Setting

Goal setting is central to the rehabilitation process and has been described as a core skill of the rehabilitation professional (Wade, 1998). It may be defined as a process of discussion and negotiation in which the patient and staff determine the key priorities for that individual and agree the performance level to be attained by the patient for defined activities within a specified time frame. There are two elements to this definition and this chapter will focus on the first element – that is, the process of discussion and negotiation.

5.3 Shared Decision Making

In medicine as a whole, many health treatment and screening decisions have no single *correct* answer. Whereas it may be clear the best way to treat appendicitis is by appendectomy, only about a third of common treatments are clearly or likely to be beneficial. These types of decisions are considered *preference sensitive*. Preference-sensitive decisions are those in which there is no clear evidence supporting one treatment option or approach over another, in which each option has different risks and benefits and therefore patients' values are important in deciding which option is best (Coulter & Collins, 2011). Preference-sensitive decisions present specific challenges to both patients and clinicians. There is explicit guidance in the UK General Medical Councils' *good medical practice* that doctors should work in partnership with patients and that this includes listening to patients; respecting their views; discussing diagnosis, prognosis, treatment and care; and maximizing patients' opportunities and ability to make decisions for themselves. In each case, the risks and benefits for an individual have to be balanced. Although in rehabilitation the treatment options are often more varied and the outcome less predictable, there are few situations in medicine when a single treatment is considered. For example, the management of hypertension may encompass some or all of weight management, dietary modification, increasing activity, smoking cessation and medication. All of these demand a behaviour change from the patient, as occurs during rehabilitation. Moreover, these behaviour changes are preference sensitive. For example, weight loss can be managed using calorie restriction or by increasing calorie expenditure through exercise. The individual can choose which they prefer and can also choose to remain overweight and accept the potential increase in morbidity and mortality associated with this. None of these decisions is intrinsically right or wrong. In rehabilitation, where any problem can be solved in a number of different ways, interventions may be regarded as quintessential preference-sensitive interventions.

In rehabilitation, the aim is to maximize activity and participation, and different patients will have different priorities. The risks associated with specific choices are often low in terms of the likely impact on disease progression. For example, for some people, independence in dressing is less important than the ability to work, and effort spent in dressing may detract from the ability to work for a chosen period. Rehabilitation may therefore be regarded as an area where preference-sensitive decisions are made regularly and where the risks are relatively easy to mitigate.

When the importance of patients' beliefs, values and preferences is ignored by clinicians, it is easy for goal-oriented programmes to become trivial or irrelevant. For example, a young woman with an intracerebral haemorrhage who wants privacy in the bathroom may not see the link between this goal and practising transfers in the gym. Similarly, a young man with multiple sclerosis who enjoyed mountain climbing may not feel that he wants to be seen walking with a frame. A 40-year-old woman with progressive neuropathy may resist doing an exercise programme because she believes exercise will weaken already weak muscles. These three examples demonstrate the range of reasons why patients may not adhere to their rehabilitation programme and probably arise from a lack of understanding of the individual patient's wishes and motivators. This frequently results in an expensive and rare resource being wasted, resulting in mutual frustration. To improve goal setting, clinicians need to embrace shared decision making.

Shared decision making is a process in which clinicians and patients work together to select tests, treatments, management or support packages based on the clinical evidence and the patient's informed preferences (Stacey et al., 2011). Key characteristics of shared decision making are that the patient and the clinician are involved, that both parties share information, that both parties take steps to build consensus about the preferred treatment and that an agreement is reached on the treatment to implement. Many elements of shared decision making are found in other areas of clinical practice including in developing self-management strategies, personalized care planning and in goal setting.

Coulter and Collins (2011) state that shared decision making is appropriate in every clinical conversation where a decision point has been reached and where the situation is not immediately life threatening. This can demand a change in behaviour from both the clinician and the patient. The clinician needs to recognize the need to share information and to develop the skills to elicit information about patient preference and values in the consultant as a prelude to decision making. They then may need to operate as a coach encouraging the patient to articulate their views about different options. The patient needs to have the motivation, information, skills and confidence to effectively make decisions about their health care. Being an engaged and active participant in one's own care is linked to better health outcomes (Bodenheimer, Lorig, Holman, & Grumbach, 2002; Lorig et al., 1999).

5.4 Patient Decision Aids

In recent years, patient decision aids have been developed. These differ from health education materials in that they make explicit the decision being considered. Typically, they contain (1) a description of the condition, (2) the treatment options including a *do nothing* option, (3) the risk of side effects with each treatment option, (4) the likely prognosis with different forms of treatment (including the *do nothing* option), (5) how strong the evidence is for different options and (6) a means of helping people clarify and communicate the values that inform their preferences. These aids can be used by patients before and during the meeting with the clinician to support them in their discussions. The aim is to have an active, informed and engaged patient.

A recent Cochrane review of 86 studies found that when patients use decision aids, they (a) improve their knowledge of the options, (b) are helped to have more accurate expectations of possible benefits and harms, (c) reach choices that are more consistent with their informed values and (d) participate more in decision making (Stacey et al., 2011).

5.5 World Health Organization International Classification of Function, Disability and Health

It is, however, clear that the shift to shared decision making and working as equals is challenging for both patients and professionals. Rehabilitation professionals may be more used to this than other types of clinicians, perhaps because the evidence base is weaker than in some specialties and because the dominant conceptual framework is the World Health Organization International Classification of Function, Disability and Health (ICF) (2001). The ICF is named as it is because of its focus on functioning. It acknowledges that every human being can experience disability. The ICF thus shifts the focus from cause to acknowledging that the experience of disability is influenced by personal factors (belief systems, cultural values, family experience, education) and environmental factors (accessible buildings and equality legislation), and this interaction is made manifest in the ability to maintain personal, social and civic roles. Thus, rehabilitation professionals acknowledge that patients not only bring to the goal-setting process their experience of illness and its impact (activity limitation and participation restriction) but that they also bring a set of values, preferences and attitudes and a unique set of conditions related to the family and social and physical environment they live within.

In contrast, clinicians bring expertise of a different type to goal setting. In traditional medical practice, they bring an understanding of diagnosis, aetiology, prognosis, treatment options and probable outcomes. In many common conditions such as hypertension, these factors can be defined with a reasonable degree of certainty. In rehabilitation, although the clinician brings knowledge of diagnosis and aetiology, prognosis is often difficult to state with certainty, and there are a multitude of treatment options. For example, a 50-year-old married solicitor with two children who had a stroke may receive 4 h of treatment a day from a multidisciplinary team composed of physiotherapy, occupational therapy, speech therapy, psychology, nursing and medicine. Treatment could be directed at impairments such as attention difficulties, activities such as walking, self-care, participation roles such as return to work or child care, or, as is commonly the case, a goal-oriented programme focused on participation but taking into account the underlying impairments. Thus, in rehabilitation, patients bring one type of expertise, and clinicians another, and potentially, the goal-setting negotiation that can take place between the professional and the patient in rehabilitation is a true negotiation in that it takes place between equals.

5.6 Barriers to Shared Decision Making and Goal Setting

Despite these different contributions from patients and clinicians, in clinical practice, shared decision making happens relatively infrequently (Holliday, Antoun, & Playford, 2005). The reasons for this have been explored from both patient and professional perspectives. On the professional side, reasons cited for this include lack of time and lack of agreement with some specific aspects of shared decision making tools, such as lack of applicability to either the clinical situation or the particular patient (Frosch, May, Rendle, Tietbohl, & Elwyn, 2012; Holliday, Ballinger, & Playford, 2007). On the patient side, patients feel they should conform to the *patient role* deferring to physicians during clinical consultations. They also report that physicians can be authoritarian and that the fear of being categorized as *difficult* prevents them from engaging in shared decision making (Frosch et al., 2012).

In rehabilitation, similar reasons for a lack of shared decision making are found when exploring professionals' and patients' views of goal setting. A survey of goal-setting practice in the United Kingdom highlighted that only in a minority of cases were patients present during the goal-setting meeting (Holliday et al., 2005). Two main barriers to patient-centred goal-setting practice described in the literature are (1) patients feeling they are not competent to actively participate in the process because they lack knowledge or skills or (2) patients feeling that the system prevents their participation and that the decision-making process is removed from them by health-care systems (Schoeb & Bürge, 2012). However, when structures are put in place that support shared goal setting, it allows patients to identify a route to functional improvement. Similarly, rehabilitation professionals may have reservations about actively engaging patients in setting goals if they perceive that patients are unable to participate effectively due to their cognitive, communication or expertise limitations. Professionals have reported that having a goal-setting tool to frame the agenda and the aims of rehabilitation was very helpful provided they had the time to go through it (Schulman-Green, Naik, Bradley, McCorkle & Bogardus, 2006). Lack of time was seen as a barrier, as were particular work patterns such as shifts influencing the nurses' ability to get involved and the lack of experience (Van de Weyer, Ballinger, & Playford, 2010). Shared goal setting was seen to demand high-level communication and negotiation skills. Clinicians also felt that some patients were not yet ready to participate in goal setting. In the language of shared decision making, they had not been *activated*.

When staff feel patients are passive or not ready to participate in goal setting, the reasons for this need to be considered. The readiness of an individual to make a behavioural change needs to be assessed, and clinicians need to develop the skills necessary to support patients in making behavioural changes. Formal training in such approaches is not an intrinsic part of medical, therapy or nurse education, but many rehabilitation services have an individual who is trained in motivational interviewing, and clinical psychologists use cognitive behavioural and other approaches to challenge beliefs which may hinder behavioural change (Medley & Powell, 2010).

5.7 Challenging Patient Groups

It is common for clinicians to argue that involving patients in goal setting or shared decision making is, in some circumstances, too difficult. Arguments are marshalled against involvement of patients in goal setting because they have a sudden disabling diagnosis such as acute stroke or because they are felt to be too cognitively impaired or because patients are not capable of setting goals that conform to the clinicians' ideas of what a rehabilitation goal should look like (e.g. conforming to *SMART* goal criteria). These issues are addressed in the next section.

5.7.1 Sudden Disabling Diagnoses

Most people have a life plan, that is, a view of themselves and their future and how they will spend it (even if this plan has never been explicitly articulated). It is within this life plan that decisions are made. The decisions they make support delivery of the life plan (or long-term goal). It is argued that when that life plan is suddenly and irrevocably altered through sudden onset illness, particularly when recovery is unlikely, selecting goals is difficult because the goal posts have shifted. Although this is often true, nevertheless, individuals can exert autonomous decision making over a simple task. For example, they can become passive and let the nurses provide all care, or they can try to do as much for themselves as possible and ask staff to support them in regaining independence. If people fail to make any active decisions about their treatment and recovery, this may be because of the way they are treated by professionals in the hospital setting. For example, nurses performing a medication round may prioritize completion of the round over teaching patients about their medication and ensuring they know when to take it. This is important because if hospital routines and professional attitudes dominate decision making, then we are at risk of diminishing our patients further and feeding in to a sense of dependence and futility. Decision making takes place at a number of levels, and patients should do so at whatever level they feel comfortable.

5.7.2 Levels of Participation

Thompson (2007), following a series of focus groups and individual interviews with patients and physicians, described five levels of decision making in which the lowest level (0) was physician-determined decisions with the patient excluded. Level 3 described shared decision making in which the professional may act as the final agent taking a decision but based on knowledge of the patient's views and preferences. At level 4, the patient is an autonomous decision-maker. Thompson observed that with increasing autonomy comes increasing responsibility for the outcomes which some patients may find insupportable.

Payton, Nelson, and Ozer (1990) offered a four-level patient participation system. The highest level is that in which the person answers open-ended questions; in the second level, the person is offered multiple-choice options and then forced choice; and finally, the lowest level is that in which the person is asked to assent or dissent. Although assessment of values and priorities is not implicit in this system, inviting a patient to witness the process staff go through when setting goals (to which they, the patient, are asked to assent) may help build trust and an understanding of the process – all of which are critical to later involvement when the patient has started to rebuild a life plan and can then identify goals for themselves.

5.7.3 Cognitive Impairment

The presence of cognitive impairment may be a reason some patients are not invited to participate in goal setting. Clearly at one extreme, a patient in a persistent vegetative state cannot participate in goal setting. In this case, disability management proceeds through a series of action plans for the staff. It is however important to involve families to try to elucidate the patient's values, beliefs and wishes. Decisions are made in the best interests of the patient and it is the responsibility of the clinician to do so, not that of the family. However, there is evidence that patients with cognitive impairment can participate in decision making and goal setting by simplifying the decision (Parsons & Parsons, 2012). If the patient is not capable of selecting one of two options, then inviting patients to witness the process invites trust.

Current structures in inpatient rehabilitation may prevent this. Guidelines suggest long-term goals should be set within 1 or 2 weeks of admission to inpatient rehabilitation and should be reviewed fortnightly (British Society for Rehabilitation Medicine, 2002). The time allocated to this may be relatively short. Involving patients in goal setting may increase the time taken to set goals. If staffing levels are fixed, increasing the time spent in goal setting diminishes the time available for therapists to deliver hands-on treatment, which staff can perhaps more easily attribute to improvements in performance. Thus, staffing levels, and the drive to deliver enough treatment sessions (often determined by insurance or health policies), can prevent there being enough time to really involve patients in sharing decisions about the best way to achieve stated goals. Given the importance attached to goal setting in rehabilitation and the growing policy context around shared decision making, the importance of goal setting may have to be reassessed and more time dedicated to it in rehabilitation services and in training rehabilitation professionals.

5.8 Judging Shared Decision-Making Processes

The International Patient Decision Aids Standards Collaboration developed a set of criteria that could be used to judge when a patient decision aid was effective in achieving a high level of patient involvement in clinical planning. Stacey et al. (2011) stated that these criteria were as follows:

- *Choice*: There is evidence that the patient decision aid improves the match between the chosen option and the features that matter most to the informed patient.
- *Decision process*: There is evidence that the patient decision aid helps patients to recognize that a decision needs to be made, know the options and their features, understand that values affect the decision, be clear about the option features that matter most, discuss values with their practitioner and understand the reasons for their preferred behaviours (Stacey et al., 2011, p. 4).

How would one judge when these criteria are met? The King's Fund report (Coulter & Collins, 2011) suggests there are a number of steps in the shared decision making consultation, including

1. Developing empathy and trust
2. Negotiated agenda setting and prioritizing
3. Information sharing
4. Communicating and managing risk
5. Supporting deliberating
6. Summarizing and making the decision
7. Documenting the decision

5.8.1 Developing Empathy and Trust

Little has been written about this topic in rehabilitation. In our service, as part of a larger study, we developed a key worker interview, which we have subsequently modified (Holliday, Cano, Freeman, & Playford, 2007). This interview started with an invitation for the patient to tell the key worker what had happened to them. Typical opening gambits might be *I understand you have recently had a stroke. Would you like to tell me about that?* This approach needs to be differentiated from a medical history. The aim is not to identify the nature of the underlying pathology (sudden onset hemiparesis equates to stroke) but to understand the individual patient's experience. This narrative is important. Greenhalgh and Hurwitz (1999) made three key observations of particular relevance to patients with chronic disabling diseases. First, they stated that 'The processes of getting ill, being ill, getting better (or getting worse), and coping (or failing to cope) with illness, can all be thought of as enacted narratives within the wider narratives (stories) of people's lives' (p. 48). They pointed out that narratives can provide a framework for approaching a patient's problems holistically, which may uncover diagnostic and therapeutic options. Narratives can also offer a method for addressing existential qualities such as inner hurt, despair, hope, grief, which are manifest in people as they struggle to come to terms with new or progressive disability.

However, for narrative history taking to be most effective, the clinician needs to be an active listener (Charon, 2001). As the patient tells their story, they are trying to contain the chaos and disorder that illness brings and give their lives shape and meaning. As the clinician listens, they imagine how the patient has experienced these events but also interpret them using the clinician's own experience, both personal and professional. Only through this engagement can the clinician work with the patient to find effective solutions to the problems presented by the patient. If the clinician does not do this work, then, although the diagnosis may be correct at an impairment and activity level, the patient will recognize that the clinician is not engaged, that the objectives of intervention (i.e. the goals) do not address their needs and that the patient will be non-adherent to treatment regimens and abandon goals the clinical team regard as important.

With this in mind, subsequent questions should focus not only on symptoms but also on activity and participation, on peoples' feelings about their performance and on the impact this has had on them and those around them. Examples of potential questions are listed in Box 5.1.

It is perhaps the first question in Box 5.1 that is most important, as it allows the patient to tell their story on their terms. Such interview questions allow patients to express their concerns, thoughts, feelings and emotions as well as explain their hopes and fears for the future. These questions are a useful basis for establishing the values that influence future decision making. Taking a narrative history differs from establishing a diagnosis which needs a focus on symptoms and signs. Doing both is time consuming, but it is the basis of the relationship within which rehabilitation and goal setting should take place. In the long term, it results in a better therapeutic relationship and better adherence to treatment and is, thus, a useful investment.

5.8.2 Negotiated Agenda Setting and Prioritizing

The Rivermead Life Goals Questionnaire was one of the earliest tools used to determine priorities for patients who were asked to grade the importance of nine life goals (Nair & Wade, 2003). These life goals were placed in order of the importance attributed to them by

BOX 5.1 EXAMPLES OF QUESTIONS TO ELICIT INFORMATION ON PATIENT'S NARRATIVES ABOUT THEIR CONDITION AND SITUATION

- I understand you have recently had (…a relapse of your multiple sclerosis/ a stroke). Would you like to tell me about that?
- What difficulties is that causing you?
- Are these difficulties affecting your key roles or responsibilities (at home/ at work/at college/in your relationships)?
- Have these difficulties had an impact on your mood or levels of worry?
- Which of your roles/responsibilities are going well?
- What is your long-term hope for your everyday life?
- What are you expecting to achieve during this admission?
- What are your strengths that you think will help you at the moment?
- What do you think may be unhelpful? (This could be based on previous experience of overcoming problems, e.g. ignoring problems, putting excess pressure on yourself or others, rushing ahead, using alcohol or drugs.)
- What do you feel the people around you expect from rehabilitation?
- What do you feel they expect from you?

patients with a progressive neurological disability, for example, relationship with my partner or my wish to have one; relationship with my family, including those not living in my home; ability to manage my personal care; leisure, hobbies and interests, including pets; residential and domestic arrangements; financial status; work, paid or unpaid; contacts with friends, neighbours and acquaintances; and religion or life philosophy.

Other structures have also been described to support negotiations during goal setting. In Payton et al.'s (1990) patient participation system, four general questions serve as the basis for developing a rehabilitation plan. The first two questions are as follows: *What are your concerns? What are your goals?* These are used to involve the patient in the processes of exploration, selection and specification of the person's concerns and goals. The last two questions are as follows: *What have you achieved? What worked?* These are addressed after the patient has participated in a period of therapy, to involve them in the evaluation of the success of the programme.

Other studies of goal setting have used the Canadian Occupational Performance Measure (COPM) as a goal-setting tool (Pollock, 1993). The COPM is administered using a semi-structured interview to allow the client to identify areas of difficulty in the areas of self-care, productivity and leisure. Following problem identification, the client rates the importance of each issue using a scale from 1 to 10 (10 being the most important). Up to five identified problems are chosen by the individual as the goals of treatment. Individuals rate their current level of performance and satisfaction with their performance on each of the five identified goals. Again, a scale from 1 to 10 is used (1 representing greatest difficulty and least satisfaction and 10 representing no difficulties and complete satisfaction). Mean scores across multiple areas of occupation are obtained for satisfaction and performance with scores ranging from 1 to 10. On reassessment, the COPM guidelines recommend that individuals review their goals and again rate their performance and satisfaction on the goals identified on initial assessment. A change score is obtained by subtracting the post-treatment score from the initial score. Doig, Fleming, Kuipers, and Cornwell (2010) reported that the COPM was used with 14 participants with traumatic brain injury to generate 53 goals that were used to inform a 12-week occupational therapy programme. They commented that the resultant goals were perceived almost unanimously as client centred, despite most participants having moderate or severe impairment in self-awareness. Similarly, in a study of preschoolers with cerebral palsy, the COPM was used by parents to set goals resulting in a 'dynamic and interactive approach of setting and implementing goals in the context of everyday activities' (Ostensjø, Oien, & Fallang, 2008, p. 252).

Since these early tools, there has been further work on negotiated agenda setting and prioritizing. In our study of goal setting, we asked patients to work through and complete a goal-setting workbook, ideally before they came to the rehabilitation unit (Holliday, Cano, et al., 2007). The workbook was in three sections, which the patients were encouraged to complete initially with support from family and friends and then, if necessary, with support from their key worker. This was to encourage people to think about activity and participation in the broadest sense, rather than focusing on *self-care* and *mobility* when it came to goal selection. The first section asked patients to prioritize activity and participation domains and the second to identify specific tasks within those domains that they wished to work on. The final section involved determining what individuals wanted to achieve within the time frame of the rehabilitation admission.

More recently, Scobbie, Wyke, and Dixon (2009) identified a number of theories of behaviour change relevant to goal-setting practice and used this to develop a theoretically informed practice framework (Scobbie, Dixon, & Wyke, 2011). The practice framework was built on seven theoretical constructs: self-efficacy, outcome expectancies, goal attributes including goal specificity and difficulty, action planning (specific plans that describe how the goal will be achieved), coping planning (plans that describe how potential barriers will be overcome), appraisal (assessment of performance in carrying out the plan and progress in relation to the goal) and feedback (feedback about performance in carrying out the plan and progress in relation to the goal). Based on these constructs, four intervention points for therapists and patients were identified: (1) developing goal intentions; (2) setting a specific goal; (3) activating goal-related behaviour through proactive planning, action planning and coping planning; and (4) appraising performance and giving feedback. At each intervention point, the patients' beliefs about achieving a successful outcome (including self-efficacy beliefs) were supported and validated by the therapists' behaviour.

Studies have also been conducted to elucidate how therapists elicit goals in the absence of a formal structure. It is clear from a number of studies, for example, Parry (2004), Schoeb (2009) and Barnard, Cruice, and Playford (2010), that this first step in the rehabilitation process can be difficult for both the patient and the therapist to negotiate and that it can take considerable time to implement. Both Schoeb (2009) and Barnard et al. (2010) highlighted the fact that patients use strategies such as minimal responses or nonresponses to maintain control over the goal-planning process, and face-saving devices, such as humour, are used to raise potentially conflicting perspectives and to express concerns if any particular goal is not considered realistic.

5.8.3 Information Sharing

The goal-setting meeting provides a formal opportunity for therapists to discuss with patients both the expected outcome and the reasons for this. Scobbie et al. (2011) described the steps that can be used to support people in developing goal intentions. These behaviours – which include encouraging patients about their capability of achieving goals, highlighting therapists' expectations for success on the basis of similar patients having achieved similar goals in the past and providing information that allay worries (e.g. that exercise will not make things worse) – are all examples of information sharing from professional to patient. However, within the framework, there are clear points in which the patient must share information with the professional, including while developing goal intentions and when activating goal-related behaviour in which the patient must identify action plans and coping strategies for when things go wrong.

Barnard et al. (2010) conducted a conversation analysis of goal-setting meetings that were attended by patients and their respective treating team to explore and describe the interaction of participants during interdisciplinary goal setting and to identify the strategies used to agree on goals. In this study, patient presence in these meetings was observed to result in increased dialogue about goals and required the treating team to explain their clinical reasoning for proposed goals.

Schoeb (2009) and Parry (2004) have also both observed that truly patient-centred goal setting is time consuming for clinicians to engage in. This may arise because patient-centred goal setting has both an educative information sharing element and possibly a *coaching* element supporting the patient to make a decision. One difficulty lies in the quality of published information materials. It has been reported that while many materials contain clear descriptions of the disease and common symptoms, factors such as the consequences of and natural history of conditions were much less well covered (Coulter, Entwistle, & Gilbert, 1999). This is a particular problem in rehabilitation when a wide variety of questions may be asked. It is unlikely that any clinician would feel confident predicting the progression of spasticity in multiple sclerosis and the impact it will have on dressing in 3 years' time. Thus, one of the roles of the clinician is supporting the patient to understand and deal with uncertainty. Uncertainty is multifactorial. It may derive from disease-related factors such as prognosis or from patient-related factors such as whether a patient wants to be treated (e.g. being unsure whether the side effects of medication are worth the benefit). Relatively little has been written on the nature of uncertainty or how to manage it, but it flavours many interactions between the patient and the clinician and needs to be acknowledged in discussions around goal setting.

5.8.4 Communicating and Managing Risk

One of the major barriers to goal setting is the time involved. Both eliciting goals and sharing information take time. This is highlighted by both patients' and professionals' experiences. However, one very specific aspect of information sharing which is rarely discussed in the literature is the sharing of information about risk. In the short term, rehabilitation interventions tend to be associated with low risk. Three types of risk may be identified: first, barriers to goal achievement which result in loss of self-efficacy; second, a risk of complications of the underlying condition; and third, a risk associated with the intervention itself. Recent goal-setting protocols have asked patients to identify potential barriers to goal achievement (Scobbie et al., 2011) and how they will be mitigated, but there is little in the literature about the prevalence and incidence of particular risks associated with specific diagnoses or treatments. Where there is potential risk, the problem often develops gradually and can be identified and treated before it becomes permanent (e.g. in the case of shoulder pain occurring during treatment of the upper limb after stroke). Of greater difficulty is predicting long-term risk. What is the risk of recurrent urinary tract infections in an individual with a post-micturition residual of 200 mL comparing intermittent self-catheterization with no treatment?

5.8.5 Supporting Deliberation

In managing the time available to make decisions, it is easy for clinicians to choose to close down a discussion prematurely. Barnard et al. (2010) identified six strategies that therapists use to close down such discussions:

1. *Framing a goal around a particular episode of care.* For example, when a patient with poor sitting balance expresses a desire to run a marathon, therapists may focus on the next 2 weeks, rather than address the idea that the goal is unlikely to be achieved. This approach enables modification of a goal without denying the possibility of its eventual achievement. It also softens unwelcome news and enables the discussion to move forward in the direction determined by the therapist. As expressed in a consensus meeting, the idea that goals have to be achievable is a source of concern for professionals as it has potential to create conflict with patients and undermine a therapeutic relationship. This approach of concentrating on the short term is interesting because it allows the patient to keep an ambitious goal in mind. It is not necessarily a bad approach. In the psychological literature, goals do not need to be achievable, and ambitious self-set goals can result in higher levels of performance. This may well be true in rehabilitation. It may be time we stopped focusing on achievable goals if it inhibits sharing and working with patients.

2. *Indicating that a goal is essentially non-negotiable.* For example, the therapists may write the goal down on a rehabilitation plan before the patient has agreed to it, thus indicating that further discussion is useless, the goal has been decided or, by indicating that if the therapist's assessment of what is achievable is wrong, the patient can exceed the performance level specified in the goal. An example of such behaviour occurs when a period of inpatient rehabilitation extends over 6 weeks and the patient wants to walk independently at the end of that time but the therapist thinks this will not be possible. Rather than spend time with the patient explaining the reasons for the therapist's concerns and allowing the patient to explain why this goal is important to them, the therapist might simply state that if things go well, then the patient may be able to walk independently (although in the opinion of the therapist, this is unlikely) before closing down further discussion on this topic. The patient may have very specific reasons for the 6-week goal of walking independently, for example, walking his daughter down the aisle as she gets married. It might have been possible to set the goal to walk with minimal assistance of one, so that he and his daughter could walk down the aisle together. A failure to explore the patient's motivations and values in a situation like this can lead to a resentful, unhappy patient.

3. *Presenting information in a stepwise fashion.* This approach is designed to elicit agreement. Patients demonstrating resistance are implicated in acceptance of the goal, by securing their agreement with each step in a process of clinical reasons, allowing the team to progress quickly through the business of the meeting.

4. *Collaborating with other team members to formulate the goals.* In this situation, a physiotherapist may formulate the goal with an occupational therapist despite a patient's resistance. This approach indicates (both to each other and to the patient) that the team will be inclined to fight for the goal the therapists want rather than the one important to the patient.

5. *Using the authority implicit in the professional role.* In this approach, clinicians draw on their status as rehabilitation *experts* to lay claim to being in the strongest position to know what is in the best interests of the patient. This may be done explicitly (such as by pointing out professional roles and years of experience in a field of practice) or implicitly (through manner and presentation).

6. *Moving on to the next goal, despite signs of patient resistance.* Here, clinicians simply ignore (or acknowledge but do not act on) expressions by patients of alternative views regarding goal selection, thus closing down a difficult discussion and preventing further challenges.

Once any of these strategies have been used, the patient is likely to feel coerced into a particular position, and shared decision making has not occurred.

Ozer, Payton, and Nelson (2000) suggested that we invite patients to specify how they know an intervention will have been successful. Perhaps critical in rehabilitation is identifying what it is about the goal that matters to the patient and considering the range of approaches that could be used to achieve the goal. For example, earlier in this chapter, a young woman with an intracerebral haemorrhage was described, who wanted privacy in the bathroom and who did not recognize the link between her goal and plinth to plinth transfers in the gym. In her eyes, her goal was not being achieved, even though the therapists were pleased with her progress and were confident she would be independent in the bathroom at discharge. A number of approaches can be considered, the first of which is the goal that in the long term she will be independent in transfers, toileting, showering and dressing. However, that goal may well start with a plinth to chair transfer in a gym and the link may seem remote. Explaining to the patient that this is a first step may help, but it may also be helpful to consider what could be done immediately to preserve her dignity in the bathroom. Can the nurses leave her for short periods? Would a larger towel help?

It is the identifying why the goal is important that matters. A grandmother may bake once a week not because she likes baking but because it provides a reason for her grandchildren to visit. Identifying a means to support the visiting that does not involve baking may be a satisfactory outcome. Reteaching baking but not ensuring that her grandchildren understand what has happened to her will result in an unsatisfactory outcome but an *achieved* goal. Describing different options and recognizing that at different times in rehabilitation different approaches may be needed are critical. In this sense, the relationship between the long-term goal and short-term goals may be more like crazy paving than stepping stones.

5.8.6 Summarizing and Making the Decision

Schoeb (2009) describes how the therapist and the patient can mutually signal that agreement has been reached. Typically, the therapist will ask whether agreement has been reached, and the patient will agree. Often, there is reference to the scheduling of a follow-up meeting.

5.8.7 Documenting the Decision

In a UK survey of goal setting in rehabilitation service, it was reported that 60% of patients were given copies of their goal (Holliday et al., 2005). It is clear that in many centres, patients do not have copies of their goals, but rather these are kept in the clinical notes. As clearly described in Holliday, Ballinger, et al. (2007), patients like having copies of their goals. It provides a point of reference and allows them to monitor change and progress. In addition to having a copy of the goals, the goal should have a review date (British Society for Rehabilitation Medicine, 2002), and the patient should be aware of how and when the goal will be reviewed. It is worth noting that goal-setting theory would suggest that evaluation of performance is initiated by patients and as a prelude to further goal setting (Locke & Latham, 2002). In this sense, it would be important to explore with a patient what worked well for them and what did not work so well before setting the next set of goals. In this way, the therapist will be seen as helpful, facilitating and receptive to ideas. This will build on the empathy and trust initiated at the first stage and also brings the patient's experience to the next round of goal setting.

5.9 Conclusion

Shared decision making and goal setting have many features in common. In both cases, clinicians need to explore patients' knowledge, understanding, values, preferences and beliefs as well as understand the underlying impairments, activity limitations, participation restrictions and environmental factors. In the context of goal setting, this means working with the patient to identify their goals and considering different routes to achieve that goal. A thorough understanding of the different steps in successful goal setting and an acknowledgement of its importance need to be embedded in the rehabilitation process. Training needs to acknowledge the range of communication skills required.

References

Barnard, R. A., Cruice, M. N., & Playford, E. D. (2010). Strategies used in the pursuit of achievability during goal setting in rehabilitation. *Qualitative Health Research, 20*(2), 239–250.

Bodenheimer, T., Lorig, K., Holman, H., & Grumbach, K. (2002). Patient self-management of chronic disease in primary care. *JAMA: The Journal of the American Medical Association, 288*(19), 2469–2475.

British Society for Rehabilitation Medicine. (2002). *British Society for Rehabilitation Medicine Standards for specialist inpatient and community rehabilitation services*. Retrieved August 2012, from http:// www.bsrm.co.uk/ClinicalGuidance/BSRMStandardsforRMServices2002.pdf.

Charon, R. (2001). Narrative medicine. *JAMA: The Journal of the American Medical Association, 286*(15), 1897–1902.

Coulter, A., & Collins, A. (2011). *Making shared decision-making a reality: No decision about me, without me*. London, U.K.: The King's Fund.

Coulter, A., Entwistle, V., & Gilbert, D. (1999). Sharing decisions with patients: Is the information good enough? *BMJ: British Medical Journal, 318*(7179), 318.

Doig, E., Fleming, J., Kuipers, P., & Cornwell, P. L. (2010). Clinical utility of the combined use of the Canadian Occupational Performance Measure and Goal Attainment Scaling. *The American Journal of Occupational Therapy, 64*(6), 904–914.

Frosch, D. L., May, S. G., Rendle, K. A., Tietbohl, C., & Elwyn, G. (2012). Authoritarian physicians and patients' fear of being labeled 'difficult' among key obstacles to shared decision making. *Health Affairs, 31*(5), 1030–1038.

Greenhalgh, T., & Hurwitz, B. (1999). Narrative based medicine: Why study narrative? *BMJ: British Medical Journal, 318*(7175), 48.

Holliday, R. C., Antoun, M., & Playford, E. D. (2005). A survey of goal-setting methods used in rehabilitation. *Neurorehabilitation and Neural Repair, 19*(3), 227–231.

Holliday, R. C., Ballinger, C., & Playford, E. D. (2007). Goal setting in neurological rehabilitation: Patients' perspectives. *Disability & Rehabilitation, 29*(5), 389–394.

Holliday, R. C., Cano, S., Freeman, J. A., & Playford, E. D. (2007). Should patients participate in clinical decision making? An optimised balance block design controlled study of goal setting in a rehabilitation unit. *Journal of Neurology, Neurosurgery & Psychiatry, 78*, 576–580.

Locke, E. A., & Latham, G. P. (2002). Building a practically useful theory of goal setting and task motivation: A 35-year odyssey. *American Psychologist, 57*(9), 705–717.

Lorig, K. R., Sobel, D. S., Stewart, A. L., Brown, B. W., Jr., Bandura, A., Ritter, P., ... Holman, H. R. (1999). Evidence suggesting that a chronic disease self-management program can improve health status while reducing hospitalization: A randomized trial. *Medical Care, 37*(1), 5–14.

Medley, A. R., & Powell, T. (2010). Motivational interviewing to promote self-awareness and engagement in rehabilitation following acquired brain injury: A conceptual review. *Neuropsychological Rehabilitation, 20*(4), 481–508.

Nair, K. P. S., & Wade, D. T. (2003). Changes in life goals of people with neurological disabilities. *Clinical Rehabilitation, 17*, 797–803.

Ostensjø, S., Oien, I., & Fallang, B. (2008). Goal-oriented rehabilitation of preschoolers with cerebral palsy – A multi-case study of combined use of the Canadian Occupational Performance Measure (COPM) and the Goal Attainment Scaling (GAS). *Developmental Neurorehabilitation, 11*(4), 252–259.

Ozer, M. N., Peyton, O. D., & Nelson, C. E. (2000). *Treatment planning: A patient centred approach.* New York, NY: McGraw Hill.

Parry, R. H. (2004). Communication during goal-setting in physiotherapy treatment sessions. *Clinical Rehabilitation, 18*(6), 668–682.

Parsons, J. G., & Parsons, M. J. (2012). The effect of a designated tool on person-centred goal identification and service planning among older people receiving homecare in New Zealand. *Health & Social Care in the Community, 20*(6), 653–662.

Payton, O., Nelson, C., & Ozer, M. (1990). *Patient participation in program planning. A manual for therapists.* Philadelphia, PA: F.A. Davis.

Pollock, N. (1993). Client-centered assessment. *American Journal of Occupational Therapy, 47*(4), 298–301.

Schoeb, V. (2009). "The goal is to be more flexible" – Detailed analysis of goal setting in physiotherapy using a conversation analytic approach. *Manual Therapy, 14*(6), 665–670.

Schoeb, V., & Bürge, E. (2012). Perceptions of patients and physiotherapists on patient participation: A narrative synthesis of qualitative studies. *Physiotherapy Research International, 17*(2), 80–91.

Schulman-Green, D. J., Naik, A. D., Bradley, E. H., McCorkle, R., & Bogardus, S. T. (2006). Goal setting as a shared decision making strategy among clinicians and their older patients. *Patient Education & Counseling, 63*, 145–151.

Scobbie, L., Dixon, D., & Wyke, S. (2011). Goal setting and action planning in the rehabilitation setting: Development of a theoretically informed practice framework. *Clinical Rehabilitation, 25*(5), 468–482.

Scobbie, L., Wyke, S., & Dixon, D. (2009). Identifying and applying psychological theory to setting and achieving rehabilitation goals. *Clinical Rehabilitation, 23*, 321–333.

Stacey, D., Bennett, C. L., Barry, M. J., Col, N. F., Eden, K. B., Holmes-Rovner, M., ... Thomson, R. (2011). Decision aids for people facing health treatment or screening decisions. *Cochrane Database Systematic Reviews, 10*, CD001431.

Thompson, A. G. (2007). The meaning of patient involvement and participation in health care consultations: A taxonomy. *Social Science & Medicine, 64*(6), 1297–1310.

Van de Weyer, R. C., Ballinger, C., & Playford, E. D. (2010). Goal setting in neurological rehabilitation: Staff perspectives. *Disability & Rehabilitation, 32*(17), 1419–1427.

Wade, D. T. (1998). Evidence relating to goal planning in rehabilitation. *Clinical Rehabilitation, 12*(4), 273–275.

World Health Organization. (2001). *International classification of functioning, disability and health.* Geneva, Switzerland: WHO.

6

MEANING as a Smarter Approach to Goals in Rehabilitation

Kathryn M. McPherson, Nicola M. Kayes and Paula Kersten

CONTENTS

6.1 Introduction

For 30 years, the acronym *SMART* has been almost ubiquitously associated with goals not just in rehabilitation (Wade, 2009) but in business (Doran, 1981; Johnson, Garriosn, Hernez-Broome, Fleenor, & Steed, 2012), education (Moeller, Theiler, & Wu, 2012), sport (Burton, Gillham, Weingberg, Yukelson, & Weigand, 2013), management (Johnson et al., 2012) and just about anywhere goals and goal setting are used. This is remarkably enduring for a concept that has significant limitations. Many reasons for its continued reign exist, including it being simple, comparatively easy to remember and at least some of its concepts being sound. However, is that really good enough? As noted in other chapters in this book, and a number of recent reviews (Levack, Dean, Siegert, & McPherson, 2006; Levack, Taylor, Siegert, Dean, McPherson, & Weatherall, 2006; Sugavanam, Mead, Bulley, Donaghy, & van Wijck, 2013), goals and goal setting remain problematic at times for both patients/clients and clinicians.

Goal setting is a core rehabilitation process that is used for multiple and varied purposes including engaging people in their rehabilitation, getting people *on board* with therapy aims, being more *person-centred* in our approach, working with others on the rehabilitation team, aiming for better outcomes, measuring progress and responding to contractual, legislative or professional requirements (Levack, Dean, Siegert, et al., 2006; Levack, Taylor, et al., 2006; Schut & Stam, 1994; Wade, 2009). Whilst the SMART acronym (commonly interpreted as *Specific, Measurable, Attainable, Relevant* and *Timely* – see Table 6.1) has certainly offered practical advice for aspects of goals that are about *task definition* or *task completion*, rehabilitation goals are also about assisting patients and clients to develop skills, abilities and strategies so they can do the things they want and need to do (Rosewilliam, Roskell, & Pandyan, 2011; Sugavanam et al., 2013). Theory development and research suggest that a more sophisticated approach to goal setting and goals in

TABLE 6.1

Range of Terms for the SMART Acronym

Letter	Frequently Used Term	Alternative Terms (Selected Examples)
S	Specific	Significant, stretching, simple, stimulating, succinct, straightforward, self-owned, self-managed, self-controlled, strategic, sensible, shared
M	Measurable	Monitored, meaningful, motivational, manageable, magical, magnetic, maintainable, mapped to goals
A	Attainable	Achievable, acceptable, action oriented, attributable, actionable, appropriate, ambitious, aspirational, accepted/acceptable, aligned, accountable, agreed, adapted, as-if-now accessible
R	Relevant	Relevant, reasonable, rewarding, results oriented, resources are adequate, resourced, recorded, reviewable, robust, relevant to a mission
T	Timely	Timely, tangible, trackable, tactical, traceable, towards what you want, many starting with *time* (e.g. limited, constrained, etc.), transparent

Sources: Bovend'Eerdt et al. (2009), Evans (2012), and Wade (2009).

rehabilitation is warranted (e.g. Barnard, Cruice, & Playford, 2010; Holliday, Ballinger, & Playford, 2007; Levack, Dean, McPherson, & Siegert, 2006; Levack, Dean, Siegert, et al., 2006; McPherson, Kayes, & Weatherall, 2009; Siegert & Taylor, 2004).

This chapter does not seek to comprehensively review the extensive literature on SMART goals. Nor does it suggest discarding SMART altogether as some of its components are worth considering at points in the goal-setting process. However, we do argue that MEANING (both the *word* itself and a series of concepts represented in it when used as an *acronym*) has more relevance and potential for goal setting in rehabilitation. Whilst allegiance to SMART goals remains strong, and some have opted for extending the acronym to SMARTER (Evans, 2012; Hersh, Worrall, Howe, Sherratt, & Davidson, 2012), we suggest an alternative word MEANING to capture a quite different approach.

This chapter contains three sections. Section 6.2 briefly outlines the rationale for rethinking the place of SMART goals in rehabilitation. Section 6.3 discusses the connection between two specific theoretical approaches and goal setting in rehabilitation: self-regulatory theory (Carver & Scheier, 1998; Locke & Latham, 1990, 2002; Mann, deRidder, & Fujita, 2013) and the theory of intentional action control (Achtziger, Martiny, Oettingen, & Gollwitzer, 2012; Gollwitzer, 1993, 1999), whilst Section 6.4 introduces the new acronym MEANING as a practical tool to support a theoretically informed focus in goal setting. Not so much *out with SMART* but definitely *in with MEANING*.

6.2 Rethinking SMART Goals in Rehabilitation

So just why have SMART goals prevailed for so long, and so widely in rehabilitation, given (a) the variability in how the acronym is interpreted (see Table 6.1) (e.g. Bovend'Eerdt, Botell, & Wade, 2009; Evans, 2012; Wade, 2009); (b) the weak (or absent) theoretical rationale for some of its components (Siegert & Taylor, 2004); (c) its origins in aiming to enhance business performance (Doran, 1981), not clinical practice, and as such failing to be informed by the impairments people experience; and finally (d) the very limited evidence that exists to suggest SMART goals are the most effective strategy to enhance the goal-setting process or improving goal-related outcomes (Rosewilliam et al., 2011; Scobbie, Dixon, & Wyke, 2011; Siegert & Taylor, 2004; Sugavanam et al., 2013). In fact, part of the longevity of the SMART approach may have been precisely because of a tendency for people to disregard research and just modify the SMART acronym to suit whatever context they happen to be working within and whichever values they wish to promote. The acronym might have stayed the same, but its interpretation has varied – a phenomena described by Rubin (2002) as *acronym drift* (para. 5).

It is important to acknowledge that SMART goals continue to be recommended in reha- bilitation (Bovend'Eerdt et al., 2009; Hersh et al., 2012; Turner-Stokes, 2009), and there is indeed support for some components. For example, it is fairly well accepted that specific goals (the usual interpretation of the S in SMART) are far more likely to be attained than vague and imprecise ones – the *do your best* goals (Strecher et al., 1995). It is also reason- able to propose that goals need to be measurable (the most common interpretation of M) as without clear definition of the goal or steps towards it, one would not know whether progress was being made or attainment achieved. However, other common interpretations of SMART are less clearly established, and that begs the question as to whether they might even be harmful. Some specific questions worth considering are as follows:

- Do goals need to be (A) achievable?

  …or does progress towards a demanding goal (while not necessarily attaining it) bring about positive outcomes and help patients/clients become more involved in the process? (Levack, Taylor, et al., 2006)

- Do goals need to be (R) realistic?

  …or do aspirational goals play an important part in sustaining motivation to keep striv- ing and working at rehabilitation? (Bright, Kayes, McCann, & McPherson, 2011; Bright, Kayes, McCann, & McPherson, 2012; Hammer, Mogensen, & Hall, 2009; Wiles, Cott, & Gibson, 2008)

- Do they need to be (T) timebound?

  …or does a fixation on short term achievement reduce the potential for long term recov- ery and adaptation – an important aim of rehabilitation? (Bright, Boland, Rutherford, Kayes, & McPherson, 2011)

Along with others, Edwin Locke and Gary Latham have driven much of the theoreti- cal and empirical progress we have seen in goal setting in the past 30 years (Locke and Latham, 1990, 2002). Whilst they have both undertaken research that supports SMART goals (particularly around *specific* goals), Latham (2003) made an observation that seems of real relevance to rehabilitation (even though it is about golf!):

  …when people have the necessary knowledge and skill to attain the goal, a perfor- mance outcome goal should be set (e.g., revenue to be earned; costs to be reduced). Goals affect choice, effort, and persistence. However, when people lack the knowledge or skill for goal attainment, a SMART learning rather than an outcome goal should be set. A learning goal, as the name implies, focuses attention on the discovery of strategies and skills necessary for goal attainment. Hence, the emphasis is on the development of procedures or systems necessary for mastering the task. Thus a good golfer with a low handicap should set a goal in terms of the desired score.

  A poor golfer should set a goal in terms of acquiring the skills necessary for using a 3 wood or a 1 driver, or in the adept use of the putter. In short, a learning goal focuses attention on skill or knowledge acquisition rather than on a specific performance outcome. Setting learning goals leads eventually to the ability to profit from setting performance goals. (Latham, 2003, p. 313)

Whilst one aim of rehabilitation is clearly to enhance performance (in both activity and participation), inevitably, many patients or clients lack the expertise required for goal attainment – otherwise rehabilitation would be redundant. Rehabilitation goals therefore need, at least in part, to focus on learning (strategy and skill) development regardless of the performance target or specific focus of therapy – as Latham (2003) said 'the discovery of strategies and skills necessary for goal attainment' (p. 313). Latham actually suggested in this paper and elsewhere (Latham & Brown, 2006) that SMART can be applied to learning goals or strategy development, but it is not clear that this approach necessarily works in rehabilitation (his paper addresses business and commercial activities where impairment is neither a factor limiting performance nor impacting on learning).

There is no doubt that SMART has something to offer if simple and straightforward task completion is *the goal* (the Specific and Measurable components anyway). But rehabilitation is rarely just about simple task completion. It might appear the case when professional treatment alone is administered (such as bandaging a sprained ankle) and the patient is considered solely to be a *recipient of care*, rather than an *active participant* in it. However, even in such cases, there is frequently a need for the patient to be involved and to do some work themselves, for optimal outcomes. For example, the patient with a sprained ankle is likely to be given exercises to do at home to improve proprioception. Moreover, following health professional advice about what the patient or client needs to do to optimize their rehabilitation in even relatively simple straightforward situations can be problematic (Chan, Lonsdale, Ho, Yung, & Chan, 2009). Furthermore, it is often problematic for people with complex disabling conditions that have lifelong sequelae, where accessing or maintaining the optimal functional, social, emotional and vocational recovery or restoration is typically challenging.

There appear three key areas where SMART goals have made few inroads in dealing with this complexity:

1. Informing strategies on how to engage patients in goal identification and goal setting
2. Helping patients (and clinicians) maintain the motivation and effort required to work towards goals in therapy or treatment
3. Preventing deterioration and promoting *carry over* or the ability to maintain or attain further progress (generalize) in activity and participation once rehabilitation has finished

Others have highlighted these as problematic areas, and a few have proposed new ways forward (Hersh et al., 2012; Scobbie et al., 2011). Optimizing our approaches to make the most of the potential that goals hold for enhancing outcomes and further research still is required, particularly in complex contexts or populations.

6.3 Two Theoretical Perspectives of Interest

Although there are multiple goal theories (Locke & Latham, 2006; Scobbie, Wyke, & Dixon, 2009; Siegert & Taylor, 2004), there are two approaches we think show promise in specifically addressing the three areas of difficulty in goals noted earlier. The first is *self-regulatory theory* (Carver & Scheier, 1998; Locke & Latham, 1990, 2002; Mann et al., 2013) and the second is a related but specific theory called the *theory of intentional action control* (Achtziger et al., 2012; Gollwitzer, 1993, 1999).

Self-regulatory theory has long been associated with neuropsychology but its concepts appear to have widespread applicability in many patient groups. Although there are a number of variants, they most commonly share these five assumptions:

1. Most human behaviour is goal directed.
2. People strive towards multiple goals.
3. Success in achieving desired goals is determined by a person's skill in regulating their own cognition, emotions and behaviour.
4. Progress or failure in goal attainment has affective or emotional consequences.
5. Goal attainment, motivation, affect and sense of self are closely related and will interact (Carver & Scheier, 1998; Locke & Latham, 1990, 2002).

These points clearly suggest a hypothesized connection between goal progress/failure and mood, motivation and sense of self – goals therefore being about more than simply task definition and completion. Goal progress in this model is influenced by meaning (e.g. sense of self relating to the very meaning of a fit with oneself), with interactions between these factors and levels of motivation being inevitable. Such a relationship has been further emphasized by Emmons and Kaiser (1996) who suggested that the most adaptive form of self-regulatory behaviour seemed to relate to the ability to select concrete, manageable goals (lower-order tasks) that are linked to personally meaningful (higher-order) representations.

Emmons went on to say that these skills are complex – being difficult to attain and hard to put into practice for anyone. However, clearly, this complexity is exacerbated for people whose self-regulatory skills are impaired. Although self-regulatory skills relate to brain function, it would be incorrect to assume difficulties only occur for people who have neurological damage to the parts of the brain responsible for executive functioning – self-monitoring and control. Whilst this is where most of our own investigation of goal-setting interventions drawing on self-regulation principles has occurred (McPherson et al., 2009; Siegert, McPherson, & Taylor, 2004; Ylvisaker, McPherson, Kayes, & Pellett, 2008), many patients experience difficulties in the key components identified earlier: goal failure, mood disorder (such as depression, anxiety), reduced motivation and challenges to a sense of who they are and how they fit in their *new* or *changed* world.

Self-regulatory theory could therefore be considered quite liberating in a number of ways by acknowledging the very real place and potential power of meaning in goals, given that they are such a routine rehabilitation process associated with almost all rehabilitation interventions. Taking the time to get to know patients and clients, and using strategies to elicit what is meaningful and important, may be not only legitimate but essential. Further, whilst at least some of the health professionals team need to be experts in eliciting what is most important for the patient/client, all health professionals could then draw on that information to reframe and make sense of the lower-order tasks they are asking patients to work on. This is relevant to the second area of goal difficulty we proposed earlier, where aligning lower-order rehabilitation goals with one's sense of self may be the very thing necessary to maintain the motivation and effort needed (Siegert & Taylor, 2004). Additionally, given that modelling behaviour has been shown to be a very useful strategy in rehabilitation (Marks, Allegrante, & Lorig, 2005), if we reference or connect to *meaningful goals* whilst working on the *lower-order tasks*, it may be that patients and clients learn and practice this skill or strategy during therapy but also beyond the clinical setting. So, for example, referencing what may be an archetypal higher-order goal (perhaps aspiring to return to a regular or special social event) whilst working on say balance may assist with a therapy goal or target that otherwise could seem far removed from what is meaningful and appear to be simply mundane practice and activity.

The theory of intentional action control originates from earlier work in social psychology and behaviour change (Achtziger et al., 2012; Gollwitzer, 1993, 1999). It is related to self-regulatory or control theory and is an extension to Gollwitzer's earlier work on the mind-set theory of action phases (Gollwitzer, 1990). The mind-set theory of action phases is one of a number of approaches developed in the early 1990s that distinguished between two core self-regulatory processes: goal *setting* and goal *striving* (*deliberation* and *implementation*; a state of *willing* and a state of *planning*; *motivation* and *volition*) (Gollwitzer, 1990; Heckhausen, 1991; Schwarzer, 1992). We refer to it here because the clear identification of the difference between the *intention* to act (thinking of an action or hoping for something one wants to achieve) and *implementation* (seeing through the planned or intended act) appears a particularly salient and relevant point of conceptual difference for rehabilitation practice in goal setting.

Earlier theories of behaviour change, such as the *theory of planned behaviour* (Ajzen, 1991, 2011), advanced thinking considerably at the time with recognition of the crucial place of *intentions* in behaviour. However, in some ways, this resulted in a tendency towards an overly simplistic assumption of an *intention* to *behaviour* continuity (Godin, Conner, & Sheeran, 2005; Godin & Kok, 1996). That is, if there is an intention to act, then the behaviour (or behaviour change) will follow. Gollwitzer and others (Orbell, Hodgkins, & Sheeran, 1997) have argued that this does not necessarily eventuate, for example, in the case where there are other conflicting goals (or intentions) or where barriers to successful implementation exist. In recognition of this, an *intention–behaviour gap* (de Nooijer, de Vet, Brug, & de Vries, 2006; Gollwitzer, Sheeran, & Zanna, 2006; Hall et al., 2008; Michie, Abraham, Whittington, McAteer, & Gupta, 2009; Ryan, 2009) has been the source of much discussion in the literature in recent years. Indeed, Hall and colleagues (Hall et al., 2008) argued that the assumption of intention–behaviour continuity only holds when

1. The behaviour in question is discrete rather than repetitive
2. The behaviour is fully under the control of the individual
3. The costs and benefits of the behaviour occur at the same point in time allowing for equal temporal weighting (p. 433)

In thinking about rehabilitation, one or all of these requirements is frequently unmet or is at least under significant challenge, perhaps helping to explain why goal failure and difficulties in maintaining gains beyond treatment are so common (Mudge, Barber, & Stott, 2009). Indeed, when thinking about one's own *intentions* to *implement* a new fitness routine or to lose weight, it does not take long to identify multiple failures of our own, very clear intention–implementation gaps!

Over recent years, attempts have been made to respond to this additional complexity by integrating behavioural strategies into self-management plans in diabetes (Nadkarni, Kucukarslan, Bagozzi, Yates, & Erickson, 2010) and other long-term conditions (e.g. Brown,

Sheeran, & Reuber, 2009; Jackson et al., 2005). Latterly, this move has been followed in rehabilitation with, for example, action–coping plans (Mudge et al., 2009; Scobbie et al., 2011) and motivational interviewing (Miller & Rose, 2009).

However, as highlighted in these publications and other reviews of incorporating psychological strategies into *physical* therapies, significant barriers have existed to implementation. Health professionals have expressed concerns that behavioural interventions seem outside their scope of practice with the level of skill and expertise required meaning the intervention is difficult to deliver without significant time demands for training (Alexander et al., 2012; Arvinen-Barrow, Penny, Hemmings, & Corr, 2010; Frerichs, Kaltenbacher, van de Leur, & Dean, 2012; McPherson et al., 2009; Woby, 2009). Given it has proven difficult to integrate such behavioural strategies in a research setting (Scobbie, McLean, Dixon, Duncan, & Wyke, 2013), it is likely to be even more difficult to deliver in the clinical setting lacking the supports for intervention integrity and an implementation *protocol*. This emphasizes the need for a practical tool to support use of such strategies (something that might rival SMART, for instance).

The *theory of intentional action control* is of particular interest with its focus primarily on the translation of intentions into behavioural action through the development of a simple (but not simplistic), very specific type of action–coping plan: an *implementation intention* in the form of an *if–then plan* (Gollwitzer & Sheeran, 2011; Gollwitzer, 1993, 1999; Gollwitzer et al., 2006). These *if–then* plans seek to address the intention–implementation gap by:

1. Explicitly identifying situations or cues that support or trigger the goal-directed behaviour
2. Explicitly identifying and planning for the things that get in the way of that activity, for example, failures in initiation or getting started or getting derailed whilst doing the activity
3. Consistently using and rehearsing the strategy of forming *if–then plans*

Goal planning in this approach is not just about the goal itself, but identifying and planning for the things that get in the way of doing the goal-related activities. For example, rather than framing an activity goal as being *to walk every day to the front gate*, one would frame a series of if–then goals that are quite *specific* (not out with SMART characteristics, just reinterpreted and fully operationalized):

- *If* it is 11 am, *then* I will walk to my front gate

  ...with additional if–then plans identified that are connected to the things (both practical and internal states) that might interrupt the likelihood that the person will do the walk, for example.

- *If* it is raining at 11 am when I have planned to do my walk to the front gate,
  - *then* I will walk around the living area in my house three times, OR
  - *then* I will go to the local shopping mall for my walk
- *If* I am tired at 11 am when I have planned to do my walk to the front gate,
  - *then* I will remind myself I am trying to get fitter to return to the golf/tennis club (or other important location/action)
- *If* there is something on the radio that I want to listen to at 11 am when I have planned do my walk to the front gate,
  - *then* I will schedule the walk in my diary for 2 pm instead

Whilst this might seem a remarkably simple strategy, evidence has indicated it is a very effective way to bridge the implementation gap in a range of health promotion interventions (Arbour & Martin Ginis, 2009; Armitage & Arden, 2010; Chapman & Armitage, 2010). Although our recent review suggests it is not yet widely used in rehabilitation (Kersten, McPherson, Kayes, Theadom & McCambride, 2012), we have tested if–then plans in a recent pilot study which highlighted that both health professionals (physiotherapists) and patients (people with multiple sclerosis and stroke in the community) largely found the approach relatively straightforward and helpful (Kersten, McPherson, McCambride, Kayes, & Theadom, 2013). It is early days in relation to evidence of effectiveness in a rehabilitation context, but *if–then* plans appear to have very real potential to assist both patients and clinicians enhance maintenance of goal-related behaviour.

In summary, self-regulatory theory and the theory of intentional action control appear to usefully inform how we might better address a number of difficulties in goal setting. Whilst evidence is accruing, and there is more work to be done, we would argue there is a strong and sufficient rationale for all practitioners in rehabilitation to at least consider or become aware of these theories and how they could enhance goal setting and indeed goal striving. However, given that we and others have noted difficulty in integrating this thinking into practice, we make a suggestion in the following section as to how to remember or operationalize these concepts.

6.4 MEANING as a Practical Tool to Support Goal Setting and Goal Striving

Determining what is meaningful for people is not the only thing that matters in goal setting and goal striving, but theory (self-regulatory theory and the theory of intentional action control), our own work (Bright, Boland, et al., 2011; McPherson et al., 2009; Ylvisaker et al., 2008) and that of many others (Emmons, 2003; Hammell, 2007; Levack, Kayes, & Fadyl, 2010) suggest it to be an important part of the process. In addition to what seems a robust human and ethical argument justifying consideration of what is meaningful to people in their rehabilitation, we are persuaded by Robert Emmons' argument:

> As far as we know humans are the only meaning-seeking species on the planet. Meaning-making is an activity that is distinctly human, a function of how the human brain is organised. (p. 105)

and

> Goals are essential components of a person's experience of his or her life as meaningful and contribute to the process by which people construe their lives as meaningful or worthwhile. (p. 107)

Hence, we propose MEANING as a key term and as an acronym to underpin, remind and support rethinking actions and activities in goal setting. Table 6.2 outlines the related terms for such an approach along with strategies that may be useful for attending to these concepts.

TABLE 6.2

MEANING: A New Acronym to Support Goal Setting and Goal Striving

Letter	Meaning	Explanation	Possible Strategies
M	Meaning	Meaningful overall goals identified – knowing what matters as the context for all goal-related activity.	1. Invite stories about what has been important in the past and what people want for their future (Bright, Boland, et al., 2011). 2. Listen to and recognize these aspirations. 3. Where people find saying what is important to them to be difficult, allowing time and perhaps introducing tools such as metaphorical identity mapping to aid reflection in this (Ylvisaker et al., 2008).
E	Engage	Engage to establish trust and communication to discuss what is meaningful.	4. Listen to and acknowledge aspirations – a common issue in reviews of quality of care is that patients do not feel *heard* hence really listening appears key to gaining trust (Bright, Boland, et al., 2011; Fadyl, McPherson, & Kayes, 2011). 5. Being present as a practitioner – that is, recognizing that as a practitioner, one can *be engaging* to facilitate *engagement* in the process (Bright, Kayes, Worrall & McPherson, in press).
A	Anchor	Anchor sub-goals to what is most meaningful for the patient/client as a tool for making sense of therapy and as modelling this as a strategy for the patient to continue to use.	6. Verbalize the connection between a meaningful goal for the patient/client to enhance connection between patient goals and therapy aims.
N	Negotiate	Negotiate levels of progress towards attainment as (1) progress may bring other self-regulatory benefits (mood/motivation/sense of self) and (2) this models another strategy of breaking down goals into sub-steps.	7. Goal attainment scaling (GAS) appears a useful strategy for acknowledging the overall aspiration whilst anchoring targets or steps that indicate progress (and appears to assist motivation) (McPherson et al., 2009).
I	Intention–implementation gap	Specific steps are frequently needed to bridge the intention–implementation gap – *if–then* plans appear a useful way to frame sub-goals to help maintain and address potential barriers to goal practice.	8. Use *if–then* plans to make explicit both facilitators and barriers to goal striving and goal activity. 9. Use *if–then* plans to make explicit the actions required to carry out the plan in relation to the facilitators and barriers. 10. *If–then* plans seem to have great potential when considering how to help people carry on goal-related activity once therapy stops (Kersten et al., 2013).
N	New goals	Rather than have 'goal attainment' itself as the objective, view goal setting abilities as a strategy that be used over time.	11. View goal setting and goal striving as part of the therapeutic process versus simply a means to an end. 12. Discussing the potential for goals to work in this way with patients and clients (Bright, Boland, et al., 2011).

(Continued)

TABLE 6.2 (*Continued*)

MEANING: A New Acronym to Support Goal Setting and Goal Striving

Letter	Meaning	Explanation	Possible Strategies
G	Goals as behaviour change	Goals are about behaviour change and therefore health professionals should be informed about behaviour change approaches.	13. Recognize that goals are an active intervention that impacts on people's actions, mood, motivation and sense of self (relating to self-regulation). 14. At the basic level, we suggest all practitioners involved in goal setting should understand basic behaviour change principles and that each centre would have *champions* to lead and support initiatives in practice. 15. Adopt a competency framework around levels of knowledge and expertise of behaviour change required (indeed, a focus on this in the area of health behaviour change exists) (Dixon & Johnston, 2010; Whifield & Machaczek, 2010).

Whilst there is further research to be done, findings from a range of our own projects and those of others suggest considering these steps may help us in three stages of goal-related work with patients in rehabilitation:

1. Pre- or early rehabilitation (identifying and valuing what is meaningful to people and providing a specific focus on our own behaviour as clinicians in regard to how we engage people in the process)

2. Early and mid-rehabilitation (connecting what is meaningful with specific therapy, strategies and steps for goal progress to keep motivation and enhance mood and a positive sense of self or identity)

3. Translation or generalization beyond the intervention period (specific consideration of bridging the intention–implementation gap using if–then plans)

Indeed, the three issues identified as being frequently problematic become a focus for a different approach as proposed in Figure 6.1.

Whilst a number of others have proposed integrating behavioural approaches with goal setting in rehabilitation (e.g. see Chapters 11 and 14), we think conceptualizing these three stages and reflecting on MEANING when working with goals in rehabilitation may be advantageous.

6.5 Conclusion

There is no doubt that there is further work to be done to empirically test different aspects of goals with MEANING. For now, we hope this chapter has provided sufficient argument, theoretical rationale and preliminary evidence, to support rethinking the place of meaning in goals in rehabilitation.

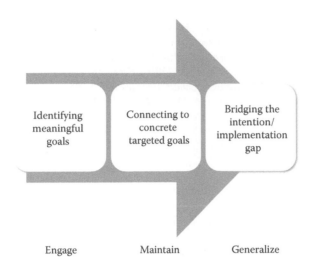

FIGURE 6.1
A three tiered approach to goals and goal setting.

Acknowledgement

A primary acknowledgement is to the late Mark Ylvisaker, collaborator and friend, who contributed so much to the thinking that has led us to proposing the centrality of MEANING in goals. However, he is in no way responsible for any inadequacy in our argument. Thanks also to the students, research assistants and participants in our research programme on goals who have similarly contributed much.

References

Achtziger, A., Martiny, S. E., Oettingen, G., & Gollwitzer, P. M. (2012). Metacognitive processes in the self-regulation of goal pursuit. In P. Brinol & K. G. DeMarree (Eds.), *Social metacognition* (pp. 121–139). New York, NY: Psychology Press.

Ajzen, I. (1991). The theory of planned behaviour. *Organizational Behaviour and Human Decision Processes, 50*, 179–211.

Ajzen, I. (2011). The theory of planned behaviour: Reactions and reflections. *Psychology & Health, 26*(9), 1113–1127.

Alexander, J. A., Bambury, E., Medoza, A., Reynolds, J., Veronneau, R., & Dean, E. (2012). Health education strategies used by physical therapists to promote behaviour change in people with lifestyle-related conditions: A systematic review. *Hong Kong Physiotherapy Journal, 30*(2), 57–75.

Arbour, K. P., & Martin Ginis, K. A. (2009). A randomised controlled trial of the effects of implementation intentions on women's walking behaviour. *Psychology and Health, 24*(1), 49–65.

Armitage, C. J., & Arden, M. A. (2010). A volitional help sheet to increase physical activity in people with low socioeconomic status: A randomised exploratory trial. *Psychology and Health, 25*(10), 1129–1145.

Arvinen-Barrow, M., Penny, G., Hemmings, B., & Corr, S. (2010). UK chartered physiotherapists' personal experiences in using psychological interventions with injured athletes: An interpretative phenomenological analysis. *Psychology of Sport and Exercise, 11*(1), 58–66.

Barnard, R. A., Cruice, M. N., & Playford, E. D. (2010). Strategies used in the pursuit of achievability during goal setting in rehabilitation. *Qualitative Health Research, 20*(2), 239–250.

Bovend'Eerdt, T. J., Botell, R. E., & Wade, D. T. (2009). Writing SMART rehabilitation goals and achieving goal attainment scaling: A practical guide. *Clinical Rehabilitation, 23*(4), 352–361.

Bright, F. A., Boland, P., Rutherford, S. J., Kayes, N. M., & McPherson, K. M. (2012). Implementing a client-centred approach in rehabilitation: An autoethnography. *Disability and Rehabilitation, 34*(12), 997–1004.

Bright, F. A., Kayes, N. M., McCann, C. M., & McPherson, K. M. (2011). Understanding hope after stroke: A systematic review of the literature using concept analysis. *Topics in Stroke Rehabilitation 18*(5), 490–508.

Bright, F. A., Kayes, N. M., McCann, C. M., & Mcpherson, K. M. (2012). Hope in people with aphasia. *Aphasiology, 27*(1), 41–58.

Bright, F. A., Kayes, N. M., Worrall, L., & McPherson, K. M. (in press). The intersection of disability and disparity: A conceptual framework. *Disability and Rehabilitation.*

Brown, I., Sheeran, P., & Reuber, M. (2009). Enhancing antiepileptic drug adherence: A randomized controlled trial. *Epilepsy and Behavior, 16*(4), 634–639.

Burton, D., Gillham, A., Weingberg, R., Yukelson, D., & Weigand, D. (2013). Goal setting styles: Examining the role of personality factors on the goal practices of prospective Olympic athletes. *Journal of Sport Behaviour, 36*(1), 23–44.

Carver, C. S., & Scheier, M. F. (1998). *On the self-regulation of behavior.* Cambridge, U.K.: Cambridge University Press.

Chan, D. K., Lonsdale, C., Ho, P. Y., Yung, P. S., & Chan, K. M. (2009). Patient motivation and adherence to postsurgery rehabilitation exercise recommendations: The influence of physiotherapists' autonomy-supportive behaviors. *Archives of Physical Medicine and Rehabilitation, 90*(12), 1977–1982.

Chapman, J., & Armitage, C. J. (2010). Evidence that boosters augment the long-term impact of implementation intentions on fruit and vegetable intake. *Psychology and Health, 25*(3), 365–381.

de Nooijer, J., de Vet, E., Brug, J., & de Vries, N. K. (2006). Do implementation intentions help to turn good intentions into higher fruit intakes? *Journal of Nutrition Education and Behavior, 38*(1), 25–29.

Dixon, D., & Johnston, M. (2010). *Health behaviour change competency framework: Competences to deliver interventions to change lifestyle behaviours that affect health.* Retrieved 3 February 2013, from http://www.healthscotland.com/documents/4877.aspx.

Doran, G. T. (1981). There's a S.M.A.R.T. way to write management's goals and objectives. *Management Review, 70*(11), 35.

Emmons, R. A. (2003). Personal goals, life meaning, and virtue: Wellsprings of a positive life. In C. L. M. Keyes (Ed.), *Flourishing: The positive person and the good life* (pp. 105–128). Washington, DC: American Psychological Association.

Emmons, R. A. & Kaiser, H. A. (1996). Goal orientation emotional well-being: Linking goals and affect through the self. In L. Martin & A. Tessler (Eds.), *Striving and Feeling: Interactions among Goals, Affect and Self-Regulation* (pp. 79–98). Hillslade, N.J.: Lawrence Erlbaum Associates.

Evans, J. J. (2012). Goal setting during rehabilitation early and late after acquired brain injury. *Current Opinion in Neurology, 25*(6), 651–655.

Fadyl, J. K., McPherson, K. M., & Kayes, N. M. (2011). Perspectives on quality of care for people who experience disability. *BMJ Quality & Safety, 20*(1), 87–95.

Frerichs, W., Kaltenbacher, E., van de Leur, J. P., & Dean, E. (2012). Can physical therapists counsel patients with lifestyle-related health conditions effectively? A systematic review and implications. *Physiotherapy Theory and Practice, 28*(8), 571–587.

Godin, G., Conner, M., & Sheeran, P. (2005). Bridging the intention–behaviour 'gap': The role of moral norm. *British Journal of Social Psychology, 44*(4), 497–512.

Godin, G., & Kok, G. (1996). The theory of planned behavior: A review of its applications to health-related behaviors. *American Journal of Health Promotion, 11*(2), 87–98.

Gollwitzer, P., & Sheeran, P. (2011). *Implementation intentions.* Retrieved 7 February 2011, from http://cancercontrol.cancer.gov/BRP/constructs/implementation_intentions/goal_intent_attain.pdf.

Gollwitzer, P. M. (1990). Action phases and mind-sets. In E. T. Higgins & R. M. Sorrentino (Eds.), *The handbook of motivation and cognition: Foundations of social behaviour*. New York, NY: The Guilford Press.

Gollwitzer, P. M. (1993). Goal achievement: The role of intention. *European Review of Social Psychology, 4*, 141–185.

Gollwitzer, P. M. (1999). Implementation intentions: Strong effects of simple plans. *American Psychologist, 54*, 493–503.

Gollwitzer, P. M., Sheeran, P., & Zanna, M. P. (2006). Implementation intentions and goal achievement: A meta-analysis of effects and processes. *Advances in Experimental Social Psychology, 38*, 69–119.

Hall, P. A., Elias, L. J., Fong, G. T., Harrison, A. H., Borowsky, R., & Sarty, G. E. (2008). A social neuroscience perspective on physical activity. *Journal of Sport and Exercise Psychology, 30*(4), 432–449.

Hammell, K. W. (2007). The experience of rehabilitation following spinal cord injury: A meta-synthesis of qualitative findings. *Spinal Cord, 45*(4), 260–274.

Hammer, K., Mogensen, O., & Hall, E. O. (2009). The meaning of hope in nursing research: A meta-synthesis. *Scandinavian Journal of Caring Sciences, 23*(3), 549–557.

Heckhausen, H. (1991). *Motivation and action*. Berlin, Germany: Springer-Verlag.

Hersh, D., Worrall, L., Howe, T., Sherratt, S., & Davidson, B. (2012). SMARTER goal setting in aphasia rehabilitation. *Aphasiology, 26*(2), 220–233.

Holliday, R. C., Ballinger, C., & Playford, E. D. (2007). Goal setting in neurological rehabilitation: Patients' perspectives. *Disability and Rehabilitation, 29*(5), 389–394.

Jackson, C., Lawton, R., Knapp, P., Raynor, D. K., Conner, M., Lowe, C., & José Closs, S. (2005). Beyond intention: Do specific plans increase health behaviours in patients in primary care? A study of fruit and vegetable consumption. *Social Science and Medicine, 60*(10), 2383–2391.

Johnson, S. K., Garriosn, L. L., Hernez-Broome, G., Fleenor, J. W., & Steed, J. L. (2012). Go for the goal(s): Relationship between goal setting and transfer of training following leadership development. *Academic Management Learning & Education, 11*(4), 555–569.

Kersten, P., McPherson, K., Kayes, N., Theadom, A., & McCambride, A. (2012). *Implementation-intentions: A strategy for longer term engagement.* Presented as part of the symposium: McPherson, K., Kayes, N., Kersten, P., Colantonio, A. Goals related activity in neurorehabilitation: Rethinking meaning, engagement and outcomes. Presented at the meeting of the seventh World Congress of NeuroRehabilitation, May 2012, Melbourne, Victoria, Australia.

Kersten, P., McPherson, K., McCambride, A., Kayes, N., & Theadom, A. (2013). *Bridging the intention implementation gap: A feasibility study of 'if-then' planning in neurorehabilitation.* Presented at the meeting of the New Zealand Rehabilitation Association Conference, Nelson, New Zealand.

Latham, G. P. (2003). A five-step approach to behaviour change. *Organizational Dynamics, 32*(3), 309–318.

Latham, G. P., & Brown, T. C. (2006). The effect of learning vs. outcome goals on self-efficacy, satisfaction and performance in an MBA program. *Applied Psychology, 55*(4), 606–623.

Levack, W. M., Dean, S. G., McPherson, K. M., & Siegert, R. J. (2006). How clinicians talk about the application of goal planning to rehabilitation for people with brain injury-variable interpretations of value and purpose. *Brain Injury, 20*(13–14), 1439–1449.

Levack, W. M., Dean, S. G., Siegert, R. J., & McPherson, K. M. (2006). Purposes and mechanisms of goal planning in rehabilitation: The need for a critical distinction. *Disability and Rehabilitation, 28*(12), 741–749.

Levack, W. M., Kayes, N. M., & Fadyl, J. K. (2010). Experience of recovery and outcome following traumatic brain injury: A metasynthesis of qualitative research. *Disability and Rehabilitation, 32*(12), 986–999.

Levack, W. M., Taylor, K., Siegert, R. J., Dean, S. G., McPherson, K. M., & Weatherall, M. (2006). Is goal planning in rehabilitation effective? A systematic review [Review]. *Clinical Rehabilitation, 20*(9), 739–755.

Locke, E. A., & Latham, G. P. (1990). *A theory of goal setting and task performance.* Upper Saddle River, NJ: Prentice-Hall.

Locke, E. A., & Latham, G. P. (2002). Building a practically useful theory of goal and task motivation. A 35-Year Odyssey. *American Psychologist, 57*(9), 705–717.

Locke, E. A., & Latham, G. P. (2006). New directions in goal-setting theory. *Current Directions in Psychological Science, 15*(5), 265–268.

Mann, T., de Ridder, D., & Fujita, K. (2013). Self-regulation of health behavior: Social psychological approaches to goal setting and goal striving. *Health Psychology: Official Journal of the Division of Health Psychology, American Psychological Association, 32*(5), 487–498.

Marks, R., Allegrante, J. P., & Lorig, K. (2005). A review and synthesis of research evidence for self-efficacy-enhancing interventions for reducing chronic disability: Implications for health education practice (part II). *Health Promotion Practice, 6*(2), 148–156.

McPherson, K. M., Kayes, N., & Weatherall, M. (2009). A pilot study of self-regulation informed goal setting in people with traumatic brain injury. *Clinical Rehabilitation, 23*(4), 296–309.

Michie, S., Abraham, C., Whittington, C., McAteer, J., & Gupta, S. (2009). Effective techniques in healthy eating and physical activity interventions: A meta-regression. *Health Psychology, 28*(6), 690–701.

Miller, W. R., & Rose, G. S. (2009). Toward a theory of motivational interviewing. *American Psychologist, 64*(6), 527–537.

Moeller, A. J., Theiler, J. M., & Wu, C. (2012). Goal setting and student achievement: A longitudinal study. *The Modern Language Journal, 96*(2), 153–169.

Mudge, S., Barber, P. A., & Stott, N. S. (2009). Circuit-based rehabilitation improves gait endurance but not usual walking activity in chronic stroke: A randomized controlled trial. *Archives of Physical Medicine & Rehabilitation, 90*(12), 1989–1996.

Nadkarni, A., Kucukarslan, S. N., Bagozzi, R. P., Yates, J. F., & Erickson, S. R. (2010). A simple and promising tool to improve self-monitoring of blood glucose in patients with diabetes. *Diabetes Research and Clinical Practice, 89*(1), 30–37.

Orbell, S., Hodgkins, S., & Sheeran, P. (1997). Implementation intentions and the theory of planned behaviour. *Social Psychology Bulletin, 23*(9), 945–954.

Rosewilliam, S., Roskell, C. A., & Pandyan, A. D. (2011). A systematic review and synthesis of the quantitative and qualitative evidence behind patient-centred goal setting in stroke rehabilitation [Review]. *Clinical Rehabilitation, 25*(6), 501–514.

Rubin, R. S. (2002). Will the real SMART goals please stand up? *The Industrial-Organisational Psychologist, 39*(4), 26–27.

Ryan, P. (2009). Integrated theory of health behavior change: Background and intervention development. *Clinical Nurse Specialist, 23*(3), 161–170.

Schut, H. A., & Stam, H. J. (1994). Goals in rehabilitation teamwork. *Disability and Rehabilitation, 16*(4), 223–226.

Schwarzer, R. (1992). Self-efficacy in the adoption and maintenance of health behaviours: Theoretical approaches and a new model. In R. Schwarzer (Ed.), *Self-efficacy: Thought control of action.* Washington, DC: Hemisphere Publishing Corporation.

Scobbie, L., Dixon, D., & Wyke, S. (2011). Goal setting and action planning in the rehabilitation setting: Development of a theoretically informed practice framework [Case Reports]. *Clinical Rehabilitation, 25*(5), 468–482.

Scobbie, L., McLean, D., Dixon, D., Duncan, E., & Wyke, S. (2013). Implementing a framework for goal setting in community based stroke rehabilitation: A process evaluation. *BMC Health Services Research, 13*(1), 190.

Scobbie, L., Wyke, S., & Dixon, D. (2009). Identifying and applying psychological theory to setting and achieving rehabilitation goals. *Clinical Rehabilitation, 23*(4), 321–333.

Siegert, R. J., McPherson, K. M., & Taylor, W. J. (2004). Toward a cognitive-affective model of goal-setting in rehabilitation: Is self-regulation theory a key step? *Disability and Rehabilitation, 26*(20), 1175–1183.

Siegert, R. J., & Taylor, W. J. (2004). Theoretical aspects of goal-setting and motivation in rehabilitation [Review]. *Disability and Rehabilitation, 26*(1), 1–8.

Strecher, V. J., Seijts, G. H., Kok, G. J., Latham, G. P., Glasgow, R., DeVellis, B., … Bulger, D. W. (1995). Goal setting as a strategy for health behavior change. *Health Education Quarterly, 22*(2), 190–200.

Sugavanam, T., Mead, G., Bulley, C., Donaghy, M., & van Wijck, F. (2013). The effects and experiences of goal setting in stroke rehabilitation – A systematic review. *Disability and Rehabilitation, 35*(3), 177–190.

Turner-Stokes, L. (2009). Goal attainment scaling (GAS) in rehabilitation: A practical guide. *Clinical Rehabilitation, 23*(4), 362–370.

Wade, D. T. (2009). Goal setting in rehabilitation: An overview of what, why and how. *Clinical Rehabilitation, 23*(4), 291–295.

Whifield, M., & Machaczek, K. (2010). *Scoping the economic case for the 'Health Behaviour Change' Competence Framework.* Sheffield, U.K.: Centre for Health and Social Care Reearch (CHSCR), Sheffield Hallam University. Retrieved 1 January 2013, from http://www.yorksandhumber.nhs.uk/document.php?o=7728.

Wiles, R., Cott, C., & Gibson, B. E. (2008). Hope, expectations and recovery from illness: A narrative synthesis of qualitative research. *Journal of Advanced Nursing, 64*(6), 564–573.

Woby, S. (2009). Targeting psychological factors: Is this a job for physiotherapists? *International Journal of Therapy and Rehabilitation, 16*(1), 6–7.

Ylvisaker, M., McPherson, K., Kayes, N., & Pellett, E. (2008). Metaphoric identity mapping: Facilitating goal setting and engagement in rehabilitation after traumatic brain injury. *Neuropsychological Rehabilitation, 18*(5–6), 713–741.

Section II

Goal Setting in Clinical Practice

7

Goal Attainment Scaling in Adult Neurorehabilitation

Stephen Ashford and Lynne Turner-Stokes

CONTENTS

7.1 Introduction

As noted previously in this book, setting goals with patients and carers has become an integral activity in clinical rehabilitation (Playford, Siegert, Levack, & Freeman, 2009; Wade, 2009). In practice, the emphasis in rehabilitation is on making goals functional and meaningful to the patient. Nevertheless, the exact approach to set and monitor goals is much debated. One approach to goal setting that has gained prominence is that of goal attainment scaling (GAS). GAS has been proposed as a person-centred outcome measure that can be used to evaluate the gains from rehabilitation in the areas that matter most to patients and their families. The purpose of this chapter is to explore the application of GAS in the context of neurorehabilitation.

GAS is a technique for quantifying the achievement (or otherwise) of individualized goals. Outcome evaluation for clinical interventions through GAS was introduced by Kiresuk and Sherman in the 1960s as a means of assessing outcomes in mental health settings (Kiresuk & Sherman, 1968). Since then, it has been modified and applied in many areas of rehabilitation including the following:

- Elderly care settings (Stolee, Rockwood, Fox, & Streiner, 1992; Stolee, Zaza, Pedlar, & Myers, 1999)
- Chronic pain (Williams & Steig, 1987)
- Cognitive rehabilitation (Rockwood, Joyce, & Stolee, 1997)
- Amputee rehabilitation (Rushton & Miller, 2002)
- Neurological rehabilitation (Bovend'Eerdt, Botell, & Wade, 2009; Khan, Pallant, & Turner-Stokes, 2008; Turner-Stokes, 2009a)
- Spasticity management (Ashford & Turner-Stokes, 2006, 2008; Turner-Stokes et al., 2010)

Several different approaches to GAS have been described in the literature. In this chapter, we discuss some of these and present a simple practical approach in order to encourage uniformity in the application of GAS in routine clinical practice. In the first half of the chapter, we present the background to GAS as a person-centred outcome measurement tool. We address some of the benefits and challenges of using GAS in clinical practice and explore some potential solutions to the issues that have been raised. In the latter half of the chapter, we describe some practical applications of GAS using two clinical exemplars – first, as a holistic outcome measure for a rehabilitation programme and, second, as a targeted approach for the evaluation of a focal intervention. Finally, we discuss the application of GAS as an outcome measure for research.

7.2 Background to GAS

7.2.1 What Is GAS?

Most patients will have more than one goal for treatment. At the simplest level, goal achievement may be recorded simply by counting the proportion of goals achieved (Macpherson, Cornelius, Kilpatrick, & Blazey, 2002). However, this does not allow for the fact that some goals may be achieved more readily than others or that some may be more important to the patient or their family. GAS provides a systematic and structured approach to the evaluation of goal attainment, which takes account of this variation. Several different approaches to GAS are described in the literature, but most incorporate the following key steps:

1. *Rigorous goal setting*: The most important feature of GAS is the a priori establishment of agreed goals for rehabilitation at the outset of treatment. Goals should be clearly defined and agreed with the patient and their family or carers before intervention starts so that everyone has a realistic expectation of what is likely to be achieved and agrees that the identified goals would be worth striving for. Goals should follow the SMART principle – that is, they should be specific, measurable, attainable, relevant and timed. Bovend'Eerdt and colleagues (2009) have provided further practical advice on goal setting in the context of rehabilitation.

2. *Goal weighting*: Some goals will be more important to the patient than others; and some goals set may be more challenging to achieve (i.e. require higher levels of effort by the individual or rehabilitation team). Goals may therefore be weighted to take account of the relative importance of the goal to the individual and the difficulty that the rehabilitation team anticipates in achieving it (Rushton & Miller, 2002; Turner-Stokes, 2009a).

3. *Baseline evaluation*: The level of function in relation to each goal is identified at the start of treatment.

4. *Rating goal attainment*: At the agreed outcome evaluation point, the level of goal attainment is recorded, in accordance with pre-defined criteria as documented during goal setting.

5. *Assimilation*: Goals may be aggregated into a single composite GAS transformation score (T-score) reflecting the overall level of goal attainment, taking into account the respective achievement of multiple goals and their differential priority.

7.2.2 Kiresuk and Sherman's Original Method for Goal Rating

The literature includes a number of different rating systems for GAS goals, each with their own advantages and disadvantages. In the original method described by Kiresuk and Sherman (1968), each goal is rated on the following 5-point scale:

- If the patient *achieves* the expected level, this is scored at 0.
- If they achieve a *better* than expected outcome, this is scored at

  +1 (somewhat better)

  +2 (much better)

- If they achieve a *worse* than expected outcome, this is scored at

  −1 (somewhat worse)

  −2 (much worse)

The baseline level of function for each goal is normally set at the −1 level to allow for the possibility of a worse condition in relation to that goal, unless there is no clinically plausible worse condition, in which case the baseline rating is recorded at −2. To support reliability and to allow for the option of an independent assessor to rate goal attainment, Kiresuk and Sherman (1968) recommended the use of a follow-up guide. This involves the development of pre-defined criteria indicating achievement at each rating level. An example of a follow-up guide is presented in Table 7.1. In this example, John, a 65-year-old gentleman, experiences problems with hand function and mobility after a stroke. Table 7.1 shows his baseline scores and achievement scores on the follow-up guide.

   The GAS T-score is calculated by applying the formula as shown in Box 7.1. The T-score is designed to convert the composite goal score (the sum of the attainment levels times the relative weights for each goal) into a standardized overall rating with a mean of 50 and standard deviation of 10. If goals are set in an unbiased fashion so that results exceed and fall short of expectations in roughly equal proportions, a normal distribution of scores is expected if GAS scores are collected for a sufficiently large number of patients.

TABLE 7.1

Follow-Up Guide for Two Different Goal Areas

Goal Area	−2	−1	0	+1	+2
Using the upper limb Baseline score: −2 Achieved: 0	Unable to use hand at all **Baseline**	Requires help to get hand around cup, unable to hold cup upright	Uses hand to grasp and stabilize cup while pouring a drink **Achieved**	Uses hand to lift cup to mouth and drink	Uses hand normally
Walking Baseline score: −1 Achieved: −1	Unable to stand and step even with maximal assistance of two people	Stands with the assistance of one person and takes 1–2 steps **Baseline Achieved**	Walks short distances indoors with a walking aid and standby supervision only	Fully independently walking indoors, with or without a walking aid	Walks independently indoors and outdoors, with or without a walking aid

BOX 7.1   CALCULATION OF GAS T-SCORE

$$\text{T-score} = 50 + \frac{10 \sum (W_i X_i)}{\sqrt{(1-\rho) \sum W_i^2 + \rho \left(\sum W\right)_i^2}}$$

where
  i is the number of goal set for an individual patient
  X_i is the GAS score for each goal (between −2 and +2)
  W_i is the weighting assigned to each goal (if equal weighs, $W_i = 1$)
  ρ is the expected correlation of the goal scales
  Σ means the *sum of* (i.e. $\sum (W_i X_i)$ is the sum of the GAS scores for all goals times
     their individual weightings)

For practical purposes, according to Kiresuk and Sherman, ρ most commonly approximates to 0.3, so the equation simplifies to

$$\text{T-score} = 50 + \frac{10 \sum (W_i X_i)}{\sqrt{0.7 \sum W_i^2 + 0.3 \left(\sum W_i\right)^2}}$$

Note: The constant for the expected correlation of goal scales assumes that all scales are equally weighted.

Within the literature, there is some debate about whether to just use the end-point T-scores when reporting on outcomes, or whether there is value in also recording the T-score at baseline and thus reporting on a *change in T-score* from baseline as the outcome. However, because change is built into the way GAS is derived, the outcome T-score is by definition a measure of change and avoids the need for computation of change scores, which may be unreliable where baseline and outcome scores are highly correlated (Becker, Stuifbergen, Rogers, & Timmerman, 2000; Khan et al., 2008). Nevertheless, some authors advocate the recording of baseline scores (Gordon, Powell, & Rockwood, 1999; Rockwood et al., 1997; Rushton & Miller, 2002). Whichever option is chosen, it is important to state explicitly the method used to inform interpretation and comparison of scores.

7.2.3 Alternative Rating Methods

The 5-point rating method described earlier is the most widely used approach for GAS scoring in the literature (Ashford & Turner-Stokes, 2006; Rockwood et al., 1997; Rushton & Miller, 2002), although other authors have proposed alternative models in an attempt to improve the sensitivity of GAS (Cusick, McIntyre, Novak, Lannin, & Lowe, 2006).

On a clinical level however, the original 5-point model can seem somewhat counter-intuitive and this may partly explain its limited uptake by clinicians. Rating of achievement and overachievement is logical – goals may be achieved or overachieved, by a lot or a little. However, in clinical practice, patients often make considerable progress towards their goal (progress which is valued by them) even though they fell short of full achievement.

From the clinical perspective, if a goal is not achieved, it is pertinent to know whether it was *partially achieved*, if there was *no change* or if the patient got *worse*. However, if a given goal is rated at '–1' at baseline (to allow for the possibility of –2 scores for worsening conditions) and if partial achievement is also rated as –1, there is no scope for distinguishing between *partial improvement* and *no change*. Alternatively, if all goals are routinely rated as '–2' at baseline, it is not possible to record a worsening of condition with respect to that goal.

Steenbeek and colleagues (Steenbeek, Gorter, Ketelaar, Galama, & Lindeman, 2011; Steenbeek, Ketelaar, Galama, & Gorter, 2007; Steenbeek, Ketelaar, Lindeman, Galama, & Gorter, 2010; Steenbeek, Meester-Delver, Becher, & Lankhorst, 2005) proposed a 6-point rating scale to address this problem. In this model, all baseline scores start at '–2', with '–1' denoting partial goal achievement and '–3' denoting a worsening condition. A disadvantage of this approach, however, is that the range of –3 to +2 means that the symmetry of the original scale is lost, so that a normal distribution of T-scores can no longer be expected (Turner-Stokes & Williams, 2010).

Turner-Stokes and Williams (2010) performed a direct comparison of the Steenbeek GAS 6-point rating model with the original 5-point rating scale in the same large dataset, to examine the effect of this model on T-scores. Although the median achieved T-scores were broadly comparable for the two methods, change T-scores were significantly greater for the 6-point rating method due to the lower baseline GAS T-scores. This point underlines the importance of stating clearly whether achievement T-scores or change scores are being reported and more importantly which version of GAS is being used.

In the same article (Turner-Stokes & Williams, 2010), the authors tested an alternative 6-point model, in which baseline goal rating followed Kiresuk and Sherman's (1968) original principles, but where goals that were partially achieved from a baseline score of '–1' were rated as '–0.5' to identify that some change had occurred. This method produced a much closer fit for the standard rating system, for both *achieved* and *change* T-scores, and further offered the possibility of retrospective conversion back to the standard scoring method simply by changing all '–0.5' scores to '–1' in the dataset.

These various debates have tended to engender amongst clinicians a mistrust of numbers where goal attainment is concerned. Clinicians can be further put off by the zero and negative numbers which some fear will discourage patients when the results are discussed with them. To address this problem, in later iterations of GAS, we introduced a verbal method for goal rating, which keeps clinicians at a distance from numerical scores (Turner-Stokes, 2009a) (see Figure 7.1). Using this method, clinicians describe goal attainment using the verbal descriptors that align with their clinical reasoning and decision making. Provided that both baseline and outcome verbal ratings are recorded, all of the aforementioned numerical rating models may be applied to these verbal ratings for the purpose of calculating T-scores. In this way, the verbal rating scale provides a common language and the datasets generated can be compared with GAS data collected using any of the three models.

7.3 Strengths and Criticisms of GAS in Rehabilitation

GAS provides a person-centred approach to outcome evaluation that focuses on the patient's own priorities. It offers both advantages and disadvantages, both in terms of clinical practice and measurement.

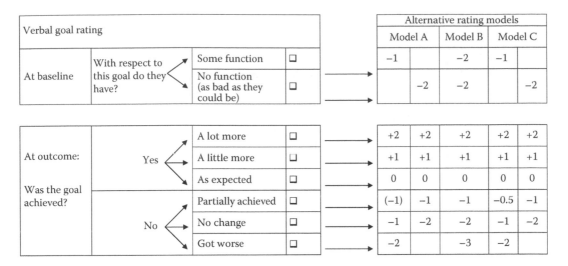

FIGURE 7.1
Verbal GAS rating scale. Model A: 5-point model as described by Kiresuk and Sherman (1968). Model B: 6-point rating model according to Steenbeek et al. (2007). Model C: 6-point rating model according to Turner-Stokes and Williams (2010).

7.3.1 Clinical Practice

At a clinical level, the major advantage of GAS is that it builds on the established practice of clinical goal setting. Providing systematic goal setting and monitoring is already embedded in the rehabilitation process. GAS provides an outcome measure that can be derived from this practice for very little extra time and effort. It also offers advantages in terms of engagement, coordination and communication:

- *Engagement*: Patients are more likely to engage positively in rehabilitation directed towards goals that are important to them (Wade, 2009), and it has been suggested that the GAS process may provide an additional therapeutic benefit by encouraging the patients to strive towards their goals (Williams & Steig, 1987).

- *Coordinated multidisciplinary teamwork*: The application of GAS supports communication and collaboration between multidisciplinary team members, providing a common language for discussing goal selection and goal attainment, encouraging the whole team to work in a coordinated fashion towards the agreed therapeutic objectives.

- *Information sharing and negotiation of realistic goals*: GAS provides a structure for the discussion of goals and expected levels of achievement with patients and their family (Hurn, Kneebone, & Cropley, 2006). Particularly in the early stages following injury, patients and their families sometimes have high expectations for recovery and resumption of their pre-injury life style, which are not always realistic. When asked to state their goals for treatment, they will usually express goals in terms of long-term aspirations. During goal setting, these are broken down by the team into medium-term objectives for the treatment programme and a series of staged goals towards those objectives (as shown in Figure 7.2). Setting SMART

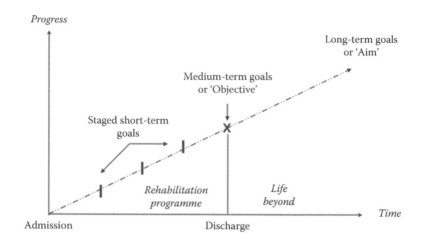

FIGURE 7.2
Short-, medium- and long-term goals.

goals via the GAS process may help establish a shared expectation of the level of achievement that is likely to be achieved for the medium-term objectives (e.g. by the end of the rehabilitation programme).

GAS, however, has some disadvantages. Common problems have been identified with the setting and subsequent evaluation of goals when using GAS in clinical practice (Kiresuk, Smith, & Cardillo, 1994). These include the following:

- Errors in the recording of goals
- Definition of goals being vague
- Multidimensional concepts within a single goal (scales that include two or more dimensions for the goal set, e.g. dressing and walking)

Rehabilitation teams need to have knowledge of the *pitfalls* and avoid these issues when setting goals. The potential impact of goals with these problems will occur when evaluating achievement and lead to ambiguity and inaccuracy in the assessment of outcome.

Many teams have also reported that applying GAS in the manner described by Kiresuk and Sherman (1968) is excessively time-consuming for routine clinical use. In particular, the time taken to draw up a full follow-up guide with robust descriptions for each level of attainment under every goal is rarely practical in a busy clinic setting.

Furthermore, as noted earlier, clinicians can be put off by numerical scores and the complicated-looking T-score formulae. Engagement of clinicians in GAS goal setting may be improved through the use of the verbal rating approach (described earlier) and computer programs to provide automated calculation of T-scores (Turner-Stokes, Williams, et al., 2012).

7.3.2 Clinical Measurement

Rehabilitation poses a number of challenges for outcome measurement. Global disability measures such as the Barthel Index (Wade & Collin, 1988) or the Functional Independence Measure (FIM) (Hamilton, Laughlin, Fiedler, & Granger, 1994) provide a valid and reliable assessment of basic physical function and are widely used as standardized outcome measures. However, they have recognized floor and ceiling effects in neurorehabilitation, where cognitive and psychosocial factors are often the main factors limiting outcome (Turner-Stokes, 1999). A variety of tools have been developed to extend the range to include psychosocial function (e.g. the Functional Assessment Measure [FIM+FAM]) (Turner-Stokes, Nyein, Turner-Stokes, & Gatehouse, 1999) or to address participation and community integration (Willer, Button, & Rempel, 1999). However, these are often more time-consuming to administer and still have significant ceiling effects (Hall et al., 1996). Standardized outcome measures can also be insensitive to small but important changes, affecting only one or two items, which can easily be subsumed (and therefore undervalued) when added to a large number of other unchanged items.

While standardized clinical measures usually comprise a battery of items or tasks, each with standardized levels, GAS takes a different approach to person-centred measurement. Tasks are individually identified to suit the patient, and the levels are individually set around their current and expected levels of performance. GAS therefore provides both qualitative information about the goals being set and quantitative information in the formal evaluation of their achievement or non-achievement. It is shown to be sensitive to changes not detected by traditional outcome measures (Ashford & Turner-Stokes, 2006, 2008; Rockwood et al., 1997; Turner-Stokes et al., 2010; Turner-Stokes, Williams, & Johnson, 2009). However, it is conceptually different. Rather than being a measure of outcome per se, it is a measure of the achievement of intention. It depends on two things: the patient's ability to achieve their goals and the clinician's ability to predict outcome. Therefore, it does not replace standardized measures but may form a useful addition to collect alongside such tools to examine the achievement of treatment intentions.

A key strength of GAS is in integrating a range of different goals into a unified evaluation of goal attainment. However, GAS has also been criticized for this very reason. In effect, when measurement is applied in rehabilitation, the expectation is that all items used for one measure should relate to a single overarching concept, often referred to as the *construct* being measured. Measurement tools, however, frequently include multiple concepts which may require that the instrument is divided into subscales. Opponents of GAS argue that the aggregation of qualitatively different goals into a single overall score is tantamount to combining apples with pears. However, GAS is not the only measure to break this rule. Other existing standardized measures also involve the pooling of scores from multiple constructs to produce total sum scores of outcome, for example, as occurs for the FIM and the Short Form-36 (SF-36) – the justification here being that these measures quantify some higher-order construct (e.g. disability or quality of life for the FIM and SF-36, respectively). Therefore, a counterargument to this criticism of GAS is that while it may combine *apples* with *pears*, these are both types of fruit (i.e. goals) and therefore may be linked by the higher-order construct of *achievement of intention*.

Critics have also highlighted the ordinal nature of the goal rating method used in GAS as undermining the validity of the calculation of the T-score, limiting the use of GAS as a standard yardstick for comparing individuals or groups (Tennant, 2007). Tennant suggested the possible development of item banks of GAS goals, using Rasch analysis, to ensure that these item banks conform to the assumptions of interval measures. This approach would produce a more standardized method of GAS and provide a better basis for comparing GAS scores between people. However, it would also undermine the bespoke nature of GAS to some extent, which others view as a core advantage of GAS. Ultimately, the extent to which these criticisms impede the use of GAS in outcome evaluation will depend on how it is applied and how the data are handled. For the reasons noted earlier, we recommend that GAS is used as an adjunct to standardized instruments rather than as an alternative.

While these criticisms have been acknowledged, the use of GAS is steadily increasing in clinical settings. Given increased use in clinical practice, the tasks ahead are now as follows:

- To make it as practical as possible to apply GAS in a time-efficient manner
- To ensure that it is applied in a consistent manner so that results are comparable across different settings

In the next section, we explore practical applications of GAS using specific examples.

7.4 Practical Applications of GAS

The procedure described in the following is based on an approach we developed in the context of upper limb spasticity (Ashford & Turner-Stokes, 2006; Turner-Stokes, 2009a). It represents an attempt to establish a more consistent method for GAS, which is practical to apply in clinical settings, and we call it the *GAS-light* method.

7.4.1 GAS-Light Method

The GAS-light method applies GAS broadly as described in Section 7.2, but with some key differences:

1. The *number of goals* is limited. GAS is not applied to every staged short-term goal but is limited to 3–4 key objectives for the rehabilitation programme.
2. *Careful definition of the goal description*: In a busy clinical setting, it is rarely practical to devote the time to pre-define all five levels for each goal. Instead, teams concentrate on pre-defining just the SMART goal description for the expected *level* 0 outcome.
3. *Wording of goals* can be time-consuming, and some goals are common. The development of goal menus is encouraged, to build up a library of pre-worded goal statements that may be adapted for the individual to avoid *starting from scratch* with each new admission.
4. Although *weighting* for *importance* has a consistent effect on overall GAS scores in the expected direction, weighting for *difficulty* can, in some circumstances, lead to a perverse bias. Overall, weighting does not make a big difference to the T-scores, and the weighted and unweighted scores are usually very closely correlated. So while it may be helpful to record the importance and difficulty of any given goals for the purpose of qualitative interpretation and team reflection on goal attainment, it is perfectly adequate to use unweighted scores in the T-score calculation or to rate for importance only. If goal weighting is used, we recommend the 3-point rating scores as shown in Table 7.2. If weighting is not used, a value of '1' is simply applied to weight in the formula.
5. *Goal rating*: At the end of the programme, the team and patient review together the progress for each goal with reference to the SMART goal description, in order to agree whether this level was achieved or not and to apply the verbal rating scale shown in Figure 7.1. Acceptable levels of agreement have been found between this approach and the use of a formal follow-up guide (Turner-Stokes & Williams, 2010).

TABLE 7.2

Weighting Scales for Importance and Difficulty

Importance	Difficulty
1 = a little (important)	1 = a little (difficult)
2 = moderately (important)	2 = moderately (difficult)
3 = very (important)	3 = very (difficult)

Readers should note that independent assessors are specifically not recommended in this approach. In this clinical context, GAS is used to enhance communication and understanding within the patient/team partnership (Turner-Stokes, Williams, et al., 2012). Patient involvement is integral to the process because learning to set, review and revise their own goals is viewed as a critical skill to enable patients to progress their own rehabilitation after they leave the programme. Provided that goals have been appropriately negotiated and SMART-ly recorded, goal review should normally be a positive experience for patients and their families that enables them to see clearly the gains that have been made towards their priority goals and thus hopefully enhance their satisfaction with the programme.

A further key element of the GAS-light approach is team reflection on results. As noted earlier, GAS depends on both the patient's ability to achieve the goals and the team's ability to predict possible gains. Some clinicians can find this threatening, but as treating professionals, it beholds us to have some idea of the expected outcome for a given intervention.

As explained earlier, if goals are set in an unbiased fashion, T-scores for any rehabilitation population should be normally distributed around a mean of 50, with a standard deviation of ±10. If a team is overcautious in goal setting, the mean score will be greater than 50. Similarly, if they are consistently overambitious, it will be under 50. It may be argued that setting more challenging goals may theoretically be associated with greater improvement (Locke & Latham, 2002) and therefore that mean scores of less than 50 are not necessarily a bad thing. However, underachievement of goals may also reflect a less than perfect understanding of the factors (including external factors) that mitigate against goal attainment, or a failure to negotiate realistic expectations for outcome (McCrory et al., 2009). Regular opportunities should be provided for the team to review their GAS results, both at the individual and population level, and to engage in discussion about the reasons for over- or underachievement of goals and so improve their experience and enhance the accuracy of future goal setting.

7.5 Use of GAS in a Rehabilitation Programme: A Clinical Case Exemplar

Jeffery was referred for rehabilitation following a high-speed road traffic accident resulting in a traumatic subarachnoid haemorrhage, cerebral contusions and diffuse brain injury. He was a university student taking a gap year from a degree in accountancy. On admission to an inpatient rehabilitation facility, he was in a minimally conscious state with an inconsistent yes/no response when given choices and was unable to follow simple one-stage commands. He presented with tetraparesis and multiple contractures in upper and lower limbs. He was also dependent on enteral feeding and was doubly incontinent.

Jeffery's initial goal setting was undertaken with his family because he was unable to participate due to limitations in his communication and level of arousal. Goals were therefore discussed between his family and the rehabilitation team. Goal areas were initially identified by the family as follows:

Initial goal areas identified for treatment were as follows:

1. To be able to communicate with his family
2. To be able to enjoy food and tastes
3. To have a shower

The GAS-light approach was used, with careful identification of goal areas and conversion of these into SMART goals by the team. Note that the GAS scoring model used was the 5-point rating scale devised by Kiresuk and Sherman (1968). A description of Jeffery's baseline, expected and achieved goal levels is shown in Table 7.3.

A summary of the goal weightings and baseline scores are shown in Table 7.4. Jeffrey's baseline scores for the three goals were −1, −2 and −1, respectively. All goals were rated as *very important* by the family. The level of difficulty for communication and being able to taste food were rated by the rehabilitation team as being *moderately difficult* (2) and *very difficult* (3), respectively.

Three months after initial admission to the inpatient service, Jeffery had made more progress than expected and had emerged from a minimally conscious state. He was able to feed himself and communicate fully verbally. He still needed the assistance of two people to wash and dress or transfer using a hoist. He was able to control an indoor powered wheelchair for mobility.

TABLE 7.3

Worked Example of Baseline, Expected and Achieved Goal Levels: Jeffrey's Initial Goals

Stated Goal	At Baseline	Expected Outcome (to Achieve Score 0)	Achieved Outcome
1. 'To be able to communicate with his family'	Unable to express himself non-verbally. No consistent means of communication	To express preference between choice of two drinks using communication aid by 3 months following admission	Able to express verbal (complex) information
	Baseline GAS *some function* (−1)	Predicted GAS *as expected* (0)	Achieved GAS *a lot more* (+2)
2. 'To be able to enjoy food and tastes'	Enteral feeding, nil by mouth	To taste for pleasure on a daily basis with no clinical signs of aspiration by 3 months following admission	Normal diet; meeting all needs orally
	Baseline GAS *no function* (−2)	Predicted GAS *as expected* (0)	Achieved GAS *a lot more* (+2)
3. 'To have a shower'	Bed bath required due to impaired sitting balance and limited ability to participate in bathing activity	To be able to shower on a standard commode chair with assistance of one carer by 3 months following admission	Able to shower on a standard commode chair with assistance of two carers
	Baseline GAS *some function* (−1)	Predicted GAS *as expected* (0)	Achieved GAS *partially achieved* (−1)

TABLE 7.4

Summary GAS Scores: Jeffrey's Initial Goals

Goal	Importance (I)	Difficulty (D)	Weight $(I \times D)$	Baseline Score	Achieved Score
Communication	3	2	6	−1	+2
Tastes of food	3	3	9	−2	+2
Have a shower	3	3	9	−1	−1

T-score calculation					
Sum weights	$\sum W_i = 6 + 9 + 9$	24			
Sum weights squared	$\sum (W_i^2) = 36 + 81 + 81$	198			
Factor	$0.7 \sum W_i^2 + 0.3 (\sum W_i)^2$ $= (0.7 \times 198) + (0.3 \times 576)$	311.4			
Square root of factor	$= \sqrt{311.4}$	17.6			
T-score	$= 50 + \dfrac{10 \sum (W_i X_i)}{\sqrt{0.7 \sum W_i^2 + 0.3 \left(\sum W_i\right)^2}}$			Baseline score 31.3	Achieved score 61.9

New goals were set for the next 3-month period of rehabilitation. Goals were discussed between Jeffery and the rehabilitation team. As with previous goal setting with his family, goal areas were initially identified by Jeffery, and from these, SMART goals were defined by the team.

The second round goal areas identified for treatment were as follows:

1. To increase the use of his left arm in functional tasks
2. To transfer from a wheelchair to a bed or car independently
3. To assess cognitive ability to be able to go back to university

A description of his baseline, expected and achieved goal levels is shown in Table 7.5. A summary of the goal weightings and baseline scores are shown in Table 7.6. His baseline scores for the three goals were all −1. All goals were rated as *very important* by Jeffery. Difficulty was rated as *moderately important* (2) for left arm use, while wheelchair transfers and assessment of cognitive ability for university were rated *very difficult* (3) by the rehabilitation team.

Jeffery's case is useful for illustrating some of the practical issues involved in the application of the GAS method. He was initially unable to participate directly in goal setting and this was therefore undertaken with his family. However, for the second round of goal setting, he was able to participate. While there is a difference between these two situations, they both address goals relevant to Jeffery's management and illustrate the different types of goal the GAS method may be applied for.

In Jeffery's case, GAS was used alongside the FIM and Northwick Park Dependency Scale to evaluate global disability and dependency (Turner-Stokes et al., 1998, 1999). Other specific instruments were used for more focal aspects of outcome evaluation within his rehabilitation programme. Of note is the fact that in the initial phase of goal setting, all goals were reflected in FIM items to some extent. However, in the second phase of goal setting, only two of the goals were reflected in FIM items, with *assessment of cognition/mental capacity regarding going back to University* not covered.

TABLE 7.5

Worked Example of Baseline, Expected and Achieved Goal Levels: Jeffrey's Second Set of Goals

Stated Goal	At Baseline	Expected Outcome (to Achieve Score 0)	Achieved Outcome
1. 'To increase use of left arm'	Assistance of two people required to facilitate trunk and left arm movement when undertaking bilateral tasks, e.g. hair gel	To use left hand to stabilize object, e.g. hair gel container, during bilateral tasks with assistance of right arm in 2 months	Achieved as predicted
	Baseline GAS *some function* (−1)	Predicted GAS *as expected* (0)	Achieved GAS *as expected* (0)
2. 'To transfer wheelchair to bed/car independently'	Assistance of two people required to transfer from wheelchair to plinth with sliding board	To transfer from wheelchair to bed or car using sliding board with assistance of 1 person in 2 months	Partly achieved. Requiring the assistance of two people for car transfers, but only one from wheelchair to bed
	Baseline GAS *some function* (−1)	Predicted GAS *as expected* (0)	Achieved GAS *partially achieved* (−1)
3. 'Assessment of cognition/ mental capacity re. going back to university'	Requiring supervision, guidance and prompting regarding prognosis and future abilities	To present (verbally or written) cognitive requirements for a university course via 15 min presentation in 2 months	Achieved as predicted
	Baseline GAS *some function* (−1)	Predicted GAS *as expected* (0)	Achieved GAS *as expected* (0)

TABLE 7.6

Summary GAS Scores: Jeffrey's Second Set of Goals

Goal	Importance (*I*)	Difficulty (*D*)	Weight (*I×D*)	Baseline Score	Achieved Score
Left arm function	3	2	6	−1	0
Wheelchair transfers	3	3	9	−1	−1
Capacity for university	3	3	9	−1	0
T-score calculation					
Sum weights	$\sum W_i = 6 + 9 + 9$		24		
Sum weights squared	$\sum (W_i^2) = 36 + 81 + 81$		198		
Factor	$0.7 \sum W_i^2 + 0.3 (\sum W_i)^2$ $= (0.7 \times 198) + (0.3 \times 576)$		311.4		
Square root of factor	$= \sqrt{311.4}$		17.6		
T-score	$= 50 + \dfrac{10 \sum (W_i X_i)}{\sqrt{0.7 \sum W_i^2 + 0.3 \left(\sum W_i\right)^2}}$			Baseline score 36.4	Achieved score 44.9

7.6 Use of GAS in Spasticity Management: A Focal Intervention Exemplar

The aforementioned example demonstrates the use of GAS in a holistic rehabilitation programme for an individual patient. However, GAS may also be applied in the evaluation of focal intervention, where global measures of function are shown to be insensitive (McCrory et al., 2009). An exemplar of this would be in the management of upper limb spasticity (Bakheit et al., 2001), where changes at the level of impairment are usually easy to measure (i.e. reduction of spasticity as measured by the Modified Ashworth Scale), but where functional gains are harder to demonstrate (Bhakta, Cozens, Chamberlain, & Bamford, 2000; Sheean, 2001). Once again, GAS can be used alongside standardized measures.

Some patients with relatively mild impairment after acquired brain injury have the potential to recover useful function such as the ability to use their hand to hold and manipulate objects (i.e. active function). Others with more severe injury will continue to have a non-functional upper limb and may require assistance from another person (or their own non-affected arm) to care for the affected limb (i.e. passive function).

Published guidelines on the use of botulinum neurotoxin (BoNT) in spasticity management for adults (Royal College of Physicians, British Society of Rehabilitation Medicine, Chartered Society of Physiotherapy, & Association of Chartered Physiotherapist Interested in Neurology, 2009) emphasize the need for multidisciplinary assessment with clearly identified goals for intervention and outcome measures to review them. They propose a battery of suggested measures for the systematic assessment of focal outcomes in addition to the use of GAS, including arm activity measures (Ashford, Slade, & Turner-Stokes, 2013a, 2013b). The proposed outcome measures assess function and disability, which can be classified according to the International Classification of Functioning, Disability and Health (World Health Organization, 2001) at either the level of *body system function* (e.g. spasticity or range of movement) or at the level of *activity* (including ease of care). However, while these standardized scales may provide an objective measure of change, they do not necessarily indicate whether the overall aim of intervention for any particular individual has been achieved or not. In addition, there is no accepted way of assimilating this multidimensional information into a single overall assessment, other than using an individualized approach such as the GAS method.

GAS has now been used in many large studies of BoNT as an intervention for spasticity and in different service settings (Borg et al., 2011; McCrory et al., 2009; Turner-Stokes, 2009b; Turner-Stokes et al., 2010; Turner-Stokes, Fheodoroff, Jacinto, Maisonobe, & Zakine, 2013). A secondary analysis of a multi-centre double-blind, placebo-controlled randomized clinical trial was conducted to examine GAS for the evaluation of treatment for upper limb post-stroke spasticity with BoNT (Turner-Stokes et al., 2010). The primary outcome for this trial was the Assessment of Quality of Life (Hawthorne, Richardson, & Osborne, 1999), which did not demonstrate a treatment effect. However, GAS T-scores were significantly higher in the active treatment group and correlated with global benefit (as rated by the researcher, patient and/or their carer) and with reduction in spasticity (as measured by the Modified Ashworth Scale).

A secondary evaluation of goals demonstrated a degree of overly optimistic goal setting for active function in this population of patients with chronic spasticity (mean duration: 6 years). Better goal attainment in the areas of passive function (i.e. caring for the affected limb), pain and mobility were also demonstrated. Other studies have corroborated these as key goal areas (Ashford & Turner-Stokes, 2006; Turner-Stokes, 2009b). In this situation, GAS not only has provided a useful outcome measure but has also offered important insights into the principal benefits of this type of treatment. One result of this work was the development of a targeted tool – the GAS-eous (Turner-Stokes, Ashford, De Graaff, & Baguley, 2012) – which has been designed to provide a more standardized approach to goal setting and GAS while still allowing for individual variation in goals, thereby maintaining this strength of the GAS process.

The key implications of the application of GAS to this area of research are as follows:

- GAS appears to be useful in demonstrating clinically important functional gains from treatment of spasticity with BoNT and physical interventions.

- GAS is feasible to apply meaningfully in clinical practice, and work has now been undertaken to establish the preliminary feasibility of GAS in a number of service settings.

- GAS appears more sensitive than *global* measures such as the Barthel Index or Assessment of Quality of Life in measuring change following focal intervention for patients with physical disability.

7.7 Research Application of GAS

The GAS-light approach was designed to make the GAS approach more practical to use in clinical practice. However, when GAS is applied as a primary outcome for research, a slightly different approach may be required to minimize the risk of bias. Careful description of unidimensional goals remains the corner stone of robust GAS application. The use of a follow-up guide to pre-define each outcome level may potentially improve reliability but, more importantly, facilitates evaluation by an independent observer not involved in treatment, which is required if blinding of outcome observers is essential to the study design.

Particularly for statistical analysis, the assumption of interval-level data inherent in the calculation of T-scores has been criticized because the procedure for follow-up guides (or GAS-light) is said to meet, at best, requirements for ordinal-level data for the actual goals (Seaberg & Gillespie, 1977). However, Kiresuk and Sherman stated that in their view, provided data are normally distributed, an assumption of interval-level measurement is justified and parametric analysis can be applied (Kiresuk et al., 1994). However, the application of parametric analysis is open to significant criticism, given that individual GAS *follow-up* guides are unlikely to produce truly interval data (and importantly this will not have been tested or demonstrated for unique GAS goals that have been developed for individual patients). We therefore advocate the use of non-parametric analysis with GAS, because individual goal scales when carefully constructed are likely to be ordinal in nature.

7.8 Summary

GAS depends on two things: the patient's ability to achieve their goals and the clinician's ability to predict outcome, which requires knowledge and experience. Some people may find this challenging, but we believe that if a clinician is providing an intervention, the ability to predict the outcome from that intervention is essential.

The GAS approach is conceptually different from standardized evaluation in that it focuses on the attainment of goals rather than on standardized items as are used in measurement instruments. We advocate the use of GAS alongside standardized instruments or measurement tools because GAS cannot replace such instruments in evaluating the direct benefit of interventions. However, GAS provides an additional indicator of the achievement of goals, which are relevant to the patient and reflective of the aims of intervention. It provides a useful reflection of outcomes that are of critical importance to the patient in the context of their own lives, which is something not provided by many measurement tools.

References

Ashford, S., Slade, M., & Turner-Stokes, L. (2013a). Conceptualisation and development of the Arm Activity measure (ArmA) for assessment of activity in the hemiparetic arm. *Disability and Rehabilitation*, 35(18), 1513–1518.

Ashford, S., Slade, M., & Turner-Stokes, L. (2013b). Initial psychometric evaluation of the Arm Activity Measure (ArmA): A measure of activity in the hemiparetic arm. *Clinical Rehabilitation*, 27(8), 728–740.

Ashford, S., & Turner-Stokes, L. (2006). Goal attainment for spasticity management using botulinum toxin. *Physiotherapy Research International*, 11(1), 24–34.

Ashford, S., & Turner-Stokes, L. (2008). Management of shoulder and proximal upper limb spasticity using botulinum toxin and concurrent therapy interventions: A preliminary analysis of goals and outcomes. *Disability and Rehabilitation*, 31, 220–226.

Bakheit, A. M., Pittock, S., Moore, A. P., Wurker, M., Otto, S., Erbguth, F., … Coxon, L. (2001). A randomised, double-blind, placebo-controlled study of the efficacy and safety of botulinum toxin type A in upper limb spasticity in patients with stroke. *European Journal of Neurology*, 8(6), 559–565.

Becker, H., Stuifbergen, A., Rogers, S., & Timmerman, G. (2000). Goal attainment scaling to measure individual change in intervention studies. *Nursing Research, 49*, 176–180.

Bhakta, B. B., Cozens, J. A., Chamberlain, M. A., & Bamford, J. M. (2000). Impact of botulinum toxin type A on disability and carer burden due to arm spasticity after stroke: A randomised double-blind placebo-controlled trial. *Journal of Neurology, Neurosurgery and Psychiatry*, 69(2), 217–221.

Borg, J., Ward, A., Wissel, J., Kulkarni, J., Sakel, J., Ertzgaard, P., … on behalf of the BEST Study Group. (2011). Rationale and design of a multicentre, double-blind, prospective, randomized, European and Canadian study: Evaluating patient outcomes and costs of managing adults with post-stroke focal spasticity. *Journal of Rehabilitation Medicine, 43*, 15–22.

Bovend'Eerdt, T. J. H., Botell, R. E., & Wade, D. T. (2009). Writing SMART rehabilitation goals and achieving goal attainment scaling: A practical guide. *Clinical Rehabilitation, 23*, 352–361.

Cusick, A., McIntyre, S., Novak, I., Lannin, N., & Lowe, K. (2006). A comparison of goal attainment scaling and the Canadian Occupational Performance Measure for paediatric rehabilitation research. *Pediatric Rehabilitation, 9*, 149–157.

Gordon, J. E., Powell, C., & Rockwood, K. (1999). Goal attainment scaling as a measure of clinically important change in nursing-home patients. *Age & Ageing*, 28(3), 275–281.

Hall, K. M., Mann, N., High, W. M. J., Wright, J., Kreutzer, J. S., & Wood, D. (1996). Functional measures after traumatic brain injury: Ceiling effects of FIM, FIM+FAM, DRS, and CIQ. *Journal of Head Trauma Rehabilitation, 11*, 27–39.

Hamilton, B. B., Laughlin, J. A., Fiedler, R. C., & Granger, C. V. (1994). Interrater reliability of the 7-level Functional Independence Measure (FIM). *Scandinavian Journal of Rehabilitation Medicine*, 26(3), 115–119.

Hawthorne, G., Richardson, J., & Osborne, R. (1999). The Assessment of Quality of Life (AQoL) instrument: A psychometric measure of health related quality of life. *Quality of Life Research, 8,* 209–224.

Hurn, J., Kneebone, I., & Cropley, M. (2006). Goal setting as an outcome measure: A systematic review. *Clinical Rehabilitation, 20*(9), 756–772.

Khan, F., Pallant, J. F., & Turner-Stokes, L. (2008). Use of Goal Attainment Scaling (GAS) in rehabilitation for persons with Multiple Sclerosis. *Archives of Physical Medicine and Rehabilitation, 89*(4), 652–659.

Kiresuk, T., & Sherman, R. (1968). Goal attainment scaling: A general method of evaluating comprehensive mental health programmes. *Community Mental Health Journal, 4,* 443–453.

Kiresuk, T., Smith, A., & Cardillo, J. (1994). *Goal attainment scaling: Application, theory and measurement.* New York: Lawrence Erlbaum Associates.

Locke, E. A., & Latham, G. P. (2002). Building a practically useful theory of goal setting and task motivation: A 35-year odyssey. *American Psychologist, 57*(9), 705–717.

Macpherson, R., Cornelius, F., Kilpatrick, D., & Blazey, K. (2002). Outcome of clinical risk management in the Glouster rehabilitation service. *Psychiatric Bulletin, 26,* 449–452.

McCrory, P., Turner-Stokes, L., Baguley, I., De Graaff, S., Katrak, P., Sandanam, J., ... Hughes, A. (2009). Botulinum toxin A for treatment of upper limb spasticity following stroke: A multi-centre randomized placebo-controlled study of the effects on quality of life and other person-centered outcomes. *Journal of Rehabilitation Medicine, 41,* 536–544.

Playford, E. D., Siegert, R., Levack, W., & Freeman, J. (2009). Areas of consensus and controversy about goal setting in rehabilitation: A conference report. *Clinical Rehabilitation, 23*(4), 334–344.

Rockwood, K., Joyce, B., & Stolee, P. (1997). Use of goal attainment scaling in measuring clinically important change in cognitive rehabilitation patients. *Journal of Clinical Epidemiology, 50*(5), 581–588.

Royal College of Physicians, British Society of Rehabilitation Medicine, Chartered Society of Physiotherapy, & Association of Chartered Physiotherapist Interested in Neurology. (2009). *Spasticity in adults: Management using botulinum toxin – National Guidelines.* London, U.K.: Royal College of Physicians, Clinical Effectiveness and Evaluation Unit.

Rushton, P. W., & Miller, W. C. (2002). Goal attainment scaling in the rehabilitation of patients with lower-extremity amputations: A pilot study. *Archives of Physical Medicine & Rehabilitation, 83*(6), 771–775.

Seaberg, J. R., & Gillespie, D. F. (1977). Goal attainment scaling: A critique. *Social Work Research and Abstracts, 13,* 4–11.

Sheean, G. L. (2001). Botulinum treatment of spasticity: Why is it difficult to show a functional benefit? *Trauma and Rehabilitation, 14*(6), 771–776.

Steenbeek, D., Gorter, J. W., Ketelaar, M., Galama, K., & Lindeman, E. (2011). Responsiveness of goal attainment scaling in comparison to two standardized measures in outcome evaluation of children with cerebral palsy. *Clinical Rehabilitation, 25*(12), 1128–1139.

Steenbeek, D., Ketelaar, M., Galama, K., & Gorter, J. W. (2007). Goal attainment scaling in paediatric rehabilitation: A critical review of the literature. *Developmental Medicine & Child Neurology, 49*(7), 550–556.

Steenbeek, D., Ketelaar, M., Lindeman, E., Galama, K., & Gorter, J. W. (2010). Interrater reliability of goal attainment scaling in rehabilitation of children with cerebral palsy. *Archives of Physical Medicine and Rehabilitation, 91*(3), 429–435.

Steenbeek, D., Meester-Delver, A., Becher, J. G., & Lankhorst, G. J. (2005). The effect of botulinum toxin type A treatment of the lower extremity on the level of functional abilities in children with cerebral palsy: Evaluation with goal attainment scaling. *Clinical Rehabilitation, 19*(3), 274–282.

Stolee, P., Rockwood, K., Fox, R. A., & Streiner, D. L. (1992). The use of goal attainment scaling in a geriatric care setting. *Journal of the American Geriatrics Society, 40*(6), 574–578.

Stolee, P., Zaza, C., Pedlar, A., & Myers, A. M. (1999). Clinical experience with Goal Attainment Scaling in geriatric care. *Journal of Aging & Health, 11*(1), 96–124.

Tennant, A. (2007). Goal attainment scaling: Current methodological challenges. *Disability and Rehabilitation, 29,* 1583–1588.

Turner-Stokes, L. (1999). Outcome measurement in brain injury rehabilitation – Towards a common language. *Clinical Rehabilitation, 13,* 273–275.

Turner-Stokes, L. (2009a). Goal attainment scaling (GAS) a practical guide. *Clinical Rehabilitation, 23*(4), 362–370.

Turner-Stokes, L. (2009b). *Upper limb intervention for spasticity (ULIS) – Botulinum toxin – A cohort survey* (pp. 1–34). London, U.K.: King's College London.

Turner-Stokes, L., Ashford, S., De Graaff, S., & Baguley, I. (2012). The GAS-eous tool – A framework for evaluation of outcome in upper limb spasticity. *Neurorehabilitation and Neural Repair, 26*(6), 695–804 (poster 649).

Turner-Stokes, L., Baguley, I., De Graaff, S., Katrak, P., Davies, L., McCrory, P., ... Hughes, A. (2010). Goal attainment scaling in the evaluation of treatment of upper limb spasticity with botulinum toxin: A secondary analysis from a double-blind placebo-controlled randomised clinical trial. *Journal of Rehabilitation Medicine, 42,* 81–89.

Turner-Stokes, L., Fheodoroff, K., Jacinto, J., Maisonobe, P., & Zakine, B. (2013). Upper limb international spasticity study: Rationale and protocol for a large, international, multicentre prospective cohort study investigating management and goal attainment following treatment with botulinum toxin A in real-life clinical practice. *British Medical Journal Open, 18*(3), pii: e002230. doi: 002210.001136/bmjopen-002012-002230.

Turner-Stokes, L., Nyein, K., Turner-Stokes, T., & Gatehouse, C. (1999). The UK FIM+FAM: Development and evaluation. Functional Assessment Measure. *Clinical Rehabilitation, 13*(4), 277–287.

Turner-Stokes, L., Tonge, P., Nyein, K., Hunter, M., Nielson, S., & Robinson, I. (1998). The Northwick Park Dependency Score (NPDS): A measure of nursing dependency in rehabilitation. *Clinical Rehabilitation, 12*(4), 304–318.

Turner-Stokes, L., & Williams, H. (2010). Goal attainment scaling: A direct comparison of alternative rating methods. *Clinical Rehabilitation, 24,* 66–73.

Turner-Stokes, L., Williams, H., & Johnson, J. (2009). Goal attainment scaling does it provide added value as a person-centred measure for evaluation of outcome in neurorehabilitation following acquired brain injury? *Journal of Rehabilitation Medicine, 41,* 528–535.

Turner-Stokes, L., Williams, H., Sephton, K., Rose, H., Harris, S., & Thu, A. (2012). Engaging the hearts and minds of clinicians in outcome measurement – The UK Rehabilitation Outcomes Collaborative approach. *Disability and Rehabilitation, 34,* 1871–1879.

Wade, D. T. (2009). Goal setting in rehabilitation: An overview of what, why and how. *Clinical Rehabilitation, 23,* 291–295.

Wade, D. T., & Collin, C. (1988). The Barthel ADL index: A standard measure of physical disability? *International Disability Studies, 10,* 64–67.

Willer, B., Button, J., & Rempel, R. (1999). Residential and home-based postacute rehabilitation of individuals with traumatic brain injury: A case control study. *Archives of Physical Medicine and Rehabilitation, 80,* 399–406.

Williams, R. C., & Steig, R. L. (1987). Validity and therapeutic efficiency of individual goal attainment procedures in a chronic pain treatment centre. *Clinical Journal of Pain, 2,* 219–228.

World Health Organization. (2001). *International Classification of Functioning, Disability and Heath.* Geneva, Switzerland: WHO.

8

Goal Attainment Scaling in Paediatric Rehabilitation

Duco Steenbeek, Jan Willem Gorter, Marjolijn Ketelaar,
Krys Galama and Eline Lindeman

CONTENTS

8.1 Introduction

Goal attainment scaling (GAS) is an individualized, evaluative outcome measurement tool that rates the extent to which goals are attained. It can be used to evaluate change in a child's and/or family's functioning in paediatric rehabilitation. GAS was first introduced in the United States in mental health care in 1968 (Kiresuk & Sherman, 1968), followed by its introduction in physical rehabilitation in 1983 (Clark & Caudrey, 1983) and in paediatric rehabilitation in 1992 (Palisano, Haley, & Brown, 1992). Since the twenty-first century, there has been renewed interest in its application in the field of paediatric rehabilitation as the demand for tools responsive to clinically important change increases. Outcome measurement using GAS can be applied for all common diagnoses in paediatric rehabilitation. GAS offers the attractive possibility to measure what one intends to measure, because the content of the scales is tailored to the individual circumstances of a child and the family. GAS can be a valuable adjunct when used alongside standardized instruments, and using only standardized measures might preclude the identification of many individual rehabilitation goals attained (Steenbeek, Gorter, Ketelaar, Galama, & Lindeman, 2011). Moreover, measurement of individual goal attainment provides information about the clinical relevance of the outcome in addition to a change score as measured by standardized measures.

Notwithstanding these positive attributes, the application of GAS in paediatric rehabilitation requires considerable effort and expertise to apply the method properly, as the measurement is highly dependent on the quality of goal setting itself. Although goal-oriented rehabilitation has become common practice, constructing proper goals remains challenging for rehabilitation professionals. Another challenge in the use of GAS is preventing so-called therapist bias, that is, the lower the goals set, the greater the improvement observed.

The purpose of this chapter is to summarize the existing knowledge of the application and measurement properties of GAS when used in interdisciplinary rehabilitation practice for children. We will discuss an adaptation of the original scoring method of Kiresuk and Sherman (1968) and provide some practical examples of GAS used with children. Moreover, we will explain the positive attributes of GAS and highlight some of the challenges faced and lessons learned by our team, and finally, we will try to provide some recommendations for implementation in practice.

8.2 Need for Goals in Paediatric Rehabilitation

Several studies in paediatric rehabilitation have shown the benefits of goal-directed therapy (Ekström Ahl, Johansson, Granat, & Carlberg, 2005; Löwing, Bexelius, & Brogren Carlberg, 2009). Setting goals appears to result in an increase in motivation and better communication of mutual expectations between therapists and children/families. The process of goal setting in paediatric rehabilitation may be more complex than in rehabilitation for adults, as children's goals need to be set against the background of their physical and emotional development, their family and school performance. All children are in a constant state of *becoming* (Rosenbaum & Gorter, 2012). In paediatric rehabilitation, goals are often set to address the child and family's present realities. Through shared goal setting, children and parents can be encouraged in a positive way to think about their expectations, dreams and future perspectives (Rosenbaum & Gorter, 2012). Satisfaction in life may be related to real-istic expectations. Although goals are often set in relatively small steps, the impact, costs and usual length in therapy periods are such that achievement of the goals should have a large impact on the children.

8.3 Relevant Goals

Rehabilitation goals should be meaningful and relevant to both children and their fami-lies. In order to use goals that truly represent a child's life interests, clinical goals should correspond to the areas of the International Classification of Functioning (ICF) at the activity and participation level (Rosenbaum & Stewart, 2004) and be based on the fam-ily's unique needs and request for help. Goals should be described and documented as explicitly as possible, and in this regard, the *SMART* acronym is frequently referred to, suggesting that goals should be specific, measurable, acceptable, realistic and time-spe-cific. When measuring outcomes with goals, it is important to consider the construct of functioning for which goals are set. Capacity, capability and performance, for example, are three related but distinct constructs within the ICF domains of activities and par-ticipation (Holsbeeke, Ketelaar, Schoemaker, & Gorter, 2009). A person's capacity can be defined as what he or she can do in a standardized, controlled environment, a person's capability as what he or she can do in his or her daily environment and a person's perfor-mance as what a person actually *does* in his or her daily environment. With this in mind, promoting activity and evaluating performance should be our primary emphasis in pae-diatric rehabilitation. A child's performance may be influenced by environmental and personal factors that need to be taken into consideration when setting and evaluating goals. Clarifying the construct chosen for GAS scales will improve the reproducibility of the measure.

8.4 How Does Interdisciplinary Goal Setting Work?

Treatment in a paediatric rehabilitation setting is typically characterized by involvement of many professionals who work together in a multidisciplinary or interdisciplinary man-ner. In this section, we will discuss our experiences with an interdisciplinary approach, including the process of team communication around goal setting and GAS.

8.4.1 Interdisciplinary Approach

Collaboration in setting SMART goals is easier said than done, as defining SMART goals that both the children and their parents and therapists agree with requires a lot of skill and practice. In paediatric rehabilitation, professionals are faced with children who all have a diversity of problems, ranging from physical impairments in body function to activity and participation restrictions. In order to address these problems, professionals from various disciplines work together in teams. One of the conditions for proper rehabilitation team goal setting is the so-called *interdisciplinary* approach (Melvin, 1980). In an interdisciplinary team approach, all team members work together, with the child and his or her parents, towards shared goals. Individual treatment is attuned to achieving these shared goals.

Several prerequisites for achieving the interdisciplinary approach are mentioned in the literature (Melvin, 1980). Classically, three prior steps in the development of the interdisciplinary approach are distinguished, including the process-oriented, result-oriented and problem-oriented approach. The *process-oriented* and *result-oriented* approaches accentuate the *multidisciplinary* working style in contrast with interdisciplinary team work. Process-oriented rehabilitation is characterized by professionals from different disciplines selecting their own treatment methods and informing other team members and the parents during team conferences. In the result-oriented approach, the professionals set their own goals for defined periods of time and inform other team members and the parents. In the problem-oriented approach, team collaboration is stronger. The team members set goals, together with the children and their parents, and inform the other therapists. What distinguishes the interdisciplinary team approach is the interaction between team members regarding their findings, objectives and recommendations, in order to formulate the problems together, create shared rehabilitation goals in a common language and work as a team on the shared goals. This interaction takes place during team conferences. Parents should always be present at and be encouraged to prepare themselves for these meetings. Good communication during team conferences is crucial for an interdisciplinary team. The interdisciplinary rehabilitation approach is regarded as the preferred model for optimal team functioning.

8.4.2 Team Communication

During the last decade, the Rehabilitation Activities Profile (RAP) has been introduced in paediatric rehabilitation in the Netherlands (Roelofsen, Lankhorst, & Bouter, 2001) to facilitate team communication and achieve an interdisciplinary team approach. The children's RAP is an instrument consisting of three team report sections: (1) basic information about the child and their proxies including personal details, family situation, educational situation, adaptations/adapted living, accommodation and aids; (2) present situation of the child and their proxies, describing their needs as well as the impairments and abilities in terms of the ICF (movement abilities, learning abilities, communication, personal care, social–emotional functioning and environmental circumstances are described; the proxies are described in terms of family, adults and peers); (3) conclusions of the team conference, consisting of a primary problem, a primary goal and discipline-specific treatment goals regarding the child and proxies.

The primary problem is formulated in terms of factors that hinder or facilitate the child's progress. The factors that hinder usually lead to discipline goals which serve the principal team goal. During the conferences, it is very important to fully agree with parents and children about the extent to which the rehab team will be able to influence these factors. Differences of opinion are negotiated during the meeting and, if relevant in extra sessions, guided by the team's social worker. Agreement is considered to be a condition for goal-directed rehabilitation. If the discussion is transparent and the parents' difficulty with acceptance is respected, disagreement is rare. The implementation of the children's RAP has improved the interdisciplinary team approach (Roelofsen et al., 2001). The method encourages team members and parents to collaborate closely and continuously discuss their findings, objectives and recommendations. This collaboration is needed to achieve shared formulation of the problems and shared, client-tailored SMART-formulated rehabilitation goals.

8.5 From Goal to GAS

There is an increasing demand to evaluate clinical outcomes in rehabilitation. However, a substantial number of relevant goals are not covered by commonly used standardized measures in paediatric rehabilitation (Engelen, Ketelaar, & Gorter, 2007; Steenbeek et al., 2011). Ideally, goals should be evaluated individually, and the children and families informed about the change in their functioning depending on the purpose. Goal attainment should also be evaluated at group or programme levels to help improve the quality of care for all children and families in a rehabilitation programme. GAS measures the extent of progress in different levels of goal attainment in order to introduce nuance in goal attainment. In its original form (Kiresuk & Sherman, 1968), GAS is a 5-point scale with '0' representing the expected level of functioning after a predefined period. If a patient achieves more than expected, a score of +1 or +2 is given, depending on the level of achievement. If the patient's progress is less than expected, a score of –1 or –2 is given. In most recent research with GAS, *equal to start* is scored as –2. Our group presented arguments in favour of using an additional score of –3 for deterioration (6-point scale), which has been included in a Dutch Consensus on GAS (2011). If –2 is defined as *much less than expected* and the possibility of rating deterioration depends on the score, Turner-Stokes introduced an alternative rating method to score deterioration (see Chapter 7). A GAS scale can potentially be constructed for any relevant SMART goal. A strong point of GAS is that the scale can be used for any diagnosis or condition. Several interdisciplinary GAS scales can be constructed for one patient and can represent both discipline-specific goals and primary team goals.

8.6 Method for Constructing GAS Scales in Paediatric Rehabilitation

Optimally, GAS scales should be ordinal with hierarchical and meaningful intervals between the levels. In order to ensure the ordinality, only a single dimension of change should be reflected in a GAS scale. Choosing only one variable is often challenging, as therapists are used to working with a pallet of variables.

The steps for constructing GAS scales include identifying goal areas, the target variable in the goal area, the level to start at and the individual scale levels. Determining the variable can be relatively easy for some physical goals but can be very difficult for other goal areas. If a child wants to jump as far as possible, the variable will be the distance. If he or she wants to jump as high as possible, the variable will be the height. If fear of jumping is the main restricting factor, the variable will be the amount of fear. If he wants to jump as elegantly as possible, the quality of performance has to be rated. If the goal is complex and the determination of the key variable is difficult, task analysis may be helpful. Task analysis describes the steps of physical and/or cognitive processes which have to be successively executed to complete the whole task. For task analysis, the therapist divides the task into sub-skills. Analysing the sub-skills provides insight into why the child does not succeed in performing the activity and may be helpful in choosing the variable for the GAS scale. Examples of scales for children with cerebral palsy are shown in Tables 8.1 through 8.6.

TABLE 8.1

GAS Scale Rating Participation in Physical Functioning

Setting	A gymnasium with a standardized obstacle course including a climbing rack against the wall
Task	Walk the obstacle course as fast as possible
Scoring Method	Observation
−3	Worse than start (deterioration)	More than 2 min
−2	Equal to start	Between 2 and 1 min and 40 s
−1	Less than expected	Between 1 min 40 s and 1 min 20 s
0	Expected goal	Between 1 min 20 s and 1 min
1	Somewhat more than expected	Between 1 min and 50 s
2	Much more than expected	Less than 50 s

Note: Example of a GAS scale constructed by a paediatric physical therapist for a 5-year-old child with spastic unilateral cerebral palsy, Gross Motor Function Classification System (GMFCS) level 2. Level 2 represents walking with limitations, but without walking aids. The primary team goal was to fully participate in school gym lessons. Hindering factors were dissociation, muscle strength, endurance in running and climbing.

TABLE 8.2

GAS Scale Rating Participation in Hand Functioning

Setting	Power wheelchair plus computer with joystick control to control a children's computer program for drawing and typing. Maximal verbal help is given.
Task	Colour as many spaces as you can in the next 10 min.
Scoring Method	Observation.
−3	Worse than start (deterioration)	None.
−2	Equal to start	Colours 1–2 spaces.
−1	Less than expected	Colours 3–4 spaces.
0	Expected goal	Colours 5–10 spaces.
1	Somewhat more than expected	Colours 11–20 spaces.
2	Much more than expected	Colours more than 20.

Note: Example of a GAS scale constructed by a paediatric occupational therapist for a 9-year-old child with spastic bilateral cerebral palsy, GMFCS level 5. Level 5 represents being transported in a manual wheelchair without self-mobility. The primary team goal was to communicate with the help of computer devices. A hindering factor was manual handling of the joystick as an alternative for a mouse.

8.7 Measurement Properties of GAS in Paediatric Rehabilitation

Many authors have attested to the value of GAS as an outcome measure, confirming the assumption that GAS could be of special value in paediatric rehabilitation medicine, with its heterogeneity of therapy goals set by interdisciplinary teams working with children with various developmental disabilities (Steenbeek, Ketelaar, Galama, & Gorter, 2007). In particular, GAS has proved to be a sensitive tool to evaluate spasticity management in children (Desloovere et al., 2012; Hoving et al., 2009; Wallen et al., 2011; Ward, Hayden, Dexter, & Scheinberg, 2009). We will discuss the inter-rater reliability, content reliability, content validity and criterion- and construct validity of GAS.

TABLE 8.3

GAS Scale Rating Participation in Social Communication

Setting	Social communication with classmates during the day. Paying attention to clear simple sentences.	
Task	General stimulation of participation at school.	
Scoring method	The opinion of the class teacher is asked with regard to simple sentences in spontaneous speech with classmates.	
−3	Worse than start (deterioration)	Speaks so garbled that she cannot be understood.
−2	Equal to start	Simple sentences are so unclear that they aren't understood. (Single words are clear enough to be understood.)
−1	Less than expected	Sentences are clear enough to be understood with a picture.
0	Expected goal	Sentences are clear enough to be understood during structured play with classmates.
1	Somewhat more than expected	Sentences can be understood during a structured conversation.
2	Much more than expected	Simple sentences are always clear enough to be understood.

Note: Example of a GAS scale by a speech therapist for a 5-year-old girl with spastic unilateral cerebral palsy and serious dysarthria. The primary team goal was social communication with peers. Facilitating factors were her self-confidence and enthusiasm for speech. Articulation was the main hindering factor.

TABLE 8.4

GAS Scale Rating Family Functioning

Setting	Session with parents without child.	
Task	Ask the parents how the child is behaving.	
Scoring method	Professional's interpretation of the insight of the parents.	
−3	Worse than start (deterioration)	The parents ask too much of the child and are not motivated to discuss the problem.
−2	Equal to start	The parents are willing to discuss the problem of asking too much of the child.
−1	Less than expected	The parents discuss the behavioural disturbance that they see at home in relationship to the problem of asking too much of the child.
0	Expected goal	The parents are motivated to make a plan to address the problem of asking too much of the child.
1	Somewhat more than expected	The parents report the results of the plan and make adjustments for the following period.
2	Much more than expected	The parents ensure that the child is not asked too much and behavioural disturbance is reduced.

Note: Example of a GAS scale by a social worker for a 3-year-old boy with a young-onset juvenile rheumatoid arthritis. The boy is cognitively impaired and there is a serious behavioural disturbance. There were several primary team goals; however, enabling the parents to control the behaviour was a precondition for starting any rehabilitation programme.

8.7.1 Inter-Rater Reliability of GAS

The inter-rater reliability of GAS is considered to be good (Steenbeek, Ketelaar, Lindeman, Galama, & Gorter, 2010). We discovered that if the construct of measurement and the scoring procedure are determined and instructed properly in a team of professionals, the child's own therapists can score GAS scales reliably (linear-weighted Cohen's kappa, 0.82;

TABLE 8.5

GAS Scale Rating Emotional Functioning (1)

Setting	Adolescent therapy session
Task	P is asked about her mood in the last month in relation to her disability. VAS scale from 0% = very bad to 100% = very good
Scoring method	The child's opinion
−3　Worse than start (deterioration)	0%–15%
−2　Equal to start	16%–30%
−1　Less than expected	31%–45%
0　Expected goal	46%–60%
1　Somewhat more than expected	61%–75%
2　Much more than expected	86%–100%

Note: Example of a GAS scale by a paediatric psychologist for a 13-year-old girl with a progressive neuromuscular disease. The primary team goal was to further accept and cope with her disability. In this perspective, the progression of her disease is a hindering factor which cannot be influenced by the rehabilitation team.

TABLE 8.6

GAS Scale Rating Emotional Functioning (2)

Setting	Adolescent therapy session
Task	Participating in a regular soccer team
Scoring method	The parents' opinion regarding the child's self-esteem
−3　Worse than start (deterioration)	No intention anymore to participate in an introduction lesson
−2　Equal to start	Intention to participate but socially too anxious to register
−1　Less than expected	Participates in an introduction lesson, but does not dare to continue taking lessons
0　Expected goal	Continuous participation in regular training sessions but remains socially too anxious to participate in league matches
1　Somewhat more than expected	Plays league matches soccer, however with doubtful self-esteem
2　Much more than expected	Plays league matches soccer and reports success experiences

Note: Example of a GAS scale constructed during team conversation with parents. The scale represents the main team goal for an 8-year-old boy with developmental coordination disorder. The primary team goal was to reverse the process of decreasing self-esteem. A facilitating factor was his sensitivity to success experiences. He wanted to play soccer in a team.

95% confidence interval, 0.73–0.91). Because the scores from the child's own therapists were lower than those from independent therapists, we learned to trust the insight of professionals, as was suggested before by Palisano and colleagues (Palisano, 1993; Palisano et al., 1992). Our data were reassuring regarding the feared therapist bias.

8.7.2　Content Validity of GAS

Content validity addresses the question of whether the content of the GAS scales covers the most important aspects or elements of the attribute of interest being measured (Streiner & Norman, 2008). Inherent to the use of GAS is the crucial question of whether it measures outcome or only describes the therapist's prediction of future functioning. The content of GAS scales is based on professional insight (Steenbeek et al., 2010). Critics of GAS believe that the development of the content of scales is too subjective. GAS measures the quantitative distance to the professional's expectation of outcome. Many influences determine the content of the scales, including cultural issues, intensity and length of the therapy period, patient motivation and knowledge of prognosis. The process of constructing a GAS scale is such that differences around the world must be accepted at face value by the user. The content validity cannot easily be proved or disproved empirically.

8.7.3 Criterion and Construct Validity of GAS

As described earlier, GAS offers the attractive possibility to measure what one intends to measure as the content of the scales is tailored to the individual circumstances of a child. Therefore, GAS is potentially promising in regard to its validity. For the development of GAS as outcome measurement, it would be helpful to administer GAS and other instruments to the same sample if scales with the same or similar attributes were available. This approach is described by several terms, including *convergent* validation, *criterion* validation and *concurrent* validation (Streiner & Norman, 2008). *Criterion* validity would address the correlation of the conclusions drawn from GAS with some other measures evaluating activity and participation in children, ideally a *golden standard*. However, a golden standard for functioning of children in rehabilitation treatment does not yet exist. It has been suggested that there is low criterion validity when comparing GAS with standardized measures, supporting the value of combining the use of both measures (Steenbeek et al., 2011; Turner-Stokes, 2009).

When no other measure exists to compare the new measure with, how can data be acquired to show that GAS is indeed measuring what is intended? The solution may be found in a broad set of approaches called *construct* validity (Streiner & Norman, 2008). This begins by linking the attribute that must be measured to some other attribute by a hypothesis or construct. This hypothetical construct should then be tested by applying GAS to the appropriate samples. For example, the GAS outcome in a sample of children could be tested by comparing the data with opinions about general goal attainment of a panel of experts. If the expected relationship is found, the hypothesis and measure are sound, supporting construct validity. As yet, no research is available on the construct validity of GAS in paediatric rehabilitation.

8.7.4 Content Reliability of GAS

When relying on professional insight for GAS scale construction, the question of whether different professionals would develop similar scales arises. Critics of GAS have rightfully noted that the reliability data primarily address the accuracy of repeated GAS scores, but not the reliability of the process of constructing the scales (Steenbeek et al., 2010). It is important to realize that content reliability has not yet been explored, implicating the need for further research. Even if the content of scales was similarly constructed by different therapists in a reliability study, in practice, we still have to consider the confidence in the professionals' objectivity. Although research results were somewhat reassuring (Steenbeek et al., 2010), the phenomenon of therapist bias has to be considered and reconsidered in each new setting when using GAS. If the trial setting has no other interest than children's and family's well-being, the content of scales is considered to be reliable.

However, service providers may want to document effectiveness for reasons other than the family's well-being alone. For example, health insurance companies or government agencies could require proof of the effects of interventions before allowing them. Clinicians are increasingly inclined to introduce measurement in clinical practice in order to demonstrate individual treatment results on which they are judged. If this were the case, professionals may be tempted to set their goals at a less challenging level in order to show a better outcome. Although we certainly support the accountability of physicians for medical interventions, in our opinion and despite our reassuring findings on therapist bias, GAS is not suitable for monitoring achievements for external interests yet. This issue, however, effects rehabilitation treatment in general and is not specific to paediatric rehabilitation.

8.8 Positive Attributes of the Use of GAS

The primary strength of GAS is the ability to evaluate individual change over time. In summary, we have seen the following advantages of using GAS regarding the quality of care and study design.

8.8.1 Grading Goal Attainment

In rehabilitation practice, the process of setting specific, measurable, acceptable, relevant and time-related goals is often an intricate part of what clinicians do. In order to determine whether a patient improved after treatment, professionals often rely on approaches such as documenting the percentage of objectives attained, while patients are generally more interested in the extent to which a goal was attained. GAS classifies levels of goal attainment to better reflect the patients' experience and preferences (Schlosser, 2004).

In contrast with standardized measures, a property of GAS at group level as well as individual level is that the score by definition describes the relevance of the change. This contributes to parents' satisfaction when using GAS with their children. In our opinion, the use of GAS should always be based on the request for help and expectations regarding the outcome, which makes it impossible to apply the procedure without involving the parents. Systematically involving parents in decision making in paediatric rehabilitation is however still challenging. We found a remarkable difference of opinion between parents and therapists about the parents' participation in GAS procedures during an intensive GAS-implementation project in a rehabilitation centre in the Netherlands (Steenbeek, Ketelaar, Galama, & Gorter, 2008). Whereas parents reported to have scarcely participated, therapists reported that the parents were involved often and intensively.

8.8.2 Facilitating the Quality of Rehabilitation Care

Several authors hypothesized that the application of GAS in paediatric rehabilitation may have a positive impact on the rehabilitation process and goal attainment (Ekström Ahl et al., 2005; Steenbeek et al., 2008). Siebes et al. (2007) recommended the use of GAS to improve transparency and coordination with parents. Kiresuk, Smith, and Cardillo (1994) had already postulated that clearly specified goals can mobilize a team to pursue relevant and feasible outcomes more coherently. Turning needs into therapy goals and evaluation of individual goal attainment is still challenging in daily practice (Nijhuis, Reinders-Messelink, deBlécourt, Boonstra, et al., 2008; Nijhuis, Reinders-Messelink, deBlécourt, Ties, et al., 2008; Siebes et al., 2007). In our opinion, the use of GAS can facilitate optimizing the quality of rehabilitation care.

8.8.3 Adaptability to the Activity and Participation Level of the ICF-Child and Youth Version

GAS can be adapted to virtually any of the domains and levels specified by the ICF-Child and Youth Version (CY). The method is applicable to measure change in body functions, activities, participation, environmental factors and personal factors of children. Measuring change over time at the activities and participation level is an important advantage and highly relevant in contemporary interdisciplinary rehabilitation care for children (Rosenbaum & Stewart, 2004). A study by Nijhuis and colleagues reported that the content of needs, problems and rehabilitation goals of children with cerebral palsy can be accurately described using the ICF-CY (Nijhuis, Reinders-Messelink, deBlécourt, Ties, et al., 2008). According to McDougall and Wright (2009), the combined use of GAS and the ICF-CY presents many benefits in all spheres for the special challenges of the child and his family, as well as for institutional systems or communities. We have also shown that goals in the activity and participation domain can be properly classified using the ICF-CY, improving the reproducibility of outcome (Steenbeek et al., 2011).

8.8.4 Comparability of Goal Attainment across Goals and Individuals

GAS allows legitimate comparison of the attainment of different goals for one individual or between different individuals. Rehabilitation research typically struggles with the dilemma of the heterogeneity of the populations in general practice. Even if changes in a homogeneous population can be proven, many results are not transferable to practice as the team has to deal with various requests for help. GAS offers a generic opportunity to measure change in heterogeneous populations under a variety of conditions. The outcome between the disciplines of a team and between multidisciplinary teams can be compared using GAS (Steenbeek et al., 2010). Moreover, the evaluation of different programmes would be a promising focus for the future.

The same is true regarding the comparison of different goals attained per patient. Goals spread over several constructs will vary, necessitating many specific instruments per patient when using standardized measures. GAS in contrast permits generic measuring of a diversity of interests and allows comparability by using only one instrument. For example, in order to measure the ability of jumping, manipulating, school skills, sports participation, independence and self-confidence, we need at least three different standardized outcome measures (e.g. the Gross Motor Function Measure, the Melbourne Assessment of Unilateral Upper Limb Function and the Pediatric Evaluation of Disability Inventory). Constructing a GAS scale for each of these issues could be an acceptable alternative and improve the transparency of the data.

8.8.5 Measuring Progress

As explained earlier, defining a major therapy goal individually offers the unique opportunity to measure exactly what one intends to measure. In general, GAS enables the measurement of the outcome of any rehabilitation intervention, including medical, therapeutic, social or educational, or any combination of these. Furthermore, GAS may generally improve the responsiveness of outcome measurement when evaluating specific medical applications, for example, supplementary management of spasticity (Desloovere et al., 2012; Hoving et al., 2009; Steenbeek et al., 2007; Steenbeek, Meester-Delver, Becher, & Lankhorst, 2005; Wallen et al., 2011; Ward et al., 2009). How can one measure the effect of multilevel surgery followed by an intensive rehabilitation programme to prevent progression of serious flexion contractures, aiming to retain a child's ability to make transfers without help from wheelchair to toilet, wheelchair into a car, etc.? Attaining this therapy goal obviously justifies the intensive and expensive treatment, as it improves the child's ability to travel and function in different environments. If a patient lift is needed, it makes family transportation much more complex. In our opinion, an individualized outcome measurement would be the first choice in enabling the measurement of the treatment effects in this example.

The use of GAS can also be recommended to measure the effect of intrathecal baclofen treatment in children with severe spasticity. In her dissertation on intrathecal baclofen, Hoving recommended that outcome measures include highly individualized measures as therapy goals for intrathecal baclofen vary greatly (Hoving et al., 2009). Too often problems with measurement during previous trials on spasticity management were solved by measuring outcome at the impairment level, for example, spasticity or range of motion (Baird & Vargus-Adams, 2010), while spasticity treatment in particular should be evaluated at the ICF levels of activity and participation. GAS provides a solution for this measurement problem.

Further examples of the added value have been discussed in comparison with standardized measures. GAS, Pediatric Evaluation of Disability Inventory and Gross Motor Function Measure have been shown to be complementary in their ability to measure individual change over time in children with cerebral palsy. If only standardized instruments are used, many individual rehabilitation goals actually attained may be missed in the outcome evaluation (Steenbeek et al., 2011). This concurs with Turner-Stokes' findings in adults (Turner-Stokes, 2009).

8.9　Lessons Learned about GAS in Paediatric Rehabilitation

We discovered that GAS in paediatric rehabilitation practice has advantages and disadvantages. Our research contributes answers to some questions about the measurement properties of GAS and provides a basis for introduction in paediatric rehabilitation practice and future research. It also highlights issues on its use that should be followed critically and evaluated as part of an on-going learning process. Although GAS could be used by itself in practice evaluations, in research projects, combining GAS with standardized measures is generally recommended. When using GAS in trials and practice, we recommend that users consider the following matters on (1) validity, (2) reliability, (3) data analysis, (4) scoring deterioration, (5) missing side effects, (6) training and (7) changing the intervention by the introduction of GAS.

8.9.1　Criteria of GAS Scales

We determined criteria for GAS scales to improve the reproducibility of our studies. Although the criteria were useful for the participants (Steenbeek et al., 2008), some need to be discussed further. SMART goal setting may be a time-consuming component of constructing GAS scales, but this competence should be required whether or not GAS is introduced. We agreed that scales should be ordinal. Therefore, only a single dimension of change should be reflected in a GAS scale. This criterion required the most practice and feedback during a training period (Steenbeek et al., 2008), as we discovered that defining six realistic, distinct levels of outcome with only one variable, and no gaps or overlap between levels, was challenging.

8.9.2 Rater Selection

In our study (Steenbeek et al., 2010), scale construction by the child's own therapist as opposed to an independent rater had a positive influence on the inter-rater reliability of the scales. In concurrence with the issues described earlier (content validity and content reliability), the ability to generalize this finding is assumed to be dependent on interest in the outcome of a study. It is interesting that in previous studies, there has been an almost unanimous agreement among promoters and critics of GAS to only use independent raters to follow-up (Cytrynbaum, Ginath, Birdwell, & Brandt, 1979; Kiresuk et al., 1994). However, over time, this criterion has changed. Particularly in the field of paediatric rehabilitation, we recommend the involvement of the child's own therapist (and the child or its parents) when designing goals for therapy. We strongly believe that one of the positive attributes and added value of GAS is the result of the interaction between child and therapist. The child's therapist has more knowledge about the needs of the child and family than an independent therapist. Moreover, collaborative goal setting and construction of GAS scales by the parents, child and therapist promotes family-centred services. In research settings in contrast to practice evaluations, the additive involvement of independent assessors can be valuable to reduce bias and improve the study's credibility.

A broad introduction of GAS as an outcome measure in a rehabilitation centre will be complicated by the implications of training and how time-consuming it is to start using GAS. We have found that inexperienced therapists usually require 45 min per GAS procedure (Steenbeek et al., 2008), although in our opinion, most of the time needed is to set the SMART goal. It is probably more practical to train a few GAS experts to carry out GAS construction and scoring for patients treated by other therapists. However, we still recommend cooperating with the child's therapists during construction and scoring of GAS scales. This introduces a dilemma of investing in training more team members versus investing in the time required for additional collaborations between therapists for the purposes of goal setting.

8.9.3 Computation and Data Analysis

Originally, the attainment levels for each goal are combined in a single aggregated *T score* by applying the following formula:

$$T \text{ score} = 50 + \frac{10 \sum (W_i X_i)}{\sqrt{0.7 \sum W_i^2 + 0.3 \left(\sum W_i \right)^2}}$$

where
  W_i is the weight assigned to the *i*th goal
  X_i is the score of the *i*th goal

This accounts for variable numbers of goals, intercorrelation of goal areas and variable weighting of goals according to importance to transform goal attainment into a standardized measure (called the *T* score) for each patient, with a mean of 50 and standard deviation of 10.

However, although this formula is typical for GAS and still widely used, it has mathematical pitfalls. First, T scores may be calculated as having several decimal places, which may give a false impression of precision and a false sensitivity to change. A fundamental problem is that in this calculation, the data are treated as interval data, using mean scores for groups, whereas they represent at best an ordinal scale of value judgments. Because of the mathematical properties of ordinal scales (which provide information about the order of particular scores, but not the extent of differences in values between scores), they should not really be added, subtracted, multiplied or divided. However, this is precisely what the T score calculation does with GAS scores.

In order to examine the impact of treating GAS scores as interval data as opposed to ordinal data, Tennant (2007) conducted a mathematical test of the T score calculation. For this test, Tennant used Rasch analysis, which is the formal way of examining the extent to which items from one scale approaches the expected pattern of an interval scale. Using randomly produced GAS data, Tennant used Rasch analysis to compare GAS scores when they were treated like ordinal data to GAS scores when they were treated like interval data. Tennant found that for almost 15% of the simulated data, the difference between two approaches to GAS scores was greater than a minimal clinically important difference for GAS scores. In other words, the GAS calculation appeared to produce evidence of a change in 15% of the simulated patient data when none should have existed.

Second, according to the originators, if goal setting is unbiased so that results exceed or fall short of expectations in roughly equal proportions, one would expect a normal distribution of scores. However, most rehabilitation studies in which GAS was used were small and expected to result in non-normal distribution, not allowing the application of parametric statistics. In our opinion, in small studies, the formula deflects the positive attributes of GAS rather than contributing to the method. Only in studies with large numbers of participants, it may fulfil its claim of being a parametric expression of non-parametric information. A study of Turner-Stokes, Williams, and Johnson (2009) concerning neurorehabilitation of adults was unique in its size ($n = 164$) and presumably met the normal distribution expected of GAS outcomes, thus legitimizing the use of parametric statistics. As far as we know, none of the studies that used GAS in paediatric rehabilitation were large enough to show normal distribution of GAS scores and therefore to permit parametric statistics.

Finally, another reason for abandoning the formula is that caution must be exercised in the interpretation of results after weighting goals (although weighting is not required but optional in the formula). In our opinion, the weighting process itself is too subjective and threatens the reproducibility of GAS outcomes. Furthermore, weighting may in fact be unnecessary as suggested by Turner-Stokes et al. (2009) in whose study weighting had no influence on the results of the analysis.

As a result of these criticisms of the T score calculation, we have introduced analysis of raw GAS scores (treating these as ordinal data) instead of the T score in our clinical practice and research. Even representing small amounts and non-normal distribution, different GAS data sets can be compared by using non-parametric statistics (which are appropriate for ordinal data). It is important to realize that non-parametric statistics are different from parametric equivalents. The differences are particularly relevant when small changes in small populations occur.

8.9.4 Scoring Deterioration

Recently, a study by Turner-Stokes and Williams (2010) was published, comparing the method we introduced for scoring deterioration and an alternative 6-point GAS rating system. They were able to transform an existing data set based on the use of the original 5-point GAS scales from the large study on neurorehabilitation in order to attain two new data sets of 6-point scales. Version 1 set all baseline scores at '−2' and added '−3' to denote *worsening*, in reference to our work. Version 2 added a '−0.5' score to denote *partial achievement* for goals starting at '−1'. While the median of the achieved *T* scores was 50.0 for all three methods, version 1 underestimated and version 2 marginally overestimated goal attainment, in comparison to standard goal rating. They recommended the use of their '−0.5' version as it provided the closest match to the standard rating. If the formula is not used, this discussion has no relevance as only the ranking of numbers matters. This study demonstrates that this is an interesting time for GAS and that sharing our findings with the world helps in the development of GAS.

8.9.5 Missing Side Effects

In general practice, GAS scales focus on the most important goals in order to represent outcome. Users should recognize that a GAS scale may be scored as +2 even if the patient regrets the treatment as a result of unexpected side effects. When side effects are expected, as in spasticity management for example (Hoving et al., 2009), one should consider combining GAS with relevant standardized measures, or questionnaires targeting the potential side effects. Professional expertise and patients' opinions might be more important in weighing individual therapy effects than any outcome measure. The opposite may happen as well. GAS may be scored as −2 even if the patient is very happy because of attaining other goals rather than the goal used for the GAS scale.

8.9.6 Training

Although test developers may demonstrate that a measure is reliable and valid in the context of a study, it does not necessarily mean that the measurement properties will be the same for all users under any condition. Regardless of who does the construction and follow-up, the degree to which the raters are trained influences the reliability and validity of GAS. As for each (new) instrument, critical questions include how much training and practice is necessary to ensure the user's competence in the administration and scoring of the measure. The question is how much training is needed and how do we know when someone is a reliable user? Although many training methods for GAS have been discussed, these questions have not yet been answered in the rehabilitation literature.

8.9.7 Changing the Intervention by Introducing an Outcome Measure

Finally, although facilitation of the quality of rehabilitation care (team spirit, transparency to patients, etc.) is considered to be a positive attribute of GAS, for research purposes, changing the quality of an intervention by the introduction of an outcome measure could also introduce a bias in outcome. For research purposes, we recommend designing controlled trials using GAS in both the intervention group and the control group, enabling a similar change in both groups. For projects evaluating interventions in rehabilitation practice, we recommend comparing different rehabilitation programmes. If measurement with GAS is introduced in both programmes, the influence on the outcome of the introduction of GAS might be considered to be equal.

8.10 Implications for Practice

Health professionals can be motivated to use GAS in rehabilitation by emphasizing the opportunity to measure group effects in heterogeneous populations and the satisfaction from working on GAS scales with patients, families and other team members. GAS is ready for introduction in various rehabilitation teams and diagnostic groups to evaluate change and compare aspects of interventions. This chapter can be used to discuss many important issues on uniformity and to stimulate further curiosity about this topic, but we are not presenting our method of GAS as the only valid approach.

Recently, a Dutch manual was published and is freely available on the Internet (www.revant.nl), and an English translation will follow soon. Hopefully an international consensus on scale construction, criteria and time needed for GAS scale construction in rehabilitation programmes will be feasible in the future. We recommend the development of an implementation programme, knowledge brokering (Russell et al., 2010), for example, to ensure that the GAS method is embedded in paediatric rehabilitation services. In our opinion, with the current knowledge, further training procedures can be promoted in paediatric rehabilitation practice. We also recommend a broad exchange of any new information on the content, intensity and amount of training necessary. Special attention should be given to the participation of parents and, if possible children and youths themselves, in the development of scales for children. Parents' and children's satisfaction should motivate their involvement and their enthusiasm should be used to improve participation. Families and children with disabilities know best what their needs are. Their involvement in goal setting and individual outcome evaluation is crucial in paediatric rehabilitation.

Future research in rehabilitation practice should include the examination of the content reliability of GAS scales and exploring the combined use of GAS with other individual outcome measures, for example, the possible benefit of combining GAS and the Canadian Occupational Performance Measure (Cusick, McIntrye, Novak, Lannin, & Lowe, 2006; Doig, Fleming, Kuipers, & Cornwell, 2010; Ostensjø, Oien, & Fallang, 2008; Wallen et al., 2011). When used in practice, the Canadian Occupational Performance Measure might help to clarify the request for help and be used as the basis for constructing GAS scales.

GAS is a useful and reliable outcome measure for children and their families in paediatric rehabilitation provided the necessary conditions are met. We hope that this chapter on GAS in paediatric rehabilitation arouses curiosity and leads to professionals introducing it in their own practice in order to improve the quality of care.

References

Baird, M. W., & Vargus-Adams, J. (2010). Outcome measures used in studies of botulinum toxin in childhood cerebral palsy: A systematic review. *Journal of Child Neurology*, 25(6), 721–727.

Clark, M. S., & Caudrey, D. J. (1983). Evaluation of rehabilitation services: The use of goal attainment scaling. *Disability and Rehabilitation*, 5(1), 41–45.

Cusick, A., McIntrye, S., Novak, I., Lannin, N., & Lowe, K. (2006). A comparison of goal attainment scaling and the Canadian occupational performance measure for paediatric rehabilitation research. *Pediatric Rehabilitation*, 9(2), 149–157.

Cytrynbaum, S., Ginath, Y., Birdwell, J., & Brandt, L. (1979). Goal Attainment Scaling: A critical review. *Evaluation Quarterly, 3*(1), 5–40.

Desloovere, K., Schörkhuber, V., Fagard, K., Van Campenhout, A., De Cat, J., Pauwels, P., ... Molenaers, G. (2012). Botulinum toxin type A treatment in children with cerebral palsy: Evaluation of treatment success or failure by means of goal attainment scaling. *European Journal of Paediatric Neurology, 16*(3), 229–236.

Doig, E., Fleming, J., Kuipers, P., & Cornwell, P. L. (2010). Clinical utility of the combined use of the Canadian Occupational Performance Measure and Goal Attainment Scaling. *The American Journal of Occupational Therapy, 64*(6), 904–914.

Ekström Ahl, L., Johansson, E., Granat, T., & Carlberg, E. B. (2005). Functional therapy for children with cerebral palsy: An ecological approach. *Developmental Medicine and Child Neurology, 47*(09), 613–619.

Engelen, V., Ketelaar, M., & Gorter, J. W. (2007). Selecting the appropriate outcome in paediatric physical therapy: How individual treatment goals for children with cerebral palsy are reflected in GMFM-88 and PEDI. *Journal of Rehabilitation Medicine, 39*(3), 225–231.

Holsbeeke, L., Ketelaar, M., Schoemaker, M. M., & Gorter, J. W. (2009). Capacity, capability, and performance: Different constructs or three of a kind? *Archives of Physical Medicine and Rehabilitation, 90*(5), 849–855.

Hoving, M. A., van Raak, E. P., Spincemaille, G. H., van Kranen-Mastenbroek, V. H., van Kleef, M., Gorter, J. W., & Vles, J. S. (2009). Safety and one-year efficacy of intrathecal baclofen therapy in children with intractable spastic cerebral palsy. *European Journal of Paediatric Neurology, 13*(3), 247–256.

Kiresuk, T., & Sherman, R. (1968). Goal Attainment Scaling: A general method for evaluating community health programs. *Community Mental Health Journal, 4*, 443–453.

Kiresuk, T., Smith, A., & Cardillo, J. E. (Eds.). (1994). *Goal attainment scaling: Applications, theory, and measurement*. London, U.K.: Lawrence Erlbaum Associates.

Löwing, K., Bexelius, A., & Brogren Carlberg, E. (2009). Activity focused and goal directed therapy for children with cerebral palsy – Do goals make a difference? *Disability and Rehabilitation, 31*(22), 1808–1816.

McDougall, J., & Wright, V. (2009). The ICF-CY and Goal Attainment Scaling: Benefits of their combined use for pediatric practice. *Disability and Rehabilitation, 31*(16), 1362–1372.

Melvin, J. L. (1980). Interdisciplinary and multidisciplinary activities and the ACRM. *Archives of Physical Medicine and Rehabilitation, 61*(8), 379.

Nijhuis, B. J. G., Reinders-Messelink, H. A., de Blécourt, A. C. E., Boonstra, A. M., Calamé, E. H. M., Groothoof, J. W., ... Postema, K. (2008). Goal setting in Dutch paediatric rehabilitation. Are the needs and principal problems of children with cerebral palsy integrated into their rehabilitation goals? *Clinical Rehabilitation, 22*, 348–363.

Nijhuis, B. J. G., Reinders-Messelink, H. A., de Blécourt, A. C. E., Ties, J. G., Boonstra, A. M., Grooth, J. W., ... Postema, K. (2008). Needs, problems and rehabilitation goals of young children with cerebral palsy as formulated in the rehabilitation activities profile for children. *Journal of Rehabilitation Medicine, 40*, 347–354.

Ostensjø, S., Oien, I., & Fallang, B. (2008). Goal-oriented rehabilitation of preschoolers with cerebral palsy – A multi-case study of combined use of the Canadian Occupational Performance Measure (COPM) and the Goal Attainment Scaling (GAS). *Developmental Neurorehabilitation, 11*(4), 252–259.

Palisano, R. J. (1993). Validity of Goal Attainment Scaling in infants with motor delays. *Physical Therapy, 73*(10), 651–658.

Palisano, R. J., Haley, S. M., & Brown, D. A. (1992). Goal attainment scaling as a measure of change in infants with motor delays. *Physical Therapy, 72*(6), 432–437.

Roelofsen, E., Lankhorst, G., & Bouter, L. (2001). Simultaneous development and implementation of the Children's Rehabilitation Activities Profile: A communication instrument for pediatric rehabilitation. *Disability and Rehabilitation, 23*(14), 614–622.

Rosenbaum, P., & Gorter, J. (2012). The 'F-words' in childhood disability: I swear this is how we should think! *Child: Care, Health and Development, 38*(4), 457–463.

Rosenbaum, P., & Stewart, D. (2004). The World Health Organization International Classification of Functioning, Disability, and Health: A model to guide clinical thinking, practice and research in the field of cerebral palsy. *Seminars in Pediatric Neurology, 11*, 5–10.

Russell, D. J., Rivard, L. M., Walter, S. D., Rosenbaum, P. L., Roxborough, L., Cameron, D., … Avery, L. M. (2010). Using knowledge brokers to facilitate the uptake of pediatric measurement tools into clinical practice: A before–after intervention study. *Implementation Science, 5*(1), 92.

Schlosser, R. W. (2004). Goal attainment scaling as a clinical measurement technique in communication disorders: A critical review. *Journal of Communication Disorders, 37*(3), 217–239.

Siebes, R. C., Ketelaar, M., Gorter, J. W., Wijnroks, L., De Blécourt, A. C., Reinders-Messelink, H. A., … Ketelaar, M. (2007). Transparency and tuning of rehabilitation care for children with cerebral palsy: A multiple case study in five children with complex needs. *Developmental Neurorehabilitation, 10*(3), 193–204.

Steenbeek, D., Gorter, J. W., Ketelaar, M., Galama, K., & Lindeman, E. (2011). Responsiveness of Goal Attainment Scaling in comparison to two standardized measures in outcome evaluation of children with cerebral palsy. *Clinical Rehabilitation, 25*(12), 1128–1139.

Steenbeek, D., Ketelaar, M., Galama, K., & Gorter, J. W. (2007). Goal attainment scaling in paediatric rehabilitation: A critical review of the literature. *Developmental Medicine and Child Neurology, 49*(7), 550–556.

Steenbeek, D., Ketelaar, M., Galama, K., & Gorter, J. W. (2008). Goal Attainment Scaling in paediatric rehabilitation: A report on the clinical training of an interdisciplinary team. *Child: Care, Health and Development, 34*(4), 521–529.

Steenbeek, D., Ketelaar, M., Lindeman, E., Galama, K., & Gorter, J. W. (2010). Interrater reliability of Goal Attainment Scaling in rehabilitation of children with cerebral palsy. *Archives of Physical Medicine and Rehabilitation, 91*, 429–435.

Steenbeek, D., Meester-Delver, A., Becher, J. G., & Lankhorst, G. J. (2005). The effect of botulinum toxin type A treatment of the lower extremity on the level of functional abilities in children with cerebral palsy: Evaluation with goal attainment scaling. *Clinical Rehabilitation, 19*(3), 274–282.

Streiner, D. L., & Norman, G. R. (2008). *Health measurement scales: A practical guide to their development and use* (4th ed.). Oxford, U.K.: Oxford University Press.

Tennant, A. (2007). Goal attainment scaling: Current methodological challenges. *Disability and Rehabilitation, 29*(20–21), 1583–1588.

Turner-Stokes, L. (2009). Goal attainment scaling (GAS) in rehabilitation: A practical guide. *Clinical Rehabilitation, 23*, 362–370.

Turner-Stokes, L., & Williams, H. (2010). Goal attainment scaling: A direct comparison of alternative rating methods. *Clinical Rehabilitation, 24*, 66–73.

Turner-Stokes, L., Williams, H., & Johnson, J. (2009). Goal attainment scaling: Does it provide added value as a person-centred measure for evaluation of outcome in neurorehabilitation following acquired brain injury? *Journal of Rehabilitation Medicine, 41*(7), 528–535.

Wallen, M., Ziviani, J., Naylor, O., Evans, R., Novak, I., & Herbert, R. D. (2011). Modified constraint-induced therapy for children with hemiplegic cerebral palsy: A randomized trial. *Developmental Medicine and Child Neurology, 53*(12), 1091–1099.

Ward, A., Hayden, S., Dexter, M., & Scheinberg, A. (2009). Continuous intrathecal baclofen for children with spasticity and/or dystonia: Goal attainment and complications associated with treatment. *Journal of Paediatrics and Child Health, 45*(12), 720–726.

9

Applying the International Classification of Functioning, Disability and Health to Rehabilitation Goal Setting

Alexandra Rauch and Anke Scheel-Sailer

CONTENTS

9.1 Introduction

In this chapter, an approach to goal setting based on the use of the World Health Organization (WHO)'s International Classification of Functioning, Disability and Health (ICF) (WHO, 2001) is presented. Goal setting is a process that includes the decision of what needs to be accomplished (the goal) and the formulation of a plan to achieve that desired result. It includes the identification of the goal areas in different hierarchical levels and clarification of the corresponding expected outcome. To do this, information that helps understand the patient's problems and needs comprehensively is necessary (Hurn, Kneebone, & Cropley, 2006). This is the essential foundation of successful goal setting (Rauch, Cieza, & Stucki, 2008).

Since the overall goal of rehabilitation usually refers to achieving an optimal level of functioning (Stucki, Cieza, & Melvin, 2007), the basic information necessary to work on the achievement of this should include information on functioning and disability (Wade, 2009). In this regard, the ICF provides a classification system that allows for the description and organization of information about functioning in persons with health conditions in a standardized language. This classification system is based on the WHO's model of functioning and disability, which provides a comprehensive understanding of these concepts. Both the model and the classification system are useful resources for rehabilitation professionals and can be applied in rehabilitation management through the use of ICF tools developed specifically for this purpose (Rauch et al., 2008).

ICF Core Sets are important components of ICF tools. While the ICF's conceptual model can be applied to explain relationships among the different components of functioning and disability and the influencing health conditions and contextual factors (Steiner et al., 2002), the classification system of the ICF as such is too comprehensive to be used in daily practice (Ustun, Chatterji, & Kostanjsek, 2004). The ICF Core Sets were thus developed in order to make the ICF classification more applicable in daily practice (Cieza et al., 2004; Grill, Ewert, Chatterji, Kostanjsek, & Stucki, 2005).

To date, various approaches have been published in which the ICF is applied in rehabilitation management, some of them specifically addressing goal setting in rehabilitation. For example, Steiner et al. (2002) developed the Rehabilitation Problem-Solving Form (RPS-Form) which is based on the conceptual model of functioning and disability and helps identify rehabilitation goals and their related target problems from information gathered through an assessment structured by the components of the ICF. Power, Anderson, and Togher (2011) applied this RPS-Form to a person with Huntington's disease and rated it as a useful tool that systematizes the assessment findings and hence offers a helpful resource for the goal-setting process. Rauch et al. (2008) developed several ICF-based documentation tools for the different steps of rehabilitation management, including the assessment and the ensuing goal-setting process, and applied these in various case studies to persons with spinal cord injury (Rauch et al., 2010). (These case studies and tools can be accessed on the Internet at the following address: http://www. icf-casestudies.org.) Martinuzzi et al. (2010) developed and implemented another ICF-based documentation tool to apply the ICF for children and youth (ICF-CY) (WHO, 2006) in rehabilitation management, specifically to children and youth in a neuropaediatric setting. This tool also facilitates the systematic description of the assessment findings in different components of the ICF and, furthermore, allows the documentation of mid- to long-term rehabilitation goals. Bornman and Murphy (2006) developed a product called Talking Mats®, which presents graphic symbols to represent the nine ICF domains from the activities and participation component and two from the contextual factors. These graphical symbols help individuals with communication difficulties to identify main topics for rehabilitation goals from their own perspective and, hence, contribute to the development of a person-centred rehabilitation programme. Harty, Griesel, and van der Merwe (2011) found that the Talking Mats® visual framework was a useful tool for communication between individuals with communication disorders and their health professionals in order to identify rehabilitation goals.

In addition to the development of practical tools for the process of goal setting, various studies have demonstrated that the terminology of the ICF classification can be utilized for rehabilitation goal setting by showing that ICF categories (1) are reliable to code therapy goals (Soberg, Sandvik, & Ostensjo, 2008) and (2) cover the broad spectrum of intervention goals addressed by physical therapists (Huber, Tobler, Gloor-Juzi, Grill, & Gubler-Gut, 2011; Mittrach et al., 2008). Furthermore, it has been demonstrated (3) that intervention goals based on the ICF can be used to determine the workload of therapists (Grill, Huber, Gloor-Juzi, & Stucki, 2010) and (4) that the ICF categories are applicable to describe patients' goals in acute hospitals (Muller, Strobl, & Grill, 2011) as well as for musculoskeletal, neurological and cardiopulmonary conditions (Lohmann, Decker, Muller, Strobl, & Grill, 2011) and geriatric patients (Kus, Muller, Strobl, & Grill, 2011) in post-acute rehabilitation care.

A variety of different approaches for implementing the ICF for goal setting in rehabilitation management in practice exist. From a more scientific perspective, it could be shown that the ICF classification provides an appropriate terminology for the description of therapists' and patients' goals. However, as yet, the classification system and in particular ICF Core Sets are rarely implemented in practice for goal setting. Hence, the aim of this chapter is to illustrate the application of ICF Core Sets by means of ICF documentation tools in rehabilitation goal setting. The approach outlined in this chapter is one that has successfully been implemented in various case studies about persons with spinal cord diseases. However, for a better understanding, the ICF and its components (the model and the classification) will be introduced briefly first, before this practical approach to applying the ICF Core Sets in rehabilitation goal setting and documentation will be illustrated.

9.2 ICF and ICF Core Sets

Following approval of the ICF by the 54th World Health Assembly in 2001, the WHO launched its universal and internationally accepted framework and classification of functioning, disability and health, the ICF (Stucki, 2005). The purpose of the ICF is to provide (1) a statistical tool for population studies and information management; (2) a research tool for outcome measurement; (3) an educational tool for curriculum design and awareness raising; (4) a social policy tool applicable to all aspects of health and disability policy, design, implementation and monitoring; and (5) a clinical tool for treatment planning, assessment and evaluation. As the ICF is fundamentally a universal classification system, it provides a common language about aspects of human functioning that can be applied across countries and health-care disciplines.

9.2.1 Model of Functioning and Disability

The model of functioning and disability (Figure 9.1) depicts interactions between a health condition and contextual factors (environmental and personal factors). These interactions

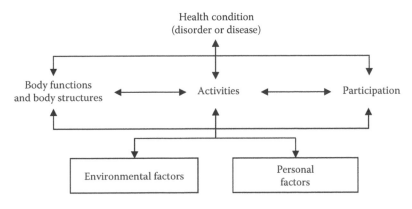

FIGURE 9.1
Model of functioning, disability and health.

result in levels of functioning in the components of body functions, body structures, activities and participation that again interact which each other. If these interactions cause impairments (in body functions and body structures), limitations (in activities) or restrictions (in participation), the result is a certain level of disability in the corresponding component.

Thus, functioning and disability are not conceptualized as the direct consequence of a health condition but rather the result of the interaction between a health condition and the contextual factors (environmental and personal factors). Since environmental and personal factors can have a positive or negative impact on functioning, they should always be taken into account when describing a person's level of functioning.

9.2.2 Hierarchical Structure of the Classification

The classification of the ICF is arranged hierarchically (Figure 9.2). The two *parts* (1) *functioning and disability* and *contextual factors* are composed of two *components* each, with letters assigned to components for the purposes of coding. Part 1 comprises *body functions* and *body structures* (given two codes, *b* and *s*, respectively) and *activities and participation* (with the code *d*). Part 2 comprises *environmental factors* (with the code *e*) and *personal factors* (which are not yet classified by the ICF and therefore not yet given a code, although some initial approaches to identify areas of personal factors as the basis for a classification have been tackled) (Geyh, Muller, et al., 2011; Geyh, Peter, et al., 2011; Grotkamp et al., 2010). Each component is composed of *chapters*, which represent the first level of the classification, and each chapter again is subdivided into *categories*. The categories are then organized in a hierarchical order of second and third levels and, in body functions and body structures, to a fourth level. In addition to the letter codes indicating the component mentioned earlier

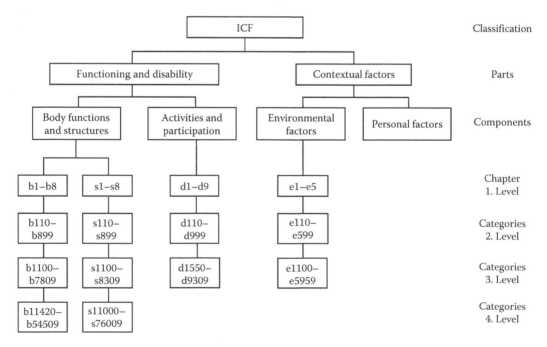

FIGURE 9.2
Hierarchical organization of the ICF.

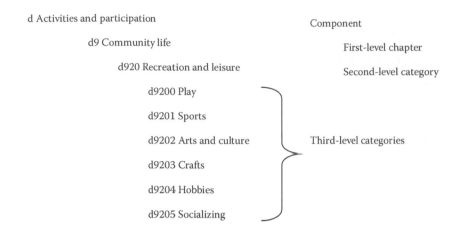

FIGURE 9.3
Example for the hierarchical organization of the ICF.

(b, s, d and e), a numeric code is applied to indicate chapters and categories, with the length of the numbers depending on the level of the category (one digit for a first-level chapter], three digits if a second-, four if a third- and five if a fourth-level category).

The hierarchical structure allows users to choose either a broader (e.g. a first-level chapter or a second-level category) or a more detailed description (e.g. a subordinated third- or fourth-level category) of a domain of functioning. The example in Figure 9.3 illustrates how the level of specificity increases with each lower level.

Due to this hierarchical structure, the number of ICF categories included in the entire classification is very large. This makes the classification on the one hand very exhaustive by covering a very comprehensive spectrum of domains of functioning and the environmental factors, but at the same time therefore difficult to use in practice. The need for practical application of the ICF led to a decision to develop user-friendly tools such as the ICF Core Sets (Stucki et al., 2002).

9.2.3 ICF Core Sets

An ICF Core Set is a selection of ICF categories from the entire ICF classification that are relevant for persons with specific health conditions at specific treatment periods. To cover the entire spectrum of relevant ICF categories, an ICF Core Set contains as many categories as necessary to be sufficiently comprehensive when describing an individual's functioning, but at the same time, with as few categories as possible to be practical (Cieza et al., 2004). In rehabilitation, ICF Core Sets can be used to describe an individual's functioning taking into account aspects from all components of functioning and the environmental factors that are typical for a person with a specific health condition. Therefore, ICF Core Sets have been developed for the long-term care primarily for single health conditions (Cieza et al., 2004) and for the acute and post-acute care primarily for condition groups covering several single health conditions (neurological, cardiopulmonary and musculoskeletal conditions) (Grill et al., 2005).

For each ICF Core Set, a brief version and a comprehensive version are available. While Brief ICF Core Sets serve as practical tools for single encounters and can be considered to be minimum data sets for the reporting of clinical and epidemiological studies and health

For acute care
Neurological conditions
Cardiopulmonary conditions
Musculoskeletal conditions
Acute inflammatory arthritis

For post-acute care
Neurological conditions
Cardiopulmonary conditions
Musculoskeletal conditions
For geriatric patients
Spinal cord injury

For long-term care in between finalized, ICF
Core Sets: Vertigo, Hearing loss, Cerebral palsy
Multiple sclerosis
Stroke
Traumatic brain injury
Spinal cord injury
Chronic ischamic heart disease
Diabetes mellitus
Obesity
Obstructive pulmonary diseases
Ankylosing spondylitis
Chronic widespread pain
Low back pain
Osteoarthritis
Osteoporosis
Rheumatoid arthritis
Bipolar disorders
Depression
Breast cancer
Head and neck cancer
Hand conditions
Inflammatory bowel diseases
Sleep disorders
Vocational rehabilitation

FIGURE 9.4
Overview of ICF Core Sets.

statistics, the Comprehensive ICF Core Sets are intended for use in multidisciplinary settings (Stucki, Kostanjsek, Ustun, & Cieza, 2008). However, another option is to use a Brief ICF Core Set as a starting point, but then to select additional ICF categories, as relevant for the description of an individual's functioning, from the corresponding Comprehensive ICF Core Set. This allows clinicians and researchers to generate an enlarged *brief* version, tailored for individual patients (Rauch, Lückenkemper, & Cieza, 2012).

Figure 9.4 provides an overview of the existing ICF Core Sets, which are available for selected health conditions at different stages. All ICF Core Sets are available at www.icf-research-branch.org/icf-core-sets-projects.html.

The use of the ICF Core Sets in clinical practice in general facilitates a comprehensive description of functioning with a common language that can inform any team member of a rehabilitation team and thus can contribute to interdisciplinary teamwork.

9.2.4 ICF Qualifiers

In addition to the ICF classification and ICF Core Sets, which organize the domains of functioning systematically, it is necessary to be able to describe the magnitude of the level of functioning in these domains. These qualifiers can be used as a way of making the ICF more applicable to clinical practice. Specifically, the ICF provides a generic scale that is graded into five qualifiers that describe the extent of the problem experienced by a person within each relevant category of the ICF. As well, in case of lack of information or inapplicability, specific qualifiers can be applied. The following overview depicts the generic scales with the qualifiers:

0	*No* problem	(None, absent, negligible, etc.)	0%–4%
1	*Mild* problem	(Slight, low, etc.)	5%–24%
2	*Moderate* problem	(Medium, fair, etc.)	25%–49%
3	*Severe* problem	(High, extreme, etc.)	50%–95%
4	*Complete* problem	(Total, etc.)	96%–100%
8	*Not specified*	(i.e. no sufficient information is available)	
9	*Not applicable*	(i.e. an evaluation is not appropriate for the category in question)	

For the extent of the positive (facilitator) or negative impact (barrier) of an environmental factor on functioning, the same scale can be applied: if an environmental factor presents a facilitator, this is displaced with a plus sign before the qualifier value.

It is important to note that an ICF category can be rated with more than one qualifier, in particular in domains of activities and participation where the first qualifier refers to *performance* and the second to *capacity*. Performance describes what an individual actually does in the light of the positive or negative impact of environmental factors (aspects of the physical, social and attitudinal world). Capacity, by contrast, describes an individual's inherent or intrinsic ability to perform a task or an action without using assistive devices, personal assistance or any other environmental factor which may either act as a facilitator or a barrier. Hence, the difference between performance and capacity reflects the impact of environmental factors on an individual's level of functioning.

A useful electronic tool to document levels of functioning based on the use of ICF Core Sets and ICF qualifiers is available for various languages at http://www.icf-core-sets.org/en/index.php.

9.3 Applying the ICF in Rehabilitation Goal Setting

In general, rehabilitation management is a structured process performed in consecutive steps (Rauch et al., 2008) (Figure 9.5): (1) assessment, (2) goal setting, (3) assignment,

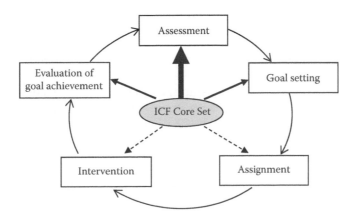

FIGURE 9.5
Cycle of rehabilitation management.

(4) intervention and (5) evaluation of goal achievement. To achieve a long-term rehabilitation goal, usually a sequence of rehabilitation cycles has to be performed in which the number of cycles may depend on the severity and stage of the underlying disease and the impact of the contextual factors.

Within any approach to goal setting in rehabilitation, the collection of information about the person and his or her level of functioning is a critical first step to inform the subsequent goal selection process (Wade, 2009). This first step impacts on all subsequent components of the rehabilitation process. Applying the ICF, and in particular the ICF Core Sets, in this step can help rehabilitation practitioners to conduct an assessment that provides the appropriate level of detail on a person's level of functioning required for decisions about goal selection. Furthermore, the ICF-based information can also contribute to planning interventions and to assigning them to different rehabilitation team members. Likewise, that same information can be later used when undertaking an evaluation of goal achievement.

As an example of how to apply the ICF in rehabilitation goal setting, consider the following: A 35-year-old woman, Lisa, admitted to an inpatient rehabilitation programme 4 months following a traumatic spinal cord injury, which resulted in complete paraplegia at the level of the eighth thoracic vertebra. The accident happened during a climb in the Swiss mountains when the team was hit by falling rocks. Beside the paraplegia, Lisa suffered several other injuries, which all healed completely during the 1st month following the accident. Before this accident, Lisa worked as a teacher of geography and sport. She was a keen sportswoman (tennis, mountain biking, hiking, climbing) and shared this enthusiasm with her boyfriend. Thus, sport was an important aspect of her life, not only in her free time but also from a professional perspective. Hence, sport would be a crucial component of her rehabilitation programme. (For more information about Lisa, go to www.icf-casestudies.org/case_studies.php?id=77&cat_id=21&k=8.)

9.3.1 Assessment of Functioning

The first step in the goal-setting process in any rehabilitation management is the assessment of functioning. ICF Core Sets facilitate the evaluation of functioning by providing a list of domains that are most likely relevant for persons with a specific health condition at a specific stage of recovery. Thus, ICF Core Sets can be used to guide the rehabilitation team through the assessment and facilitate a comprehensive description of functioning (Rauch et al., 2012).

Depending on the stage of the disease, an ICF Core Set can be selected for assessment for patients in the acute, post-acute or long-term care stage. Depending on the setting (single health discipline or multiprofessional team), either the Brief or Comprehensive ICF Core Set may be appropriate, or an enlarged brief version can be developed. If no ICF Core Set is available for the individual's particular health condition, the rehabilitation team can select ICF categories from the entire classification. In Lisa's case, an enlarged brief version based on the ICF Core Set for persons with spinal cord injury in the post-acute care stage (Kirchberger et al., 2010) was created. All ICF categories from the Brief ICF Core Set and additional ICF categories from the Comprehensive ICF Core Set are then entered into the ICF Categorical Profile (see Figures 9.6 and 9.7), which was developed to document an individual's level of functioning and rehabilitation goals (Rauch et al., 2008).

To describe the level of functioning, each ICF category contained in the selected ICF Core Set or selected from the ICF is assessed by the different team members either in a clinical examination, a technical investigation, an observation by a health professional or an interview with the patient or, if necessary, his or her proxy (e.g. a close family member). To perform the assessment, standardized measures can be applied by the experts in the

	Assessment 4 months post-trauma	
Global goal: Independent participation in community, part-time work in former profession		1
Programme goal: Independent living at home		0
Cycle goal 1: Independence in self-care d5		0
Cycle goal 2: Independence in mobility d4		0
Cycle goal 3: d920 Recreation and leisure		1

ICF categories		ICF qualifier	Goal relation	Goal value
		Impairment 0 1 2 3 4		
Body functions and body structures				
b130	Energy and drive functions			
b134	Sleep functions			
b152	**Emotional functions**		PG	1
b260	Proprioceptive functions*			
b265	Touch functions*			
b270	Sensory functions related to temperature and other*			
b280	**Sensation of pain**		CG2	0
b415	Blood vessel functions			
b420	Blood pressure functions		CG2	0
b440	**Respiration functions**			
b445	Respiratory muscle functions			
b455	Exercise tolerance functions		CG3	0
b525	**Defecation functions**			
b530	Weight maintenance functions			
b550	Thermoregulation functions			
b620	**Urination functions**			
b640	Sexual functions			
b710	Mobility of joint functions		CG2	0
b715	Stability of joint functions			
b730	**Muscle power functions**			
b7300	Power of isolated muscles and muscle groups		CG2, 3	0
b7303	Power of muscles in lower half of the body			
b735	**Muscle tone functions**			
b7353	Tone of muscles of lower half of the body		CG2, 3	1
b740	Muscle endurance functions*		CG3	0
b750	Motor reflex functions*			
b760	Control of voluntary movements*			
b7603	Supportive functions of arms		CG2	0
b810	**Protective functions of the skin**			
s120	**Spinal cord and related structures**			
s430	**Structure of respiratory system**			
s610	**Structure of the urinary system**			
s810	Structure of areas of skin		CG1	0

ICF categories marked in bold letters are contained in the Brief ICF Core Set, all other ICF categories are selected from the Comprehensive ICF Core Set for spinal cord injury in the post-acute context.

*Below the level of injury.

CG1, CG2, CG3, PG, GG = relationship with Cycle Goal 1, 2 or 3, Programme Goal or Global Goal.

FIGURE 9.6

ICF Categorical Profile for body functions and body structures created as the enlarged brief version of the ICF Core Set for spinal cord injury for the early post-acute care. (From Kirchberger, I. et al., *Spinal Cord*, 48(4), 297, 2010.)

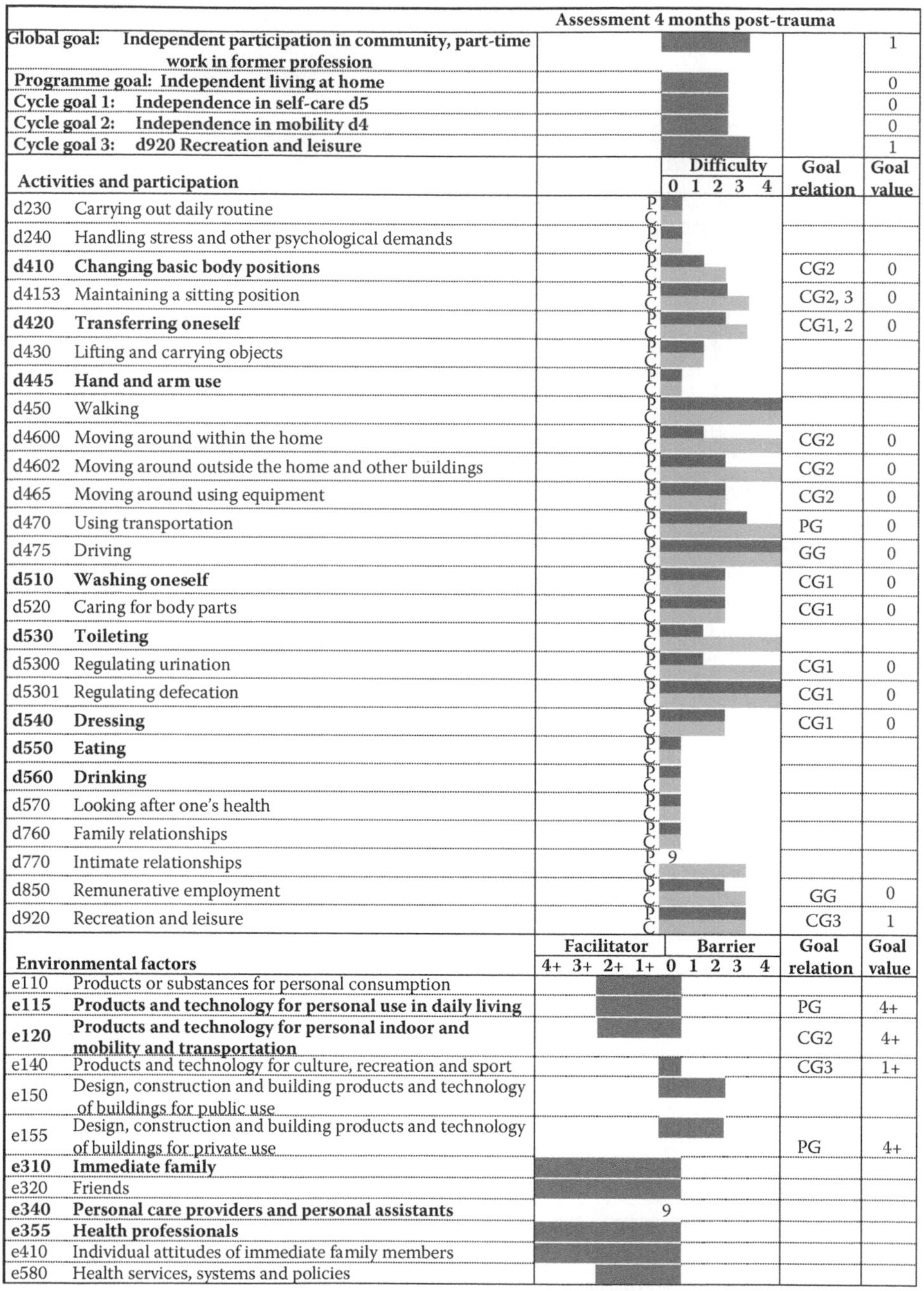

	Assessment 4 months post-trauma	
Global goal: Independent participation in community, part-time work in former profession		1
Programme goal: Independent living at home		0
Cycle goal 1: Independence in self-care d5		0
Cycle goal 2: Independence in mobility d4		0
Cycle goal 3: d920 Recreation and leisure		1

Activities and participation	Difficulty 0 1 2 3 4	Goal relation	Goal value
d230 Carrying out daily routine			
d240 Handling stress and other psychological demands			
d410 Changing basic body positions		CG2	0
d4153 Maintaining a sitting position		CG2, 3	0
d420 Transferring oneself		CG1, 2	0
d430 Lifting and carrying objects			
d445 Hand and arm use			
d450 Walking			
d4600 Moving around within the home		CG2	0
d4602 Moving around outside the home and other buildings		CG2	0
d465 Moving around using equipment		CG2	0
d470 Using transportation		PG	0
d475 Driving		GG	0
d510 Washing oneself		CG1	0
d520 Caring for body parts		CG1	0
d530 Toileting			
d5300 Regulating urination		CG1	0
d5301 Regulating defecation		CG1	0
d540 Dressing		CG1	0
d550 Eating			
d560 Drinking			
d570 Looking after one's health			
d760 Family relationships			
d770 Intimate relationships	9		
d850 Remunerative employment		GG	0
d920 Recreation and leisure		CG3	1

Environmental factors	Facilitator 4+ 3+ 2+ 1+	Barrier 0 1 2 3 4	Goal relation	Goal value
e110 Products or substances for personal consumption				
e115 Products and technology for personal use in daily living			PG	4+
e120 Products and technology for personal indoor and mobility and transportation			CG2	4+
e140 Products and technology for culture, recreation and sport			CG3	1+
e150 Design, construction and building products and technology of buildings for public use				
e155 Design, construction and building products and technology of buildings for private use			PG	4+
e310 Immediate family				
e320 Friends				
e340 Personal care providers and personal assistants	9			
e355 Health professionals				
e410 Individual attitudes of immediate family members				
e580 Health services, systems and policies				

ICF categories marked in bold letters are contained in the Brief ICF Core Set, all other ICF categories are selected from the Comprehensive ICF Core Set for spinal cord injury in the post-acute context.

*Below the level of injury.

P = Performance; C = Capacity.

CG1, CG2, CG3, PG, GG = indicates relationship with Cycle Goal 1, 2 or 3, Programme Goal or Global Goal.

FIGURE 9.7

ICF Categorical Profile for activities and participation and environmental factors created as enlarged brief version of the ICF Core Set for spinal cord injury for the early post-acute care. (From Kirchberger, I. et al., *Spinal Cord*, 48(4), 297, 2010.)

different specialties. In Lisa's example, for the description of *b7300 Power of isolated muscles and muscle groups*, a manual muscle test was performed by the physical therapist; to assess the patient's capacity and performance in *d4153 Maintaining a sitting position* the respective activity was observed, and to assess *e310 Immediate family* information regarding the support of her family was gained through an interview with the patient and her family. In addition, more comprehensive standardized measures were performed, such as the Spinal Cord Independence Measure (Itzkovich et al., 2007) to assess independence in self-care and mobility. After the assessment of functioning, each result is rated with an ICF qualifier. The respective value is entered for each ICF category into the ICF Categorical Profile in the column *ICF qualifier*. Both the specific assessment results and the corresponding rating with the ICF qualifier are critical for the later definition of goal values, which describe the level of functioning that should be achieved for each intervention target in a given period.

Once all ICF categories are rated with ICF qualifiers, a profile arises out of it, which easily allows the identification of those domains that present mild, moderate, severe or complete problems and those that present full functioning. Thus, the ICF Categorical Profile provides a comprehensive overview of an individual's functioning state in all domains of functioning which is easy to understand and, hence, is useful to inform all persons involved in the goal-setting process, including patients and their families. While specific information from discipline-specific clinical measures may be too technical for the average team member (let alone patient or family members) to understand, the ICF approach to assessment can make the key points arising from these measures available to all participants in the rehabilitation process.

9.3.2 Goal Setting

The goal-setting process includes the selection of the most important goal areas and afterwards the definition of the goal value that should be achieved in a determined time frame. The ICF Categorical Profile facilitates this process by providing the required information at a glance.

9.3.2.1 Selection of Rehabilitation Goal Areas

Using the ICF approach to goal setting, rehabilitation goals should be set in order according to the time frame in which they should be achieved and should refer to domains of functioning provided with the ICF framework (Playford, Siegert, Levack, & Freeman, 2009; Wade, 2009). Based on the description of the levels of functioning provided with the ICF Categorical Profile which summarizes the underlying specific results from the assessment, and taking into account the individual's stage of a disease (acute, post-acute, long term), goals can be identified for the different stages of recovery (long term, midterm and short term) (see Figure 9.8).

The goal setting is a joint process between the rehabilitation team and the patient. In particular, the definition of the current goals must meet the needs of the patient. Therefore, a team meeting with the patient is held; the assessment results depicted with the ICF Categorical Profile provide the necessary information that facilitates the definition of the goals for the different time frames:

1. Within this approach, *long-term goals* refer to goals that need to be achieved by the end of a series of rehabilitation programmes. Therefore, the long-term goal is also called the *global goal* and, most of the time, targets achievement at the level of participation (e.g. community or work integration). However, in the later stages

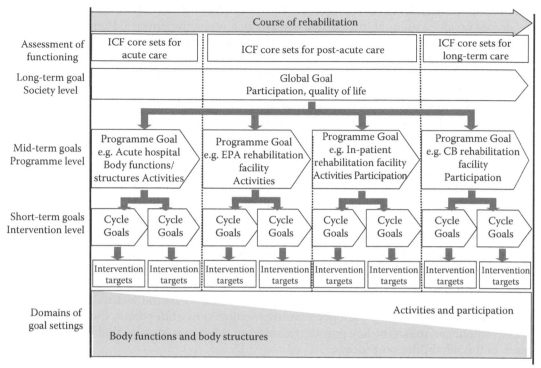

EPA: Early post-acute; CB: community-based.

FIGURE 9.8
Process of the assessment and goal setting and shifting of goal domains over the course of rehabilitation.

of more severe, chronic diseases, in which an improvement of functioning cannot be expected, a global goal may also be defined in terms of the maintenance of health, prevention of secondary conditions or as aspects related to quality of life and well-being. For Lisa, the *Independent participation in community, and part-time work in former profession* were defined as the global goals.

2. *Midterm goals* refer to the end of any specific rehabilitation programme. Over the course of rehabilitation, a person is usually assigned to a sequence of different programmes such as care in an acute hospital early after the onset of a disease, inpatient rehabilitation programmes in the early post-acute or later stage and outpatient rehabilitation programmes in long-term care. Therefore, the midterm goal is also called a *programme goal*. Usually, the achievement of a sequence of programme goals is intended to lead to the achievement of the global goal. The definition of the programme goals usually shifts from areas in body functions and body structures in the acute stage to activities in the post-acute and participation in the long-term stage of a disease. For example, while in most situations of the acute phase of a disease the goal of a treatment may be to restore impaired body functions and structures and to improve basic activities, in the long-term phase, rehabilitation goals concentrate on an individual's integration and participation in various life situations and, generally speaking, on community integration. For Lisa, the midterm goal referring to the actual inpatient rehabilitation programme targeted on the achievement of *Independent living at home.*

3. *Short-term goals* refer to goals to be achieved at the end of a single rehabilitation cycle. Therefore, the short-term goal is also called *cycle goal*. The length of a rehabilitation cycle varies. The more acute the health condition, the faster the functioning level may change and therefore the shorter a single cycle may be. In contrast, in a more chronic stage of a health condition, the length of rehabilitation cycles may increase due to the slower changes of the levels of functioning. Usually, the achievement of a sequence of cycle goals leads to the achievement of a programme goal, and it is not uncommon for a rehabilitation team to be pursuing more than one cycle goal concurrently. Therefore, several cycles will be performed within one and the same programme. The goal areas of cycle goals shift in a similar way to the programme goals, from body functions and body structures in the acute stage to more participatory goals in the late stage. For Lisa, the actual cycle goals were defined as *Independence in self-care d5*, *Independence in mobility d4* and *d920 Recreation and leisure* that addressed the reintegration into sport activities.

To document the global, programme and cycle goals, the ICF Categorical Profile provides space accordingly in the upper part of the documentation form (see Figures 9.6 and 9.7).

4. *Intervention targets* are the smallest unit in the hierarchy of rehabilitation goals. They are aspects of functioning that have to be addressed within specific interventions to achieve a cycle goal or sometimes a programme or global goal. The list of ICF categories in the ICF Categorical Profile whose level of functioning has been rated with a qualifier provides the basis for the selection of the intervention targets. Once identified, intervention targets give the description of those aspects of functioning for which the specific interventions have to be defined. Therefore, intervention targets describe aspects of functioning on a more specific level than it might be necessary for a cycle, programme or even for a global goal as it is shown in Figure 9.9. Consequently, the selection of the most relevant intervention targets

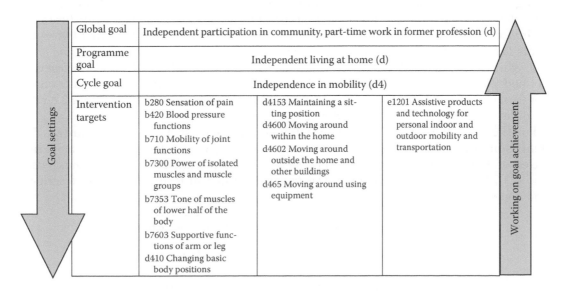

FIGURE 9.9
Relationships between the goals on the different hierarchical levels (selected for cycle goal *Independence in mobility d4*).

that are directly related to the goals is a critical step for successful intervention planning. An overview of all intervention targets summarizes the rehabilitation needs, which is also helpful for resource allocation.

To document the selected intervention targets in the ICF Categorical Profile, a link to the related goal (cycle, programme or global goal) is entered into the column *Goal relation* (see Figures 9.6 and 9.7).

It is important to emphasize that the goals and the intervention targets in the different hierarchical levels are closely related to each other as shown in Figure 9.9. In this example, the goal achievement in all intervention targets contributes to the achievement in the cycle goal *Independence in mobility (coded as d4)*. The achievement of *Independence in mobility*, again, is a prerequisite to achieve the programme goal *Independent living at home (coded as d)*, which, again, is the qualification for the achievement of the global goal *Independent participation in community, part-time work in former profession (coded as d)*.

9.3.2.2 Defining the Nature and Scope of Expected Outcomes

For each of the identified goal areas, the expected outcome has to be defined. Here, the word *define* refers to stating or describing the exact nature or scope of the expected level of functioning. The ICF approach to goal setting frequently follows the SMART rule in this regard, documenting goals that are specific, measurable, achievable, realistic and timed (i.e. with a stated time frame for achievement or re-evaluation) (Bovend'Eerdt, Botell, & Wade, 2009). Only by explicitly defining the expected outcome will the subsequent evaluation of goal achievement be possible, and hence, operationalization of goals in such a way is indispensable for the examination of the successful implementation of the specific interventions. An ICF category itself can only describe the goal area, while the expected outcome in this domain of functioning has to be defined by means of a more specific description or a goal value. In the ICF Categorical Profile, a goal value is expressed by using ICF qualifiers for the goals on all hierarchical levels. In the example of Lisa, the expected outcomes for the global goal *Independent participation in community, part-time work in former profession*, the programme goal *Independent living at home* and the first two cycle goals *Independence in self-care d5* and *Independence in mobility d4* were all set at 0 = *no problem*, while for Cycle Goal 3 *d920 Recreation and leisure*, a goal value of 1 = *mild problem* was defined. Also, goal values for each of the intervention targets were defined, such as a qualifier 0 = *no problem* for *b280 Sensation of pain* would mean an improvement of about 2 on the qualifier scale from 2 = *moderate problem* to 0 = *no problem*.

For the definition of goal values, additional options exist. First, to standardize the definition of rehabilitation goals, Rentsch and Bucher (2005) developed goal categories based on the ICF for the domains (A) *Habitation*, (B) *Participation in a sociocultural context* and (C) *Working*. For example, for *A Habitation*, six different levels have been described and coded:

A1	Integration into nursing home, maintenance of health
A2	Supported living in an institution
A3	Living at home with support by persons living in the same household
A4	Independent living at home with professional support
A5	Independent living at home
A6	Independent living at home with additional tasks

For each of the levels, the minimal requirements that are necessary to achieve the according level are defined in the components of body functions and body structures and activities and participation and with respect to environmental factors. These goal categories can be combined with ICF qualifiers as is illustrated in the ICF Categorical Profile (see Figures 9.3 and 9.4) for the definition of the programme goal.

In combination with the goal values expressed as ICF qualifiers, the expected outcome may also be described as values from specific measures. For example, the more specific description of the goal value (in ICF qualifier 0 = *no problem*) for the intervention target *b7300 Power of isolated muscles and muscle groups* (in areas above the level of the spinal cord lesion) could additionally be described with the expected outcome for specific muscles from the Oxford scale for grading muscle strength (e.g. 5 = *active movement, full range of motion, against gravity and provides normal resistance* for the triceps or deltoids). The same procedure can be performed using more comprehensive measures, such as the Spinal Cord Independence Measure, which measures an individual's independence in activities related to self-care (e.g. feeding, bathing and bladder and bowel management) and mobility (transferring, indoor mobility, etc.) in persons with spinal cord injury. While the measures for the different specific items of the Spinal Cord Independence Measure (SCIM) related to self-care and mobility activities can be used to define the goal values in the according intervention targets, the summary score of the entire measure can be used to define the rather broad cycle and programme goals.

However, since this information is sometimes very specific and can therefore only be understood by the experts from the different specialties, this may be too specific for the shared documentation available for all team members. Therefore, ICF qualifiers provide a common language for the levels of functioning for the rehabilitation team as a whole. Nevertheless, the specific values should always be available for those who are responsible for the evaluation of the goal achievement in the different domains of functioning.

9.3.3 Evaluation of Goal Achievement

The evaluation of goal achievement will be performed at the end of a defined time frame, in other words at the end of a rehabilitation cycle. This evaluation is important to check if the expected outcome in the defined domains of functioning was achieved or not and hence if the completed rehabilitative interventions were effective. Goal attainment scaling (GAS) is one common method for the evaluation of level of goal achievement (Levack, Dean, Siegert, & McPherson, 2006), but this ICF-based method of goal setting provides an alternative approach to evaluation of goal achievement, which could in fact be easily combined with the GAS approach if preferred.

For the evaluation of goal achievement, a reassessment in the domains of functioning that were defined as a goal or intervention targets has to be performed. To document the results and allow the evaluation of goal achievement, the ICF Evaluation Display is available (see Figure 9.6). In this documentation form, only those ICF categories are listed which were identified as intervention targets during the goal-setting process. The reassessment procedure is the same as in the assessment performed in the beginning, with investigations, examinations, observations or an interview again being performed for each goal and intervention target and rated with an ICF qualifier. These values are then entered into the ICF Evaluation Display as a bar. The results of the goal value (documented in the according column) and the assessment result (ICF qualifier bar) can now be compared and the goal achievement recorded in the column *goal achievement* by using a '✓' for *achieved* or a '-' for not achieved. Thus, the success and failure of goal achievement in the different goals and intervention targets can easily be read (Figure 9.10).

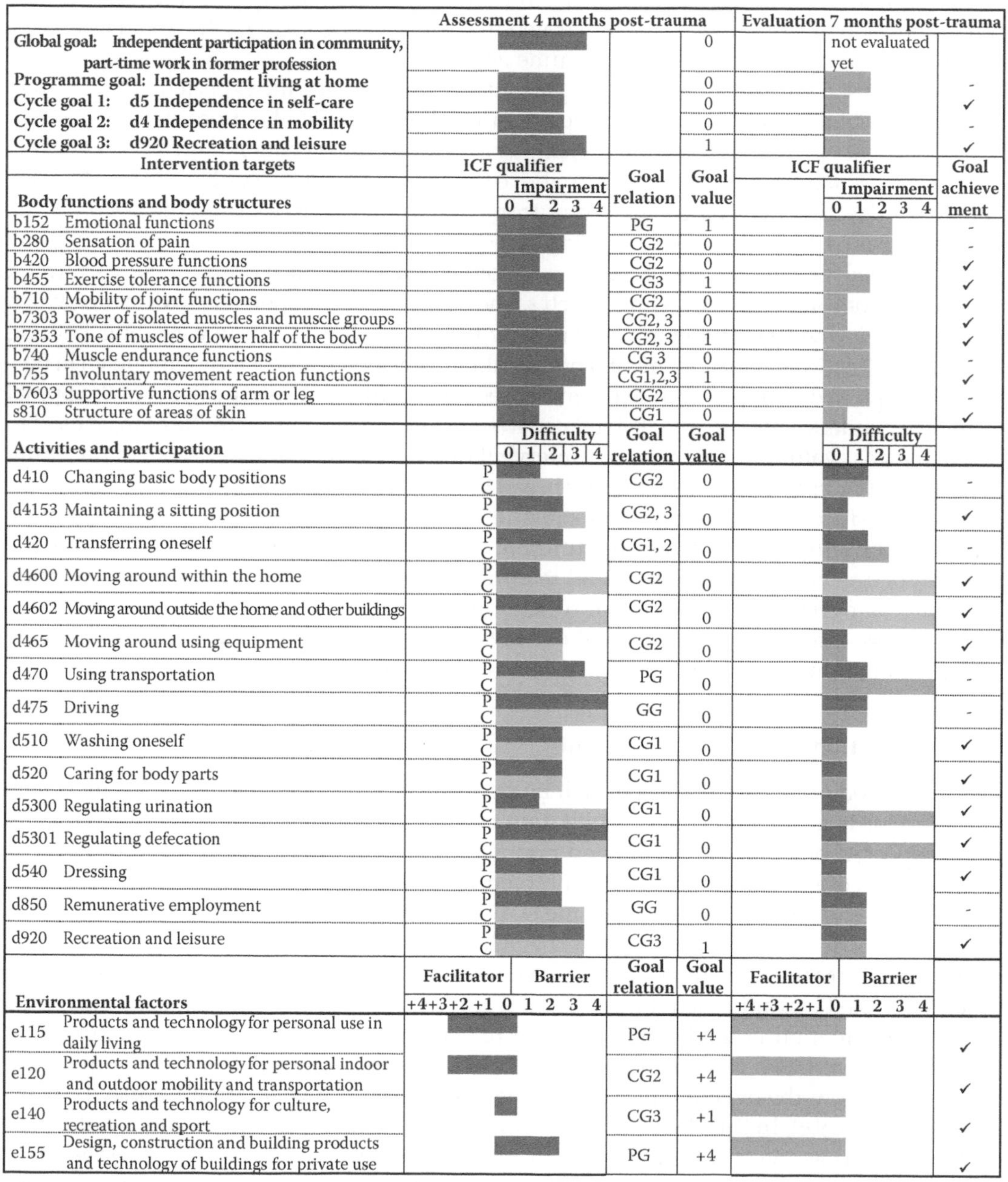

	Assessment 4 months post-trauma		Evaluation 7 months post-trauma	
Global goal: Independent participation in community, part-time work in former profession		0	not evaluated yet	
Programme goal: Independent living at home		0		-
Cycle goal 1: d5 Independence in self-care		0		✓
Cycle goal 2: d4 Independence in mobility		0		-
Cycle goal 3: d920 Recreation and leisure		1		✓

Intervention targets	ICF qualifier Impairment 0 1 2 3 4	Goal relation	Goal value	ICF qualifier Impairment 0 1 2 3 4	Goal achievement
Body functions and body structures					
b152 Emotional functions		PG	1		-
b280 Sensation of pain		CG2	0		-
b420 Blood pressure functions		CG2	0		✓
b455 Exercise tolerance functions		CG3	1		✓
b710 Mobility of joint functions		CG2	0		✓
b7303 Power of isolated muscles and muscle groups		CG2, 3	0		✓
b7353 Tone of muscles of lower half of the body		CG2, 3	1		✓
b740 Muscle endurance functions		CG 3	0		-
b755 Involuntary movement reaction functions		CG1,2,3	1		✓
b7603 Supportive functions of arm or leg		CG2	0		-
s810 Structure of areas of skin		CG1	0		✓
Activities and participation	Difficulty 0 1 2 3 4	Goal relation	Goal value	Difficulty 0 1 2 3 4	
d410 Changing basic body positions	P / C	CG2	0		-
d4153 Maintaining a sitting position	P / C	CG2, 3	0		✓
d420 Transferring oneself	P / C	CG1, 2	0		-
d4600 Moving around within the home	P / C	CG2	0		✓
d4602 Moving around outside the home and other buildings	P / C	CG2	0		✓
d465 Moving around using equipment	P / C	CG2	0		✓
d470 Using transportation	P / C	PG	0		-
d475 Driving	P / C	GG	0		-
d510 Washing oneself	P / C	CG1	0		✓
d520 Caring for body parts	P / C	CG1	0		✓
d5300 Regulating urination	P / C	CG1	0		✓
d5301 Regulating defecation	P / C	CG1	0		✓
d540 Dressing	P / C	CG1	0		✓
d850 Remunerative employment	P / C	GG	0		-
d920 Recreation and leisure	P / C	CG3	1		✓
Environmental factors	Facilitator +4 +3 +2 +1 0 Barrier 1 2 3 4	Goal relation	Goal value	Facilitator +4 +3 +2 +1 0 Barrier 1 2 3 4	
e115 Products and technology for personal use in daily living		PG	+4		✓
e120 Products and technology for personal indoor and outdoor mobility and transportation		CG2	+4		✓
e140 Products and technology for culture, recreation and sport		CG3	+1		✓
e155 Design, construction and building products and technology of buildings for private use		PG	+4		✓

The ICF Evaluation Display lists only ICF categories that were identified as intervention targets.

P = Performance; C = Capacity.

CG1, CG2, CG3, PG, GG = indicates relationship with Cycle Goal 1, 2, or 3, Programme Goal or Global Goal.

FIGURE 9.10

ICF Evaluation Display.

Based on the information contained in the ICF Evaluation Display, the relationships between goal achievement in a goal and an intervention target can be analyzed. This is particularly helpful in those cases when a superior goal was not achieved. In the illustrated case, for example, the goal value in the Cycle Goal 1 *Independence in self-care* was successfully achieved. Furthermore, the analysis of the related intervention targets (marked with CG1 in the column *Goal relation*) shows that all intervention targets related to Cycle Goal 1 were achieved. In contrast, the goal value in Cycle Goal 2 *Independence in mobility* was not achieved. Rehabilitation providers can then consider the reason for this non-achievement and speculate about whether another type of intervention should be attempted or whether the target goals in this or other dimensions of functioning should be revised. The analysis of the related intervention targets (marked with CG2) shows that in the domains *b280 Sensation of pain, b7603 Supportive functions of arm or leg* and *d410 Changing basic body positions*, the goal was not achieved. This analysis provides useful information for future intervention planning.

9.4 Conclusion and Future Development

There is an increasing interest in applications of the ICF in rehabilitation goal-setting practice. The approach presented in this chapter shows how the standardized classification and terminology of the ICF can be applied in rehabilitation management and, in particular, how the use of the ICF Core Sets facilitates a systematic and patient-centred assessment of functioning and, hence, provides meaningful information required for rehabilitation goal setting. For the goal-setting process, practitioners can make use of this functioning-oriented information for the selection of goals from different hierarchical levels and describe these goals again using the ICF terminology. This method helps practitioners to not overlook relevant domains of functioning and thus ensures a functioning-oriented approach to rehabilitation management. However, to optimize the implementation of the ICF for rehabilitation goal setting, some future developments may be helpful.

Standardized goal categories, as developed by Rentsch and Bucher (2005), facilitate the selection of goals and the collection of data regarding rehabilitation goals and, thus, more insights into rehabilitation goals. From this perspective, the development of additional goal categories based on the ICF terminology for the different hierarchical levels and, tentatively, for specific ICF Core Sets could ease the time demand involved in the goal-setting process. However, the individuality and patient centredness of rehabilitation goals should still be taken into account, even when applying standardized rehabilitation goals.

The use of ICF qualifiers for describing levels of functioning and goal values for rehabilitation goals, as illustrated in this chapter, presents both benefits and challenges. The possibility to create profiles of an individual's level of functioning across various domains provides a helpful overview and helps identify the main areas of problems and needs. However, the rating of an assessment result within an ICF qualifier has not yet been operationalized, let alone empirically tested for all ICF categories, and hence lacks empirical evidence of reliability and validity (Grill, Mansmann, Cieza, & Stucki, 2007; Starrost et al., 2008). A first attempt towards an operationalization of ICF qualifiers was performed by Grill, Gloor-Juzi, Huber and Stucki (2011) for ICF categories related to physiotherapeutic intervention targets. Such an operationalization is a promising approach towards the reliable use of ICF qualifiers for describing levels of functioning and defining goal values for specific goal areas and intervention targets.

In conclusion, while future work will contribute to the optimization of the implementation of the ICF in rehabilitation goal setting, this chapter has demonstrated that the ICF, and in particular ICF Core Sets, provides a useful conceptual framework, classification and tools for the identification and description of rehabilitation goals and ones that are ready for application to rehabilitation now. In the future, there is also the need to evaluate this and other approaches of the ICF implementation into clinical practice as this is done only rarely to date (Wiegand, Belting, Fekete, Gutenbrunner, & Reinhardt, 2012). This chapter has addressed some of the main aims of the ICF in the practice of rehabilitation goal setting, that is to say to apply the ICF as a clinical tool for treatment planning, assessment and evaluation and as a research tool for outcome measurement and for information management.

Acknowledgement

The authors thank Annette Frischmann for reviewing this chapter.

References

Bornman, J., & Murphy, J. (2006). Using the ICF in goal setting: Clinical application using Talking Mats. *Disability and Rehabilitation: Assistive Technology, 1*(3), 145–154.

Bovend'Eerdt, T. J., Botell, R. E., & Wade, D. T. (2009). Writing SMART rehabilitation goals and achieving goal attainment scaling: A practical guide. *Clinical Rehabilitation, 23*(4), 352–361.

Cieza, A., Ewert, T., Ustun, T. B., Chatterji, S., Kostanjsek, N., & Stucki, G. (2004). Development of ICF Core Sets for patients with chronic conditions. *Journal of Rehabilitation Medicine,* (44 Suppl.), 9–11.

Geyh, S., Muller, R., Peter, C., Bickenbach, J. E., Post, M. W., Stucki, G., & Cieza, A. (2011). Capturing the psychologic-personal perspective in spinal cord injury. *American Journal of Physical Medicine and Rehabilitation, 90*(11 Suppl. 2), S79–S96.

Geyh, S., Peter, C., Muller, R., Bickenbach, J. E., Kostanjsek, N., Ustun, B. T., ... Cieza, A. (2011). The Personal Factors of the International Classification of Functioning, Disability and Health in the literature – A systematic review and content analysis. *Disability and Rehabilitation, 33*(13–14), 1089–1102.

Grill, E., Ewert, T., Chatterji, S., Kostanjsek, N., & Stucki, G. (2005). ICF Core Sets development for the acute hospital and early post-acute rehabilitation facilities. *Disability and Rehabilitation, 27*(7–8), 361–366.

Grill, E., Gloor-Juzi, T., Huber, E. O., & Stucki, G. (2011). Assessment of functioning in the acute hospital: Operationalisation and reliability testing of ICF categories relevant for physical therapists interventions. *Journal of Rehabilitation Medicine, 43*(2), 162–173.

Grill, E., Huber, E. O., Gloor-Juzi, T., & Stucki, G. (2010). Intervention goals determine physical therapists' workload in the acute care setting. *Physical Therapy, 90*(10), 1468–1478.

Grill, E., Mansmann, U., Cieza, A., & Stucki, G. (2007). Assessing observer agreement when describing and classifying functioning with the International Classification of Functioning, Disability and Health. *Journal of Rehabilitation Medicine, 39*(1), 71–76.

Grotkamp, S., Cibis, W., Behrens, J., Bucher, P. O., Deetjen, W., Nyffeler, I. D., … Seger, W. (2010). Personbezogene Faktoren der ICF – Entwurf der AG "ICF" des Fachbereichs II der Deutschen Gesellschaft für Sozialmedizin und Prävention (DGSMP) [Personal contextual factors of the ICF draft from the Working Group "ICF" of Specialty Group II of the German Society for Social Medicine and Prevention]. *Gesundheitswesen, 72*(12), 908–916.

Harty, M., Griesel, M., & van der Merwe, A. (2011). The ICF as a common language for rehabilitation goal-setting: Comparing client and professional priorities. *Health and Quality of Life Outcomes, 9*, 87.

Huber, E. O., Tobler, A., Gloor-Juzi, T., Grill, E., & Gubler-Gut, B. (2011). The ICF as a way to specify goals and to assess the outcome of physiotherapeutic interventions in the acute hospital. *Journal of Rehabilitation Medicine, 43*(2), 174–177.

Hurn, J., Kneebone, I., & Cropley, M. (2006). Goal setting as an outcome measure: A systematic review. *Clinical Rehabilitation, 20*(9), 756 772.

Itzkovich, M., Gelernter, I., Biering-Sorensen, F., Weeks, C., Laramee, M. T., Craven, B. C., … Catz, A. (2007). The Spinal Cord Independence Measure (SCIM) version III: Reliability and validity in a multi-center international study. *Disability and Rehabilitation, 29*(24), 1926–1933.

Kirchberger, I., Cieza, A., Biering-Sorensen, F., Baumberger, M., Charlifue, S., Post, M. W., … Stucki, G. (2010). ICF Core Sets for individuals with spinal cord injury in the early post-acute context. *Spinal Cord, 48*(4), 297–304.

Kus, S., Muller, M., Strobl, R., & Grill, E. (2011). Patient goals in post-acute geriatric rehabilitation – Goal attainment is an indicator for improved functioning. *Journal of Rehabilitation Medicine, 43*(2), 156–161.

Levack, W. M. M., Dean, S. G., Siegert, R. J., & McPherson, K. M. (2006). Purposes and mechanisms of goal planning in rehabilitation: The need for a critical distinction. *Disability and Rehabilitation, 28*(12), 741–749.

Lohmann, S., Decker, J., Muller, M., Strobl, R., & Grill, E. (2011). The ICF forms a useful framework for classifying individual patient goals in post-acute rehabilitation. *Journal of Rehabilitation Medicine, 43*(2), 151–155.

Martinuzzi, A., Salghetti, A., Betto, S., Russo, E., Leonardi, M., Raggi, A., & Francescutti, C. (2010). The International Classification of Functioning Disability and Health, version for children and youth as a roadmap for projecting and programming rehabilitation in a neuropaediatric hospital unit. *Journal of Rehabilitation Medicine, 42*(1), 49–55.

Mittrach, R., Grill, E., Walchner-Nonjean, M., Scheuringer, M., Boldt, C., Huber, E., & Stucki, G. (2008). Goals of physiotherapy interventions can be described using the International Classification of Functioning, Disability and Health. *Physiotherapy, 94*(2), 150–157.

Muller, M., Strobl, R., & Grill, E. (2011). Goals of patients with rehabilitation needs in acute hospitals: Goal achievement is an indicator for improved functioning. *Journal of Rehabilitation Medicine, 43*(2), 145–150.

Playford, E. D., Siegert, R., Levack, W., & Freeman, J. (2009). Areas of consensus and controversy about goal setting in rehabilitation: A conference report. *Clinical Rehabilitation, 23*(4), 334–344.

Power, E., Anderson, A., & Togher, L. (2011). Applying the WHO ICF framework to communication assessment and goal setting in Huntington's disease: A case discussion. *Journal of Communication Disorders, 44*(3), 261–275.

Rauch, A., Cieza, A., & Stucki, G. (2008). How to apply the International Classification of Functioning, Disability and Health (ICF) for rehabilitation management in clinical practice. *European Journal of Physical and Rehabilitation Medicine, 44*(3), 329–342.

Rauch, A., Escorpizo, R., Riddle, D. L., Eriks-Hoogland, I., Stucki, G., & Cieza, A. (2010). Using a case report of a patient with spinal cord injury to illustrate the application of the International Classification of Functioning, Disability and Health during multidisciplinary patient management. *Physical Therapy, 90*(7), 1039–1052.

Rauch, A., Lückenkemper, M., & Cieza, A. (2012). Use of ICF Core Sets in clinical practice. In J. Bickenbach, A. Cieza, A. Rauch, & G. Stucki (Eds.), *ICF Core Sets – Manual for clinical practice*. Göttingen, Germany: Hogrefe.

Rentsch, H. P., & Bucher, P. O. (2005). *ICF in der rehabilitation.* Idstein, Germany: Schulz-Kirchner Verlag.

Soberg, H. L., Sandvik, L., & Ostensjo, S. (2008). Reliability and applicability of the ICF in coding problems, resources and goals of persons with multiple injuries. *Disability and Rehabilitation, 30*(2), 98–106.

Starrost, K., Geyh, S., Trautwein, A., Grunow, J., Ceballos-Baumann, A., Prosiegel, M., … Cieza, A. (2008). Interrater reliability of the extended ICF core set for stroke applied by physical therapists. *Physical Therapy, 88*(7), 841–851.

Steiner, W. A., Ryser, L., Huber, E., Uebelhart, D., Aeschlimann, A., & Stucki, G. (2002). Use of the ICF model as a clinical problem-solving tool in physical therapy and rehabilitation medicine. *Physical Therapy, 82*(11), 1098–1107.

Stucki, G. (2005). International Classification of Functioning, Disability, and Health (ICF): A promising framework and classification for rehabilitation medicine. *American Journal of Physical Medicine and Rehabilitation, 84*(10), 733–740.

Stucki, G., Cieza, A., Ewert, T., Kostanjsek, N., Chatterji, S., & Ustun, T. B. (2002). Application of the International Classification of Functioning, Disability and Health (ICF) in clinical practice. *Disability and Rehabilitation, 24*(5), 281–282.

Stucki, G., Cieza, A., & Melvin, J. (2007). The International Classification of Functioning, Disability and Health (ICF): A unifying model for the conceptual description of the rehabilitation strategy. *Journal of Rehabilitation Medicine, 39*(4), 279–285.

Stucki, G., Kostanjsek, N., Ustun, B., & Cieza, A. (2008). ICF-based classification and measurement of functioning. *European Journal of Physical and Rehabilitation Medicine, 44*(3), 315–328.

Ustun, B., Chatterji, S., & Kostanjsek, N. (2004). Comments from WHO for the Journal of Rehabilitation Medicine special supplement on ICF core sets. *Journal of Rehabilitation Medicine* (44 Suppl.), 7–8.

Wade, D. T. (2009). Goal setting in rehabilitation: An overview of what, why and how. *Clinical Rehabilitation, 23*(4), 291–295.

WHO. (2001). *International classification of functioning, disability and health.* Geneva, Switzerland: World Health Organization.

WHO. (2006). *The international classification of functioning, disability and health, children and youth version: ICF-CY.* Geneva, Switzerland: World Health Organization.

Wiegand, N. M., Belting, J., Fekete, C., Gutenbrunner, C., & Reinhardt, J. D. (2012). All talk, no action?: The global diffusion and clinical implementation of the international classification of functioning, disability, and health. [Review]. *American Journal of Physical Medicine and Rehabilitation, 91*(7), 550–560.

10

Occupation-Based, Client-Centred Approach to Goal Planning and Measurement

Emmah Doig and Jennifer Fleming

CONTENTS

10.1 Introduction

Goal planning is a commonly used practice in rehabilitation; however, approaches vary with no *gold standard*. Despite its widespread use in rehabilitation, research on the effectiveness of goal-planning approaches is still an emerging area (Levack et al., 2006). This chapter seeks to describe and discuss a client-centred, occupation-based approach to goal planning, as well as present recent evidence related to the clinical utility and effectiveness of this approach with clients in a rehabilitation setting. By the end of this chapter, it is expected that the reader will have knowledge about what *occupation* is and the potential benefits of occupation-based goal planning, how occupational therapists use occupation as a therapeutic tool in rehabilitation, how occupation can form the basis for goal planning in rehabilitation, client-centred practice, the Canadian Occupational Performance Measure (COPM) and the clinical utility of the combined use of the COPM and goal attainment scaling (GAS) to plan goals and structure a rehabilitation programme. This chapter will also discuss the application of and challenges to applying client-centred goal planning in teams, challenges of goal planning in different rehabilitation environments and strategies to enhance consideration of environmental factors when goal planning.

10.2 Occupation

Occupation means paid employment to most people; however, the *occupation* in occupational therapy means something more. Occupation has been variously defined as

- 'Activities that people engage in through-out their daily lives to fulfil their time and give life meaning' (Hinojosa & Kramer, 1997, p. 865).
- 'Activities… of everyday life, named, organised, and given value and meaning by individuals and a culture. Occupation is everything people do to occupy themselves, including looking after themselves… enjoying life… and contributing to the social and economic fabric of their communities' (Law, Polatajko, Baptiste, & Townsend, 1997, p. 32).
- 'Goal-directed pursuits that typically extend over time, having meaning to their performance, and involving multiple tasks' (Christiansen, Baum, & Bass-Haugen, 2005, p. 548).

Occupational performance has furthermore been described as a product of the interaction between the environment or context (i.e. cultural, physical, social) of the client, the demands of the activity (i.e. required space, tools, skills) and client or person factors (i.e. bodily functions, values and beliefs) (Roley et al., 2008). Occupational performance is 'the dynamic experience of a person engaged in purposeful activities and tasks within an environment' (Law et al., 1996, p. 16). This interdependent relationship between person, environment and occupation is fundamental to occupational therapy theoretical models such as the Canadian Model of Occupational Performance (Townsend & Polatajko, 2007). Since occupational performance encompasses activities in the areas of self-care, productivity and leisure and is influenced by environmental and societal factors (Reed & Sanderson, 1980), occupational performance is unique to each person and requires individualized measurement tools sensitive to varying needs and situations (Pollock, 1993). These principles provide the framework of an occupation-based, client-centred approach to goal planning.

10.2.1 Occupation in Occupational Therapy

Since the founding of the profession after World War I, the concept of using meaningful occupations or purposeful activities as therapeutic modalities has underpinned the philosophical basis of occupational therapy (Golledge, 1998). The selection of and engagement in meaningful occupations as *therapy* is a core intervention typically used by occupational therapists. Occupational therapy frameworks break down occupations into categories or occupational performance areas including activities of daily living (i.e. self-care, mobility, meal preparation, shopping), work and productive activities (i.e. paid work, volunteering) and play or leisure activities (i.e. socializing, play or recreational activities) (Roley et al., 2008). When problems are identified in areas of an individual's occupational performance, these areas can provide the basis for rehabilitation goals. Occupation, used as a framework for formulating rehabilitation goals, offers a formalized, structured approach to individualized goal planning allowing the practitioner to categorize what people do in their everyday lives and gain an insight into what activities characterize individuals' lives and give their life meaning.

The occupational therapy process (illustrated by Figure 10.1) in a rehabilitation context typically involves assessment of what occupations are important and meaningful to a person in the context of their life roles. It is a client-centred process which endeavours to consider problems in occupational performance from the client's perspective. Standardized testing relevant to the client's injury or illness is used in conjunction with assessment of occupational performance to plan treatment. An initial focus for occupational therapists in

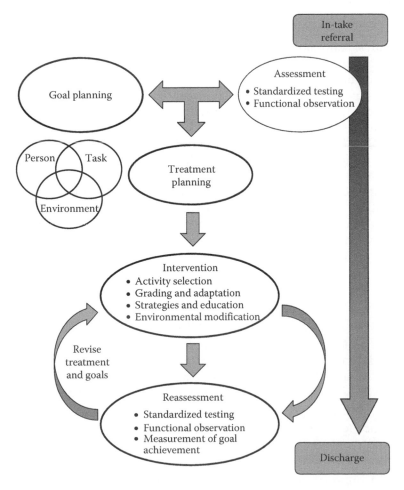

FIGURE 10.1
Summary of occupational therapy process.

rehabilitation is to determine any limitations in performing the tasks which constitute participation in valued occupational roles usually through assessment of the client performing these activities. To further define occupational roles and performance components, consider the case where a young woman has acquired an upper limb amputation. She tells the practitioner she is most concerned about how the loss of her non-dominant hand is impacting on her ability to look after her baby including carrying, positioning, washing and changing the baby. She is having difficulties with many of the activities which enable her to fulfil her occupational role of *mother*. These activities or *occupations* then become the basis for her rehabilitation goals.

An occupational therapist would carry out an *activity analysis* or *task analysis* during an observational assessment of the client performing the tasks to assist with treatment planning. Task analysis enables an occupational therapist to determine how to appropriately grade and adapt or modify tasks and environments to achieve a client's goals. Task analysis involves observation and examination of an activity to determine the components or steps (i.e. listing the steps), the level of capability needed (i.e. abilities needed for successful accomplishment) as well as environmental and task constraints (Trombly, 1995). Task analysis aids a practitioner to target treatment efforts and use tasks therapeutically as it shows where and why performance is breaking down. One example of a formalized assessment employing task analysis methodology is the Perceive, Recall, Plan and Perform (PRPP) system of task analysis developed by Chapparo and Ranka (2002). The PRPP uses a process-oriented, criterion-referenced system to determine problems with cognitive information processing during task performance (Chapparo & Ranka, 2002). Task analysis also assists with goal planning by applying the same process to break down client goals, which may be stated very broadly as end goals (i.e. return to driving, living independently, returning to work), into smaller tasks or short-term goals. Furthermore, this skill aids the practitioner to consider what gradual steps are needed in order to reach the end goal. This facilitates the use of *grading* and *adaptation*, which are techniques used by occupational therapists to assist clients in achieving desired task performance.

To illustrate an occupational therapy approach to using occupation incorporating grading and adaptation, consider further the case of the mother who has a traumatic below-elbow amputation. When working on the goal of her being able to independently change her baby's nappy, an occupational therapist may use direct involvement in the activity to achieve desired performance of the task by

- Modifying the environment (i.e. setting up necessary items in the environment so they can be accessed with the available hand)
- Modifying the task or method of accomplishing the task by using
  - *Adaptation* (e.g. doing some steps in an adapted way such as adding a prosthetic device to aid with grasp on the affected side or compensating by eliminating some task steps such as using a restraint strap on the change table to secure baby whilst changing to eliminate the need for bilateral use of hands)
  - *Grading* or pacing the activity appropriately to gradually maximize performance (e.g. aiming for increasing speed of performance with practice or gradually reducing the number of steps of the tasks that are assisted whilst learning new techniques)
- Aiming to improve performance components or to address impairments that may be contributing to poor occupational performance (i.e. working on reducing hypersensitivity of the skin on the affected upper limb)

Whilst this illustration demonstrates the mechanics of what occupational therapists may do in a therapeutic context, the main focus driving the rehabilitation efforts and therapeutic activities is founded during initial goal planning with the client. Using an occupation-based, client-centred approach to goal planning means that the tasks worked on and the skills and performance components restored during rehabilitation efforts are the ones that the client wants to work on and needs to be able to do to fulfil their most important, meaningful and valued daily occupations.

10.2.2 Determining Meaningful Occupational Goals

Due to the interaction of person, environment and activity factors which make up occupational performance, the nature of occupations that individuals engage in are unique to each person's life situation. Therefore, understanding the occupations that a person engages in and how they are unique to that person (i.e. performance level, environmental barriers and facilitators, activity factors) can only be determined by understanding the client's perspective and experience of their life. The nature of occupation and what it means to a person can only be determined by talking to the client about how they feel and think about the occupation – as occupation is subjectively experienced. For example, the occupation of *being a worker* for one person may be *enriching* and *pleasurable* whilst for another may be *a chore*. Hence, what is involved in how each person fulfils their roles and daily occupations needs to be determined in consultation and partnership with clients. If goals are assigned based on your assumptions of what a rehabilitation client needs to achieve with little or no consultation with the client about his or her life circumstances and what is important to him or her, how do you know if the goals will be meaningful to that person? Will the client understand what they are working toward and will they be motivated to participate in rehabilitation? How will you know if those goals will make a difference to their performance in their daily occupations and how will you know if the goals are relevant to the client's environmental context (i.e. will they be able to carry over improvements in their real-life environment)?

Clients are experts regarding their own occupations, and in order for rehabilitation practitioners to understand what constitutes meaningful occupations for their clients, clinicians need to practise in a client-centred manner.

10.2.3 Client-Centredness

A client-centred approach involves using goals that are set by the client where they define the problems. This enables a sense of self-determination and control, enhancing the potential for active participation of the client (Pollock, 1993). Client-centred rehabilitation has also been described from the perspective of people with long-term physical disability as involving individualization of programmes to meet needs including preparation for life in the real world, mutual participation with health professionals in decision making and goal setting, meaningful outcomes and family involvement throughout the rehabilitation process (Cott, 2004). The use of goals in rehabilitation can facilitate a client-centred approach as goals can be uniquely adapted to define and measure each individual's occupations and levels of performance.

There is a growing body of research evidence that supports the effectiveness of client-centred approaches to goal planning and rehabilitation with adults undergoing neurological rehabilitation. Gagne and Hoppes (2003) found a collaborative, goal-focused approach to rehabilitation of self-care skills resulted in better outcomes in upper body dressing for an inpatient rehabilitation group compared to a control group. Bodiam (1999) also found improvement in self-rated performance and satisfaction in goal areas for a group of 17 participants with a variety of neurological disorders receiving an inpatient occupational therapy programme. Ownsworth, Fleming, Shum, Kuipers, and Strong (2008) found gains in performance and satisfaction in goal areas when client-centred goal planning was used with 35 community-dwelling participants with traumatic brain injury (TBI) undergoing group and individual occupation-based therapy. Similarly, a client-centred goal-planning approach in two separate studies of participants with TBI undergoing outpatient rehabilitation indicated improvements in self-rated performance, satisfaction and goal attainment between admission and discharge (Trombly, Radomski, & Davis, 1998; Trombly, Radomski, Trexel, & Burnet-Smith, 2002). Furthermore, a group of participants with TBI ($n = 38$) and stroke ($n = 117$) receiving a short-term (up to 12 weeks) client-centred, goal-directed outpatient occupational therapy programme made significant gains in self-perceived performance and satisfaction in goal areas (Phipps & Richardson, 2007). Similar gains in goal achievement were demonstrated in a case description of a man who sustained a severe TBI followed by a stroke who received goal-directed multidisciplinary, inpatient rehabilitation (Wilson, Evans, & Keobane, 2002).

Studies have shown that clients achieve better outcomes and participation in rehabilitation when they are involved in goal planning. Webb and Glueckauf (1994) found that direct involvement in individualized goal planning resulted in better maintenance of treatment gains for a group of outpatients with acquired brain injury. Wressle, Eeg-Olofsson, Marcusson, and Henriksson (2002) compared a group ($n = 88$) whose rehabilitation goals were formulated using a client-centred approach (the COPM) with a control group ($n = 55$) and found that the client-centred approach resulted in greater perceived participation in goal planning and higher self-perceived ability to manage after rehabilitation. Holliday, Cano, Freeman, and Playford (2007) used a structured, joint goal-planning model to increase participation in goal planning in patients in an inpatient neurorehabilitation unit. They found this approach led to increased satisfaction with rehabilitation, more participation level goals, greater perceived autonomy and perception that goals were more relevant compared to a usual care model characterized by a therapist-assigned approach to goal planning. Whilst the concept of client-centredness has been endorsed in the literature, recent studies investigating the goal-planning process in inpatient hospital settings have indicated that, in practice, goal planning appears to be predominantly therapist-led (Leach, Cornwell, Fleming, & Haines, 2010; Levack, Dean, Siegert, & McPherson, 2011).

The effectiveness of rehabilitation based on client-centred, occupation-based goal-planning approaches has mainly been investigated in the field of occupational therapy. There has been a large body of clinical research related to the use of a well-established, client-centred, occupation-based assessment tool: the COPM.

10.3 Canadian Occupational Performance Measure

The COPM, based on the Canadian Model of Occupational Performance, is an individualized, client-centred tool, developed for use by occupational therapists in the assessment of outcomes of clients with a wide range of disabilities at any developmental stage (Law et al., 1998). The COPM is designed to identify problems in occupational performance areas that are of importance to individuals and to measure change in occupational performance (Law et al., 1998). A literature review conducted 13 years after the COPM was first published demonstrated the COPM to be a reliable, valid, clinically useful and responsive outcome measure that has been used with a wide range of client groups in varied settings (Carswell et al., 2004). The review also found that the COPM has been used to demonstrate the effectiveness of occupational therapy interventions, to enhance client-centred practice by providing a foundation for goal selection and to facilitate individualized and meaningful interventions (Carswell et al., 2004).

The COPM is a self-rated tool which is administered by interviewing the client to identify occupational performance problems, concerns or issues in three occupational performance domains: self-care, productivity and leisure. The self-care domain is concerned with personal care (e.g. dressing, hygiene), functional mobility (e.g. transfers) and community management (e.g. transport, shopping). The productivity domain is concerned with work and household management (e.g. cleaning, cooking) and play or school (e.g. homework, study). The leisure domain is concerned with quiet recreation (e.g. hobbies, reading), active recreation (e.g. sport, travel) and socialization (e.g. visiting, parties). Clients are asked to identify activities that they would typically perform and any activities which are difficult to perform to their satisfaction. Clients are then asked to rate the importance of each activity on a scale from 1 (not important at all) to 10 (extremely important). This enables the practitioner to determine which occupational performance areas are of highest priority to the client, and this information is used to formulate the client's goals. Finally, clients are asked to rate themselves according to their perception of their *performance* of each task on a scale from 1 (not able to perform) to 10 (able to perform extremely well), as well as their *satisfaction* with their performance in each area on a scale from 1 (not satisfied at all) to 10 (extremely satisfied). Total performance and satisfaction scores are generated by dividing the sum of performance and total satisfaction scores, respectively, by the number of occupational performance areas. A change equal to or more than two points in performance or satisfaction scores post-intervention is deemed to be a clinically significant change. Importantly, the COPM is a *client-centred* tool because it is designed to generate a list of occupational performance problem areas from the client's perspective and subsequent outcomes are measured according to the client's own perception of their performance and their self-rated satisfaction with performance.

10.3.1 Benefits and Limitations of the COPM

A limitation of the COPM involves its validity when used with clients with reduced insight or self-awareness (Doig, Fleming, Cornwell, & Kuipers, 2010; Tryssenaar, Jones, & Lee, 1999) as the success of the COPM in client-centred goal planning is contingent on the client being able to self-identify problem areas. Furthermore, the success of the COPM to measure rehabilitation outcomes relies on the person's ability to accurately and realistically self-rate changes in performance over time. To overcome this limitation, proxy COPM ratings by significant others have been used to reliably gather information where clients cannot accurately report on their own occupational performance. For example, studies have used proxy ratings from significant others of clients with severe TBI (Doig et al., 2010), family caregivers of people with Alzheimer's disease (McGrath, Meuller, Brown, Teitelman, & Watts, 2000) and caregivers of young children (McGavin, 1998; Pollock & Stewart, 1998).

A benefit of the COPM is its motivational value. Conducting a successful initial assessment using the COPM as a goal-planning tool is enhanced when the practitioner is a skilled interviewer who enlists motivational interviewing techniques including empathetic listening and collaborative decision making which values client autonomy (Miller & Rollnick, 2002). A client-centred goal-planning approach is itself a motivational technique, as client-centredness is aligned with the core philosophies of motivational interviewing including joint decision making, upholding the client's perspective and drawing on the client's own goals and values to evoke motivation and autonomy where the client is free to make their own decisions about change (Miller & Rollnick, 2002; Rollnick, Miller & Butler, 2008).

The COPM may often be the starting point of therapeutic contact with a client and lay the foundations for a trusting therapeutic alliance. Using a client-centred approach means conducting the interview in the spirit of mutual, collaborative decision making where the practitioner is committed to client autonomy. A positive, supportive relationship between the therapist and client has been identified as a facilitator of goal planning, particularly where the client is directing and the therapist is supportive in goal achievement (Kuipers, Carlson, Bailey, & Sharma, 2004). However, when translating the client's stated desires in occupational performance areas into therapeutic goals, users of the COPM need to be cautious about imposing their beliefs about what constitutes a relevant goal for an individual. The COPM provides a framework to guide a semi-structured interview with clients, and therefore, the exchange between the therapist and client and resulting goal planning may be mediated by the values of the therapist. The therapist comes to the interview with knowledge of a range of contextual issues (e.g. therapeutic resources or time available to work on a goal) and may have an impression of a client's ability from reports, assessment and observations or may conduct further assessment post goal planning. This may lead to the therapist making judgements about the *achievability* or *relevancy* of the client's goals. For example, goals may be perceived as unachievable given the client's assessed limitations, which may lead to redirection or modification of client goals, or goals may not be able to be worked on due to a range of contextual issues.

A qualitative study which used conversation analysis of audio- and videotaped goal-setting meetings in an inpatient neurological rehabilitation unit showed that decision making about goal formulation was heavily shaped by professional influences (Barnard, Cruice, & Playford, 2010). Notably, the treating team never agreed to goals that they did not consider achievable within the time frame of the admission (Barnard et al., 2010). Playford, Siegert, Levack, and Freeman (2009) summarized significant areas of consensus about goal setting based on findings of a systematic review and presentations given and discussions held during a conference attended by 24 invited rehabilitation professionals working in the field of goal setting. One of the conclusions that was reached about the process of goal setting was that concern about achievability may inhibit application of a client-centred care philosophy and that ambitious or difficult-to-achieve goals may be important to incorporate (Playford et al., 2009).

Steering a client away from ambitious goals for whatever reason, be it to prevent a client from experiencing a potential likely failure or pursuing an alternative goal that the therapist or family member may perceive as a higher priority should be weighed alongside the potential negative consequences. These may include a potential negative impact on the therapeutic relationship, client hopes, client level of empowerment and the client's level of motivation to pursue goals that may not be as important or meaningful for them. The therapeutic value of the journey in pursuing a goal that may be perceived by the therapist to be an *ambitious* goal that subsequently may not be achieved should be considered. For example, the process may provide an opportunity for the client to make their own judgements and adjust their perceptions of what may be relevant and achievable, within a supportive therapeutic context. A supportive therapeutic context includes building self-efficacy and includes action planning and coping strategies to increase resilience in the face of setbacks as well as use of goal performance as feedback to make adjustments to goal plans (Scobbie, Dixon, & Wyke, 2011). The challenge for clinicians is to strive to practise in a client-centred manner despite the obvious barriers in different contexts and to be conscious of how our belief systems may influence the client-centred process. We need to consider that a client-centred process can be a facilitator of a strong therapeutic alliance and that this is important for the rehabilitation process, especially where clients have impaired self-awareness such as in neurorehabilitation settings (Schonberger, Humle, & Teasdale, 2006).

There are unique challenges to client-centred goal planning when working with clients who have impaired self-awareness. Individuals with impaired self-awareness commonly experience difficulty understanding the impairments resulting from their injury as well as the impact of these impairments on their ability to function (Fleming, Strong & Ashton, 1996; Mateer, 1999; Sherer et al., 1998). Impaired self-awareness manifests as a discrepancy between actual and self-perceived performance whereby the client perceives less limitations or difficulties in their performance than are observed or reported by others. Therefore, impaired self-awareness may lead to difficulties with goal planning due to the client not identifying problems or underestimating the impact of problems. Clinicians working with clients who have difficulty identifying goals and engaging in rehabilitation can work at building a therapeutic alliance where clients arrive at a point where they may be willing to negotiate and trust suggestions that a therapist may make. This may involve the client taking some risks or having a go at working on goals that they may not at first be fully engaged in, in order to participate in rehabilitation programmes. This concept highlights an interesting tension between client-centredness and the therapeutic relationship where the client is supposed to *trust* the therapist's opinion. The experience of participating in a rehabilitation programme and achieving goals (even if they are therapist-led) has shown promise for enhancing self-awareness (Doig et al., 2010), which subsequently may enable clients to more accurately identify problems with occupational performance and participate in further goal planning.

10.3.2 Top-Down versus Bottom-Up Assessments

Many of the assessment approaches used in the field of rehabilitation are *bottom up* in nature, meaning, they assess skills or components of skills using screening tests or questionnaires designed to confirm the presence of an impairment and measure changes in impairments. Top-down assessments are concerned with assessing functional performance through observation of tasks, which reveals the implications of impairments. The COPM is a *top-down* assessment. Rather than considering the presence of individual impairments and making presumptions about the impact of those impairments on function, the COPM framework asks the practitioner to think broadly about occupational performance or everyday functioning of a person within the context of his or her life. Therefore, the implications of any impairments uncovered using *bottom-up* assessments are considered subsequently in terms of 'how might these impairments be influencing my client's occupational performance within their environmental, social and personal context'.

Impairment-based assessments are necessary and valuable in a rehabilitation context and both bottom-up and top-down assessments should be used in conjunction to reliably determine the presence of impairments and understand how the person's functional abilities may have changed (Grieve & Gnanasekaran, 2008). Subsequent to intervention, top-down and bottom-up assessments can reliably assess change in impairments and functional abilities. Top-down assessments are particularly valuable in rehabilitation settings as they usually involve observation of task performance, which enables the therapist to see the impact that impairments have on occupational performance and, subsequently, inform treatment. For example, consider a person who exhibits impairment of executive functions on standardized assessment of cognitive abilities. They also demonstrate some intellectual awareness of their cognitive impairment when describing difficulties with cooking meals. However, it is only when you see the person cooking a meal that you can determine whether the person is safe to cook independently (i.e. whether they demonstrate anticipatory awareness and use compensatory strategies to overcome their impairments in executive functions or whether they make errors and are unaware of the errors until they are prompted). Thus, assessment of occupational performance, ideally observational assessment of tasks in the person's real-life environment, indicates where it is necessary to intervene and how to intervene to improve performance.

Using a *top-down* or occupation-based approach to guide goal planning means the language of the goals is more likely to be in terms of occupational performance. Goals stated using *occupation* or functional performance (i.e. independence in walking) rather than impairment-based goals (i.e. lower limb strength) are potentially more motivating as they have more personal and practical meaning to the client. Where rehabilitation efforts aim to improve individual impairments, the framing of the goals using an occupation-based process to goal planning ensures that the client understands and can see the link between rehabilitation efforts and their rehabilitation goals.

Consider the case of goal planning with a man who has had a stroke where his main impairment is a dominant side hemiplegia with weakness and increased hypertonicity, impacting on the functional use of his hand. First, consider the scenario where a bottom-up approach to goal planning is taken rather than a client-centred, occupation-based approach to plan goals. A typical initial assessment of impairments related to the upper limb (i.e. assessments of strength, degree of hypertonicity, coordination, dexterity, etc., according to norms) and function of the hand (i.e. standardized and observational assessments of hand function) may be conducted. The practitioner may use this information, in conjunction with information about the person's history (i.e. living circumstances, previous level of function, work status), to formulate goals with the client to improve their abilities in the areas of deficit. Goals may involve improving strength, coordination and dexterity, reduction of hypertonicity and improving purposeful use of the hand. These goals and the therapeutic efforts that follow may improve the person's subsequent occupational performance.

Now consider if goal planning evolved using a top-down, occupation-based approach where you first gain an understanding of what are meaningful occupations to the person within the context of their life from their perspective via an interview (e.g. administering the COPM). The initial standardized and observational assessments of upper limb impairment and function are then considered within the context of those meaningful occupations. The importance of areas of occupational performance, according to the COPM assessment, would guide the practitioner as to what observational assessment is necessary in order to further determine the impact of the upper limb impairments on occupational performance.

An occupation-based, client-centred approach has some benefits. From the practitioner's perspective, the broader impact and meaning of the impairments and functional implications seen on an initial assessment, such as loss of strength, coordination, dexterity and inability to hold a cup or toothbrush, can be understood. From the client's perspective, the rehabilitation activities following goal planning using an occupational framework will make sense because the goals will relate to their valued occupations and activities. If the language of the goals is not the language of occupation (i.e. about everyday performance of and/or participation in a meaningful, practical tasks) and is instead written in the language of impairment (i.e. about increasing strength, dexterity, reducing hypertonicity), the client may be less likely to *own* the goals. However, if the client can see a link between the impairment-based rehabilitation goal (i.e. reducing hypertonicity in the upper limb) and what are meaningful occupational goals for the client (i.e. feeling confident about their ability to use a knife and fork so they can eat out at a restaurant), this is likely to improve their motivation to participate in rehabilitation. These motivational concepts are supported by goal planning theory.

Locke and Latham (2002) in their *goal-setting theory* asserted that the rationale for the goal must be clear to direct a person's effort and persistence towards achieving the goal. Furthermore, the concept of achievement of better outcomes and participation in rehabilitation when the client is involved in goal planning is supported by research evidence (Holliday et al. 2007; Webb & Glueckauf, 1994). The words of participants who took part in a client-centred, goal-directed rehabilitation programme for individuals with TBI (Doig, Fleming, Cornwell, & Kuipers, 2009) also provide an insight into how occupation-based goals can be a motivational tool in rehabilitation:

> It could become pretty boring if you aren't aware that hey this is all going to lead to something. (Significant other of participant with TBI)
>
> The goals helped me *focus*. (Participant with TBI)
>
> If you've mastered this one well you want to go onto the next one. (Significant other of participant with TBI)
>
> It gave you targets to achieve and once you achieved them you'd go well dust it up, that was done and you know that you can do it and you can continue to do it. (Participant with TBI)

That is, if the goals are *clear*, they help focus and motivate people towards an endpoint, and if they are *achievable*, they help the person see what he or she has achieved to enhance motivation for subsequent goals (Box 10.1).

BOX 10.1 OCCUPATION-BASED GOAL-PLANNING CHECKLIST

Understandable. Are the goals written in a way that can be understood by the client so they know what they are working towards and how the therapy tasks relate to the goal?

Environment focused. Are the goals relevant to the client's environmental context? Are the details of the goal and the specified outcome realistic in terms of the individual's real-life environment?

Client-centred. Are the goals the client's own goals? Do they want to work on them or are they what the therapist or their family members want them to work on? Are the goals meaningful to the client and individualized to reflect the client's unique circumstances?

Objective. Are the goals objective and specific? Are the outcomes able to be measured by observing/assessing the client's behaviour? Will improvement in goal performance be demonstrable to the client and provide them with meaningful feedback?

10.3.3 Combined Use of COPM and GAS

GAS and the COPM have both been used to plan goals and measure goal achievement in occupational therapy programmes for outpatients with brain injury (Lannin, 2003; Trombly et al., 1998, 2002). Building on this earlier research, we used the COPM and GAS concurrently to plan goals and measure goal outcomes in a research project that was undertaken to explore the process of a client-centred, occupation-focused, goal-directed approach to rehabilitation (Doig et al., 2009). This research investigated the clinical utility of the combined use of the COPM and GAS (Doig et al., 2010), as well as the effectiveness of the programme (Doig, Fleming, Kuipers, Cornwell, & Khan 2011). Furthermore, the research explored the experience of the goal-planning approach and rehabilitation programme from the perspectives of the participants, their significant others and their therapists (Doig et al., 2009). Participants were 14 individuals with severe TBI living in the community who were recently discharged from inpatient brain injury rehabilitation. The procedure for using the COPM and GAS concurrently to plan goals will now be summarized and is also outlined in detail elsewhere (Doig et al., 2010).

GAS has already been discussed in detail in Chapters 7 and 8; therefore, the following is a brief summary. GAS is a well-established, well-recognized tool in which individualized goals can be objectively quantified to measure client progress over time (Kiresuk, Smith, & Cardillo, 1994). GAS, originally developed for use in the field of mental health (Kiresuk & Sherman, 1968), has subsequently been used to measure the outcomes of rehabilitation programmes in a wide variety of settings across the spectrum from inpatient to community, with varying client groups of varied ages (Malec, 1999). GAS has reported high inter-rater reliability and good concurrent validity with other outcome measures (Malec, 1999). One additional benefit attributed to GAS is that although it is primarily designed to evaluate within-subject longitudinal change, GAS also allows the calculation of a standard T-score. The T-score can be used to compare performance between groups and individuals, provided the predictions made at initial evaluation and assessments made at follow-up evaluations are reliable (Ottenbacher & Cusick, 1989). Although the validity of calculating T-scores for GAS has been debated due to the ordinal nature of the data it produces (Tennant, 2007), the T-score provides a means of quantifying goal attainment scores across all of the client's goals to give one outcome score, which is especially useful in research.

The mechanics of using GAS involve several steps; however, the key is to identify objective, specific behaviours that define goal performance to enable objective and reliable measurement of performance. GAS uses an ordinal measurement scale, requiring the user to break down performance on a five-point scale ranging from –2 (much less than expected performance) to +2 (much more than expected performance) where the middle or zero level of performance is the *expected level of performance* towards which rehabilitation efforts are targeted.

The specific process for using the COPM and GAS in combination to plan goals in the study by Doig et al. (2010) involved a seven-step process:

1. *Identification of objectives and problem areas.* The COPM was administered by an occupational therapist and involved interviewing the client and their significant other. During this process, the interviewer prompted participants, using task analysis (Pedretti & Wade, 1996) and motivational interviewing techniques (Miranti & Heinemann, 2004), to break broader, long-term goals into specific problem areas to be targeted.

2. *Identification of specific goal behaviours* for each problem area was achieved by assessment and discussion. For example, for a handwriting problem, the therapist would

clarify whether the client's goal was to improve legibility or writing speed after observing writing performance.

3. *Determination of methods for goal measurement.* Procedures for measuring performance on each goal were documented using objective and measurable terms to ensure a consistent approach. The guidelines by Ottenbacher and Cusick (1989) were used to develop GAS scales for each goal area. Box 10.2 provides an example of a client's goal to take a taxi independently. This illustrate not only the process for ensuring valid, objective measurement of goal performance but also highlights the importance of in-depth task analysis to ensure successful and thorough scaling of goals and to plan treatment.

BOX 10.2   GOAL TO TAKE A TAXI INDEPENDENTLY

After individual assessment of the task procedures and environmental factors relevant to taking a taxi, a list of 11 specific steps defining this task was documented. Assessment indicated that factors impacting on performance included (1) reduced mobility (i.e. use of a walking aid), (2) cognitive deficits impacting on communication and executive functions including problem solving and planning and (3) environmental factors (i.e. steep sloping driveway impacting on access). To objectively measure performance, the assessor determined the percentage of the task performed independently, by dividing number of task steps needing supervision and/or assistance by the total number of steps.

GAS goal. Taking a taxi independently

GAS Performance Levels	Definition of Performance for Each Level
Much more than expected (+2)	Takes cab to unfamiliar destination independently
Somewhat more than expected (+1)	Takes cab to familiar destination independently
Expected level of performance (0)	Takes cab to familiar destination (1%–33% assistance)
Somewhat less than expected (−1)	Takes cab to familiar destination (34%–66% assistance)
Much less than expected (−2)	Takes cab to familiar destination (>66% assistance)

Specific task steps for taking a taxi

1. Booking the taxi (negotiating for the driver to assist with the wheel walker, giving directions, instructing where to stop to avoid having to negotiate a sloping driveway)
2. Walking to the cab with walking aid
3. Opening the car door (with walking aid) and transferring into the car
4. Giving the driver instructions regarding destination, instructing the driver appropriately about where to stop so that the destination can be negotiated on foot independently (i.e. on a flat surface within able walking distance)
5. Transferring out of the car

Return trip: As per steps 1–5, with variation for step 1 (directing driver to stop at an appropriate place in terms of distance and accessibility) and additional step 6 (walking from cab to the house with walking aid).

4. *Selection of expected level of performance.* Realistic outcomes were determined by observational assessment and input from and negotiation with the participant, their significant other and familiar rehabilitation practitioners to ensure the set expected level of performance (i.e. the 0 level) was realistic and the correct level of challenge (not too challenging or too easy) for achievement within the treatment time frame.

5. *Identification of the levels of performance.* The current level of function (set at either −1 or −2 depending on the level of function) for each goal was determined by observational assessment and, where necessary, supplemented from information from participants, significant others and familiar treating therapists. Most and least favourable levels were scaled around the expected level of performance.

6. *Review of goals to ensure validity.* Goals were checked to ensure there were equal gaps between levels, to avoid instances of performance being rated at more than one level and to avoid performance falling between levels.

7. *Assignment of a weight to each goal to enable calculation of GAS T-score.* Participants' COPM *importance* ratings were used to rank goals in order of priority. For example, where a participant identified four goals, their most important goal was weighted 4 and the least important goal weighted 1. If participants reported their goals to be equally important, all goals were given the same weight when calculating the T-value.

To incorporate assessment of environmental factors in the goal-planning process, the Environment and Person Factors Questionnaire (see Box 10.3) was developed. This scale was administered to participants and family members to determine not only how they felt changes since their injury might impact on achievement of the planned goals but also what they felt were barriers and facilitators to goal achievement in their real-life environment (i.e. physical environment characteristics, surrounding support, services). This questionnaires could be particularly valuable where a therapist is unable to see the client's environment (i.e. by conducting a home visit) and may be carrying out a goal-planning interview elsewhere (i.e. in a hospital or day hospital setting). As well as barriers and facilitators to goal achievement, practitioners working with clients in clinic or hospital settings also need to consider, when goal planning, whether the level of outcome and goal specifications are relevant to the person's real-life situation and, when planning treatment, how they can maximize *carryover of skills* to the person's real-life context.

To check whether the planned goals were client-centred, from the client's perspective, a simple rating scale was developed specifically to measure the client-centredness of the rehabilitation goals. The Client-Centredness of Goal Setting Scale (C-COGS) was designed to determine the extent to which participants perceived that their planned rehabilitation goals were important and meaningful to them (see Box 10.4). The ratings on the C-COGS indicated that there was a high degree of client-centredness of the programme goals from the perspectives of the participants and their family members (Doig et al., 2010).

Many of the statements made by the participants in follow-up qualitative interviews were reflective of the philosophies of client-centredness, primarily the importance of *goal ownership* (Doig et al., 2010): 'They were from me, they were to do with me and they were for me' (participant with TBI); 'I really wanted to do them so I would do all the steps' (participant with TBI); 'If you just set the goal to two steps forward to what you think they'll achieve they won't accept it and therefore may not engage in it' (occupational therapist) and 'I think if you'd set the goals for him and it wasn't really what he thought he needed he

BOX 10.3 ENVIRONMENT AND PERSON FACTORS QUESTIONNAIRE

Version (Tick One)	Patient (P)	Significant Other (SO)

Date

(P)　How do you feel you have changed since your injury (e.g. memory, strength, fatigue)?
(SO)　How do you feel your relative has changed since their injury?

(P)　How do you think the changes you identified will impact on how you achieve your goal/s?
(SO)　How do you think the changes you identified will impact on them achieving their goal/s?

Goal 1:

Goal 2:

Goal 3:

(P)　What things do you have around you to help you achieve your goal/s (e.g. physical environment, people, services)?
(SO)　What things does your relative have around them that you feel may help them achieve their goal/s (e.g. physical environment, people, services)?

Goal 1:

Goal 2:

Goal 3:

(P)　What things do you have around you that you feel currently prevent you from achieving your goals?
(SO)　(What does your relative have around them that you feel currently prevents them from achieving their goals (i.e. physical environment, services, people)?

Goal 1:

Goal 2:

Goal 3:

wouldn't have worked as hard at it' (significant other of participant with TBI). These sentiments were similar to themes of an earlier qualitative study (Doig, Fleming, & Kuipers, 2008) which interviewed practitioners about successful elements of community-based brain injury rehabilitation, for example, 'appreciate their expertise in the situation... and *valuing their knowledge of their own situation* and of what the brain injury means to them in their situation' (therapist participant), as well as 'I think letting the person really explain to you and tell you about what the injury means to them in their own situation and the difficulties they have and *helping them to set their own goals*' (therapist participant).

BOX 10.4   CLIENT-CENTREDNESS OF GOAL SETTING SCALE (C-COGS)

Thinking about the agreed goals that have been set with you, please *circle* the number below which
shows how important these goals are to you personally.

5	4	3	2	1
Totally important	Mostly important	Moderately important	Slightly important	Not important

Thinking about the goal-setting session that you just completed in order to arrive at your agreed goals,
circle a number which indicates how strongly you agree or disagree with the following statements:

The goal/s is what *I want* to work on

5	4	3	2	1
Strongly agree				Strongly disagree

The goal/s is *what my friend/relative wants* me to work on

5	4	3	2	1
Strongly agree				Strongly disagree

The goal/s is *what my therapist wants* me to work on

5	4	3	2	1
Strongly agree				Strongly disagree

The combined use of the subjective COPM and objective GAS scales has potential to
overcome some of the typical challenges to goal planning and measurement when the
measures are used in isolation. The COPM facilitates a client-centred goal formulation
process; however, it has limitations where clients have impaired self-awareness and a tendency to under-report impairments (Toglia & Kirk, 2000) that limits accurate self-ratings
of performance. When using GAS in conjunction with the COPM, the practitioner is able
to objectively measure change in performance using GAS via observation of performance.
Furthermore, occupational performance goals generated using the COPM may be at first
stated in very broad terms, and the subsequent use of GAS to operationalize those goals
requires the practitioner and the client to thoroughly consider what the specific goal or
goals are for the occupational performance areas. Therefore, a client may have several GAS
goals for one COPM goal (e.g. handwriting performance may involve a GAS goal for speed
of handwriting and another for accuracy or neatness of handwriting, depending on what
aspects of the task the client is wanting to work on).

Consider the case of Mr M which demonstrates the process of individualized goal planning using the COPM and GAS.

Background: Mr M is a young man undergoing outpatient rehabilitation after having a
severe TBI. Prior to goal planning with Mr M, standardized assessments by a multidisciplinary rehabilitation team indicated that he had mild impairment of functional memory
and mild high-level cognitive language deficits, with the main impairments being in the
physical domain. These were primarily upper limb and lower limb ataxia impacting on
coordination and speed of movement when moving and doing activities, especially tasks
involving fine motor skills and coordination of the upper limb. Mr M appeared to be very
motivated to participate in rehabilitation and demonstrated no deficit in self-awareness on
formalized assessment. Goal planning was guided by the combined use of the COPM and
GAS using the seven-step process described earlier:

1. *Identification of objectives and problem areas.* During the COPM interview conducted with Mr M and his mother, Mr M was able to identify a number of occupational performance problems which formed the basis for the goals he wanted to work on in his community occupational therapy programme. These goals, and their corresponding importance rating out of 10, were to be able to handwrite more neatly (10), to be able to take a taxi independently (8) and to be able to perform self-care tasks more quickly (7).

2. *Identification of specific goal behaviours for each problem area.* For illustration purposes, we will focus on the goal of wanting to perform self-care tasks more quickly. To start to break down this broad goal into objective performance areas that could be operationalized using GAS, there was further discussion about specific problem areas under the domain of self-care from which a list of difficulties with specific self-care tasks was generated. Specific goals related to self-care were *brushing teeth faster, shaving with a manual razor, eating with a knife and fork faster* and *putting on jeans faster,* for which each area was assigned a new importance rating. Consider the goal of *putting on jeans faster.* The client told the therapist that this goal was about the *speed* of performance, the subsequent assessment undertaken to further plan the goals and treatment needed to show how fast the client was performing the task currently (to provide the baseline or –1 or –2 GAS performance levels), as well as start to indicate how the therapist might work with the client to achieve this goal. Therefore, an observational assessment of the client donning his usual pair of jeans was undertaken and the speed of performance from start to finish was measured, which was 6 min and 25 s.

3. *Determination of methods for goal measurement.* Like all occupational performance, the way in which people perform tasks and the factors impacting on task performance are different for everybody. In this case, Mr M had a preference for wearing jeans with a buttoned-up fly and he used a specific procedure for donning the jeans using his bed for postural support as his ataxia impacted on his standing balance. Therefore, to ensure validity of the outcome measurement on each assessment occasion, the procedure for donning the jeans was clearly documented to ensure a consistent approach with a consistent task complexity. This documentation outlined the conditions for assessment on each occasion, which in this case included the set-up of the task (i.e. placement of jeans, type of jeans, with walking aid in front for support as needed), situational factors (i.e. standing with bed behind for safety and support) as well as when to start timing (i.e. when set up in a seated position on the bed).

4. *Selection of expected level of performance.* The GAS goal was scaled so that the baseline level of performance (6 min and 25 s) fell within the bounds of the –1 level, as it was possible that performance could decline and this could then be reflected by a rating of –2. Clinical judgement was necessary to determine a realistic zero level, which was the speed at which we expected Mr M might be donning his jeans at the end of our block of treatment. The therapist collaborated with previous therapists about the client's rate of recovery and response to impairment level interventions such as strengthening, the likelihood of resolution of ataxia, as well as considering the impact of treatment strategies trialled during the observational assessment (i.e. use of compensatory strategies such as proximal weights, adaptation of the task and environment such as positioning to

improve proximal postural stability). Since there were no normative data for the speed at which the general population dons a pair of jeans with a buttoned-up fly, the therapist decided to take a timed measurement under similar conditions with a person without TBI. This measure (i.e. 20.20 s) provided a guideline for the +2 or much more than expected level of performance.

5. *Identification of the levels of performance.* All other levels were scaled around these levels with equal gaps between each level. The GAS levels for *buttoning up jeans faster* were therefore

   2+ To be able to complete task in less than 1 min

   1+ To be able to complete task between 1 and 2 min, 59 s

   0 To be able to complete task between 3 and 4 min, 59 s

   −1 To be able to complete task between 5 and 6 min, 59 s

   −2 To be able to complete task in more than 7 min

6. *Review of goals to ensure validity.* This goal was checked to ensure that the gaps between each level were equal (e.g. an equal amount of improvement was required to go from a −1 to a 0 as to go from a 0 to a 1+) and to avoid instances of performance being rated at more than one level (i.e. there was no overlap between levels in the timings) and to avoid performance falling between levels (i.e. all possible timings were accounted for within the likely range).

7. *Assignment of a weight to each goal to enable calculation of GAS T-score.* The client's COPM *importance* ratings were used to rank goals in order of priority. As the client ended up identifying four goals, his most important goal was weighted 4 and the least important goal was weighted 1. However, if the client had reported his goals to be equally important, all goals would have been given the same weight when calculating the *T*-value.

In the case of Mr M, he achieved his expected level of performance on all GAS goals and perceived clinically significant improvements according to post COPM performance and satisfaction ratings. Mr M attained a 1+ post-intervention for his speed of buttoning jeans goal.

10.3.4 Clinical Utility of the Combined Use of the COPM and GAS

The combined use of the COPM and GAS for the 14 participants with TBI undergoing the community-based occupational therapy programme resulted in 51 COPM goals and 53 GAS goals that were perceived as almost unanimously client-centred, despite the majority of participants demonstrating moderate or severe impairments of self-awareness (Doig et al., 2010). Both measures were found to be sensitive to change and there was generally agreement in the direction of change on the COPM and GAS post-intervention (i.e. for 70% of the COPM performance ratings, there was agreement between participants and their significant others on the direction of change in performance in the direction that corresponded to improvements in GAS ratings). On occasions where the COPM participant and significant other ratings did not agree in terms of the direction of change, the majority of occasions could be accounted for by two participants who demonstrated severe self-awareness impairments. However, the COPM self-ratings of performance by other participants with moderate or severe impairments of self-awareness were consistent with the observed performance and significant other ratings. Nevertheless, the use of GAS in conjunction with the COPM was important to enable an objective, behavioural assessment of outcomes in occupational performance areas, thereby minimizing the limitations of using self-report measures to measure goal behaviours with clients with impaired self-awareness.

Further results of the clinical utility study indicated that on average, the time required to plan goals using the COPM and scale goals using GAS in this context (i.e. for use in a 12-week outpatient occupational therapy programme) was approximately 4.5 h per participant, where the participants set, on average, four GAS goals for the programme. Although this is a significant time investment in goal planning, qualitative analysis of interviews with participants, family members and therapists conducted at the end of the rehabilitation programme indicated several further benefits of the goal-planning approach. First, from the therapist's perspective, due to the environmental assessment and involvement of family members in the goal-planning process, there was a high likelihood of the treatment resulting in changes that would carry over to *real-life* functioning. Second, the approach was valuable as treatment planning was occurring in concert with goal planning, which meant that the GAS goal-planning approach itself naturally structured and organized the treatment programme by clearly defining the target behaviours. Third, the approach resulted in clear objectives in real-life terms that could be understood by the client, and once progress was measured, this could be shown very clearly, in behavioural terms, for feedback to the clients. As the determination of goal levels was undertaken thoroughly, the zero level on the GAS scale (i.e. the expected level of achievement) was accurate and realistically achievable and was set at the appropriate level of challenge for the client. Therefore, this process of concrete, meaningful, objective feedback was extremely valuable in terms of providing motivation for clients to continue to work at rehabilitation efforts, set further goals and to build self-awareness. Finally, the objective terms used to define goals ensured that expectations for the achievement of goals within the rehabilitation time frames were clearly defined for all parties. Therefore, although the process may be time-consuming and, in fact, the time involved in using such a process within a team setting may be even more time-consuming, there are many benefits to be reaped from this initial time cost.

It is clear that there are factors which can pose challenges to clients self-identifying and owning goals, particularly with clients with brain injury. These include reduced self-awareness resulting in under-reporting of impairments (Toglia & Kirk, 2000) and subsequent poor understanding of the need for therapeutic intervention (Fischer, Gauggel, & Trexler, 2004), as well as amotivation and passivity effecting participation in the process (Siegert & Taylor, 2004), and cognitive impairment such as memory impairment (Kuipers, Foster, Carlson, & Moy, 2003). All of these factors can affect a person's ability to participate in goal planning and engage in rehabilitation efforts. However, an occupation-focused, goal-directed approach to intervention has some benefits to potentially overcome some of these difficulties.

10.4 Key Elements of an Occupation-Based Client-Centred Goal-Focused Intervention

Thus far, this chapter has described the use of occupation to guide goal planning and a specific approach to goal setting using the COPM and GAS. This section explains how this approach was used to guide treatment in an outpatient brain injury rehabilitation programme (Doig, Fleming, Kuipers, et al., 2011) focusing on the key elements of its use in rehabilitation. The rehabilitation programme described involved 12 weekly occupational therapy sessions, where the therapist used an occupation-based approach to rehabilitation as well as a range of occupational therapy treatment techniques including grading and adapting tasks, trial of compensatory strategies to achieve goals and the provision of appropriately timed feedback on performance to enhance awareness of errors and self-monitoring and demonstrate improvement. There were three main principles underpinning the programme, which are described in the following.

10.4.1 Goal Based

First and foremost, the intervention was entirely goal based. The client's goals became the focus of all rehabilitation interventions. Short-term goals relating to each programme goal were set at the beginning of each session, focusing each session on the goal/s. This clearly defined expectations and enabled the client to understand that what was going to be worked on in the session related to their goal/s. The link between the goals and the therapeutic tasks was understood by the client, thereby providing the motivation to participate in rehabilitation. This concept is in line with the theory of self-efficacy and behaviour change. Schwarzer's health action process model (Schwarzer, 1992) asserts that if a person perceives that their actions (i.e. participating in rehabilitation activities) will result in treatment outcomes, he or she will be more confident and motivated to participate in rehabilitation. To this end, provision of goal-specific feedback is important to build client self-efficacy. The use of client-centred, specific goals to engage clients in rehabilitation may be of even greater value when working with clients with significant memory impairment, who may be unable to recall their goals and consequently not understand why they are participating in therapy. In these cases, goals can be valuable tools to refocus the client on what is important and why it is important to them thereby enhancing engagement in therapy.

10.4.2 Structured

The therapy process was highly structured. First, the client-centred programme goals and weekly short-term goals provided the structure on which each therapy session was based. Goal prioritization determined which goals were focused on first and goal achievement dictated when new short-term goals were to be introduced. Second, planning and memory aids (i.e. client diaries, weekly timetables) were incorporated to assist with short-term goal achievement. For example, weekly activities or targets based on the weekly short-term goals were written in client diaries or timetables. Homework tasks specific to each goal were set and were provided on a structured, written homework sheet. Third, feedback on goal performance was structured and specific and given at regular intervals. Feedback about positive gains in goal areas was timed to be most clinically advantageous in terms of client motivation (i.e. at the end of every session, at the end of the rehabilitation time frame). Lastly, the COPM importance scale not only was used to determine the most important goals at initial goal planning but, in some cases, was also used to regularly check client priorities and goal relevance over time. For example, at the beginning of each treatment session, therapists briefly checked the importance of each goal using the COPM importance scale to focus the treatment session on what was most motivating for the client at that time.

A structured, client-centred goal-planning process where the therapist structures the rehabilitation process around specific, objective, functional goals can be particularly useful when working with clients with executive dysfunction. This has been previously described in studies on goal management training (Levine et al., 2000; McPherson, Kayes, & Weatherall, 2009). Goal management training is based on Duncan's goal theory, which asserts that people with intact executive function have internal goal lists, which govern behaviour when carrying out goal-directed activity, leading to goal achievement (Duncan, 1986). According to Duncan, the disorganized behaviour and inability to focus on and achieve goals commonly seen in people with executive dysfunction can be explained by the impaired construction of goal lists (i.e. incorrect goal lists or absence of lists) or poor use of goal lists. Goal management training aims to prevent goal failure using a self-instructional technique and provides a structured framework for error prevention in attempting task performance (McPherson et al., 2009). Goal management training focuses the person on a list of steps to avoid errors in performance and assists the person to execute the steps of a task successfully to achieve a discrete goal. In the same way, a structured, specific, functional goal set out in objective, behavioural terms directs the person's awareness towards their goal. This facilitates a therapy process that is structured by defined targets and, like goal management training, focuses the client on the steps needed to achieve the desired level of performance.

10.4.3 Environment Focused

Some therapy sessions were carried out in a day hospital clinic and some in the clients' homes. However, regardless of treatment setting, therapy considered and incorporated the person's environment in the treatment. This involved including the significant other where possible and if appropriate. When therapy occurred in the day hospital, the Environment and Person Factors Questionnaire was revisited to consider the environmental barriers and facilitators in the real-life setting that may impact on goal achievement. Where appropriate to the person and their goals, clients were asked to bring in relevant equipment from home or work for use in therapy. In the absence of being able to perform tasks in the person's real-life environment, therapy involved simulation of relevant tasks and/or discussion about how participants could and did apply skills learned in their real-life situation. When therapy occurred in the person's home setting, the therapy was carried out in the context that was directly relevant to the goal/s set. For example, if the participant's goal was related to grocery shopping, some sessions took place at the participant's local shopping centre. If the participant's goal was related to making their breakfast, the intervention took place in the person's home kitchen.

10.4.4 Case Example Illustrating the Treatment Approach

As outlined, goal planning and intervention can be challenging with clients who are experiencing impaired self-awareness. This case example demonstrates the benefits of an occupation-based, client-centred approach to goal planning and rehabilitation for someone with severe impairment of self-awareness. Mr A was a 29-year-old man with a severe TBI who had recently been discharged from the inpatient brain injury rehabilitation. Prior to his brain injury, he worked full time as a builder's labourer.

Background: Prior to goal planning with Mr A, standardized assessments by a multi-disciplinary rehabilitation team indicated mild functional memory impairment, reduced speed of processing, executive dysfunction presenting as disorganized, higher-level language deficits and depressed mood. Mr A scored 7/9 on the Self-Awareness of Deficits Interview (SADI) (Fleming, Strong, & Ashton, 1996), indicating a severe impairment of self-awareness. Mr A had been discharged earlier than advised from inpatient rehabilitation as his family reported that he was not engaging in the rehabilitation sessions and was amotivated.

Goal planning: Mr A was unable to identify any occupational performance problem areas when the COPM interview was administered and although appearing disengaged with the prospect of further outpatient rehabilitation, with encouragement from his mother, agreed to involve his family by having them participate in the goal-planning process with him. Mr A agreed to the therapist identifying problems in occupational performance areas by interviewing a family member as well as his inpatient occupational therapist using the COPM and discussing specific goals for further refinement using GAS. Therefore, goals were based on the perceived problem areas of other people who were familiar with Mr A. The goals identified were

1. Understanding written information
2. Writing down information accurately (to assist with aiding memory)
3. Participating in a range of activities each day (Mr A was currently not engaged in prior work and leisure activities which contributed to his low mood)
4. Improving memory for everyday events and conversations

Each of the goal areas were presented to and discussed with Mr A, with his family member present, and although Mr A did not agree to the presence of changes in all of the goal areas or the degree of change in other areas, he agreed to sign up to working on the goals in the programme. GAS scales were developed for each goal area following observational assessment of performance in each of the areas and discussion with Mr A and his family member as well as relevant familiar therapists. The GAS example for the goal of participating in a range of everyday activities is outlined in the following (see Table 10.1) and incorporates strategies to assist with organization and memory (i.e. structuring week, use of a written timetable). Mr A identified that he would like to achieve something in this area as he was getting bored because he was currently not medically cleared to return to work or drive his motorcycle (his two main valued occupations prior to his injury). Mr A's family reported that he was having difficulty initiating ideas and getting motivated for alternative activities and that he tended to dwell on returning to work and driving without acknowledging that current impairments meant that it was not yet safe for him to do so.

Intervention and outcomes: Mr A participated in the 12-week occupational therapy programme with encouragement to attend due to low motivation. In relation to the example goal given earlier, Mr A achieved a level 0, indicating that he achieved his goal of planning and participating in a variety of daily activities. His pre- and post-intervention scores on the SADI, total COPM performance scores and GAS standard score are outlined in Table 10.2.

The SADI indicated a severe impairment of self-awareness on initial assessment, and at that time, Mr A self-perceived his overall performance on the COPM to be slightly higher than his family member. Following the intervention period, Mr A did not perceive any improvements in overall performance on the COPM. However, his family member perceived a clinically significant improvement in performance on the COPM and objective assessment of his goal performance using GAS indicated significant improvements

TABLE 10.1

GAS Goal for Planning and Participating in a Range of Activities for Mr A

GAS Level	Description
2+	Independently generates ideas for daily activities to fill in his or her time (i.e. leisure, rehabilitation homework, visiting friends, involvement in household chores), organizes his participation (i.e. researches leisure options, phones to find out about participation in an activity, organizes time for leisure around other commitments/appointments) and writes a weekly timetable that he follows through with independently
1+	Able to identify activities to fill in his time when given a checklist or prompted by others with ideas. Needs prompting to initiate organization of activities (i.e. needs to be reminded to research activities) and needs prompting to write a weekly timetable, but once this is in place is able to organize and follow the plan and participate in the activities
0	Able to identify activities to fill in his time when given a checklist or prompted by others for ideas. Needs assistance with organizing activities and writing a weekly timetable, but once this is in place is able to follow the plan and participate in the activities
1−	Has difficulty identifying activities to fill in his time even with prompting for ideas and a checklist, but with encouragement and coaxing is willing to try other activities and can see the value of doing things other than work and driving. Needs someone else to organize activities and someone else to write a weekly timetable with proposed activities, and once this is in place is able to follow the plan and participate in the activities
2−	Has difficulty identifying activities to fill in his time even with prompting for ideas and checklists and is reluctant to try suggested activities. Focuses primarily on the loss of valued activities (i.e. work and driving) and does not see the value of doing other things at present. Even with a proposed plan of activities, does not participate in them

TABLE 10.2

Pre- and Post-Intervention Scores for Mr A

	Pre-Intervention	Post-Intervention
Mr A (SADI) (range 0–9)	7	3
Mr A (COPM total) (range 0–10)	4.25	4
Family (COPM total) (range 0–10)	2	7.1
GAS standard score (range 0–100)	24.6	42.7

approaching zero levels for all goals. If the COPM performance self-ratings for all the goals were the only outcome measure administered in this case, the improvements made would not have been reflected. It was evident that Mr A had given an inflated self-rating on the COPM at initial assessment due to reduced self-awareness, and by the end of the rehabilitation programme, his self-awareness had improved according to the SADI, and thus, his COPM rating was reflecting this improvement in self-awareness rather than improvement in goal performance.

A therapist participant in an earlier qualitative study (Doig et al., 2008) on effective community-based brain injury rehabilitation stated, 'I think giving ownership to the client even if initially you are doing a lot of that goal setting but getting the client to agree to them is really important and usually things don't work unless they are on side with those goals too'. This sentiment was true of Mr A's case in respect to having Mr A agree to the goals and own some of them, even though he did not initially contribute to the goal-setting process. Mr A participated in the programme and experienced some specific, positive feedback about his progress in goal areas. It is possible that his experience of task performance and feedback on task performance contributed to the development of his self-awareness.

Mr A was one of two participants (out of 14) who presented with a severe impairment of self-awareness, both of whom were unable to generate their own programme goals using the COPM (Doig et al., 2010). In both cases, a *therapist-led* approach was used to identify goals, as outlined in the case of Mr A. Although the perceived client-centredness of goals and perception of improvement post-intervention was lower for these participants, the subsequent GAS standard scores post-intervention were similar regardless of severity of impairment to self-awareness, indicating that reduced self-awareness and reduced perceived client-centredness and ownership of goals was not a barrier to goal achievement in this rehabilitation programme (Doig et al., 2010).

In summary, this client-centred intervention approach had the key elements of being goal based, structured, and environment focused. An intervention study with 14 individuals with TBI where the majority demonstrated either moderate (5/14) or severe (4/14) impairment of self-awareness demonstrated the effectiveness of the programme. Results indicated that significant improvements were made in goal achievement and occupational performance following the intervention compared to baseline (Doig, Fleming, Kuipers, et al., 2011). In relation to client-centred goal planning with clients with reduced self-awareness, the following key elements are recommended:

- Inclusion of significant others in goal planning, where appropriate, and their recruitment to encourage participation in the rehabilitation programme, especially if there is little initial ownership of goals initially.
- A therapist-led approach may be necessary initially to identify goals.
- An initial focus on building a strong, therapeutic alliance so that the client may be willing to take on-board goal suggestions and try things with encouragement.
- Recognition that self-awareness may improve with experience, and this may lead to a need for goal reprioritization or revision.
- Attention to the sensitivity and timing of any feedback about errors in performance or lack of improvement in goal areas (i.e. avoid or minimize emotional distress by seeking support for the client).
- Focus on giving feedback about improvements that is specific, objective and meaningful.
- With experience of improvement in goal areas, increased participation in client-centred goal planning may be possible due to increased awareness and/or motivation.

10.5 Client-Centred Goal Planning in Different Rehabilitation Settings

The goal-planning and treatment approach that has been outlined in this chapter was developed for and its efficacy researched in the context of a community-based outpatient occupational therapy programme for clients with TBI. This section contrasts the application of client-centred goal planning in different settings (i.e. inpatient settings and in teams) including challenges as well as potential strategies to encourage client-centred goal planning in these situations.

10.5.1 Community Rehabilitation Settings

In community settings, occupation-based, client-centred goal planning may be facilitated with greater ease due to a move away from an impairment focus in hospital settings to focus more on functional abilities and community integration. This has been demonstrated in relation to people with brain injury, where goals after discharge from hospital become broader and more complex (Siegert & Taylor, 2004) and move from a focus on physical rehabilitation towards a greater emphasis on reintegration over time (Kuipers et al., 2003). Characteristics of goal planning with clients in community settings are that there are more natural opportunities for involvement of family members, goals are more about *participation* and *reintegration*, and clients and families have had varying opportunities to experience the impact of any changes in the real world; therefore, a client-centred, occupation-based approach to goal planning may be easier to facilitate. This has been supported by our research with a community dwelling sample (Doig et al., 2010).

10.5.2 Inpatient Rehabilitation Settings

Qualitative evidence suggests that in hospital inpatient rehabilitation settings, there may be more challenges to using a client-centred, occupation-based approach to goal planning than in community settings. Several qualitative studies have investigated the process of goal planning, with groups of patients in a geriatric rehabilitation setting (Wressle, Oberg, & Henriksson, 1999), a neurological rehabilitation setting (Barnard et al., 2010) and following stroke (Leach et al., 2010; Levack et al., 2011). Leach et al. found that therapist-directed and therapist-led approaches were more commonly described in practice than client-centred approaches. A therapist-led approach was characterized by the therapist suggesting appropriate goals with regards to assessment findings and seeking agreement from the client and family regarding goals (Leach et al., 2010). Levack et al. found that goal planning was influenced by what the therapists perceived as *privileged goals* where privileging of goals was seen to be driven largely by financial and organizational factors (i.e. discharge time frames). Similarly, outcomes of goal-planning meetings were observed to be heavily shaped by professional influences in the context of an inpatient neurological rehabilitation unit with 'rarely a straightforward translation of patient wishes into agreed-on written goals' (Barnard et al., 2010, p. 239). Wressle et al. also found that participation of patients in the goal-setting process was lacking in an inpatient geriatric stroke setting.

There can be many service delivery context factors that pose challenges to client-centred approaches to goal planning in rehabilitation. These include the following:

- The length of the rehabilitation programme may govern what is achievable, meaning priority goals become discharge priorities and preclude some goals clients may wish to work on.
- Funding, availability of specific equipment, space or resources may mean some goals are unable to be worked on.
- Goals may be greatly influenced by organizational (and presumably economic and political agendas) as well as reflective of the staffing and orientation of the service (Kuipers et al., 2004).

Despite service system factors posing some barriers to client-centred goal planning, there may be room for negotiation to find some middle ground between what the client wants and what is possible within a service delivery system. Therapists can still seek to listen to clients about what their occupations are in life and what they mean to them. Even if the goals agreed to be worked on are not the goals wished to be worked on by the client, the core philosophies of client-centredness can still be applied in these circumstances by the following:

- Conducting a client-centred, goal-planning approach
- Communicating with the client about why some goal preferences can be worked on within the system and why others cannot
- Seeking to negotiate with the client and come to an agreement so that the client has ownership of the goals
- Finding the link between the agreed-upon goals (which may not be preferred) and those goals preferred by the client and not worked on, to enhance motivation and engagement in therapy as well as ownership of goals
- Realizing the importance of the therapeutic relationship in enabling the therapist and client to have open communication where there is an atmosphere of mutual respect and joint decision making and where the client may be more willing to make some concessions and take on-board suggestions
- Advocating for change in aspects of a service delivery environment that are barriers to client-centred goal planning and rehabilitation

Further potential strategies to enhance the clinical hospital environment to facilitate an environment-focused approach may include home visiting and early overnight stays for the client where appropriate. This may assist with understanding and awareness of the impact of injury or illness on functioning in the real world (Playford et al., 2000). Additionally, increased awareness by staff about the influence of the environment on the perceived roles of those involved may enhance client-centredness. Research has shown that hospital environments can evoke a role set where clients feel like *patients*, family members feel like *intruders* and patients and family members perceive therapists as *experts and teachers* compared to the home environment where patients reportedly feel more like *partners* and *experts* on more equal footing with therapists who are perceived as a *friend* and *visitor* (Doig, Fleming, Cornwell, & Kuipers, 2011; Von Koch, Wottrich, & Widen-Holmqvist, 1998). Potential ways a hospital environment can be adapted to avoid or minimize this include the following:

- Modifying the design of the environment to appear less formal and clinical and more home-like.
- Providing equipment, resources and environments that facilitate an occupation-based approach to goal planning and rehabilitation by enabling clients to participate in everyday tasks (i.e. homelike kitchens, bathrooms, offices, leisure resources) which are characteristic of activity- and participation-level goals.
- Ensuring the culture is one of inclusion of families (i.e. provision of adequate nearby car parking, opportunities for participation in goal planning and treatment). Ensure regular systems of two-way feedback and communication between families and therapists.

- Changing, where necessary, the perceived role set to be one where therapists, clients and significant others are partners in the process, which may require a shift in values of the people working in the organization.

10.5.3 Goal Planning in Teams

The dynamics and complexities of inpatient multidisciplinary or interdisciplinary teams may influence the goal-planning process as inpatient rehabilitation teams typically involve a number of therapists in formulating client goals. In contrast, the dynamics of a community-based therapy team are likely to be less complex, especially in community teams where members may be more dispersed with involvement of fewer therapists (i.e. likely one case manager) in the goal-planning process. A unified client centred, goal-planning approach for clients receiving rehabilitation from a team of therapists requires a structured procedure for the team goal-planning process to ensure the team members are all working towards the same client goals. Some team variables that adversely influence goal setting include a lack of understanding about the philosophy and process of goal setting, poor writing of goal statements, failure with leading goal-setting meetings, absence of staff at meetings and a lack of clarity about the goal-setting process (Elsworth, Marks, McGrath, & Wade, 1999).

Holliday et al. (2007) put forward a team goal-planning model which advocates the use of a key worker system for goal planning in an inpatient rehabilitation team setting. The key worker, which can be likened to the role of a case manager in a community model of service delivery, assists the client to identify priority goals and acts as an advocate to facilitate participation in goal planning. Parallel to this goal facilitator role of the key worker, therapists conduct initial multidisciplinary assessments and then meet with the client to discuss their goals in the light of assessment outcomes. This enables the goals to be refined and set collaboratively. Furthermore, the concept of life goals has been described in the literature as a principle for assisting with identifying rehabilitation goals, and this has potential for goal planning in teams (Sivaraman Nair, 2003). Sivaraman Nair described life goals as hierarchical with the lowest goals being immediate actions (e.g. reading, writing) through to higher-level goals approximating idealized self-images (e.g. scholar), whereby fulfilment of lower goals leads to realizing higher goals closer to idealized self-image. Life goals can be used to identify rehabilitation goals and influence a person's motivation to participate in treatment if there is concurrency between life goals and rehabilitation goals (Sivaraman Nair, 2003).

In summary, in relation to client-centred goal planning in teams,

- A formalized, joint goal-planning process may ensure team members work towards the same goals
- Shared goals encourage interdisciplinary working in teams
- A process of documenting goals is required so progress can be evaluated and team members and patients and families know what is expected
- A key worker system can be valuable for identifying goals in teams
- Staff training is needed to ensure an understanding of the philosophy of client-centredness in goal planning and to ensure consistency in goal-planning processes including documentation and measurement
- The process can be time-consuming, however should be considered for its benefits

10.6 Conclusion

It is currently unclear, in terms of research evidence, what is the most effective approach to goal planning. Current qualitative evidence indicates that the ease with which client-centred goal planning can be applied varies across clients and across settings. Therefore, the method of goal planning may need to be varied somewhat for different individuals within different rehabilitation environments. However, there is evidence that client-centred, occupation-based approaches to goal planning have benefits in terms of motivation and participation in rehabilitation as well as leading to goal achievement. If the core ideals of client-centredness and occupation form the foundations for goal-planning processes as central, unifying philosophies in the consciousness of rehabilitation practitioners, the process of goal planning regardless of setting would, at a minimum, be characterized by listening to clients about what they do (which makes them who they are) and what they want to achieve as an entree to rehabilitation practitioners applying their knowledge, skills and experience to assist clients to achieve their goals. The specific processes and mechanics of how goal planning is implemented may vary according to systematic influences such as the rehabilitation setting, team structure and resources, as well as individual circumstances such as injury or illness characteristics, stage of recovery, goal orientation and preference. The challenge for rehabilitation practitioners is to strive to practise goal planning and rehabilitation in a client-centred, occupation-focused way, regardless of the context in which services are delivered.

References

Barnard, R. A., Cruice, M. N., & Playford, E. D. (2010). Strategies used in the pursuit of achievability during goal setting in rehabilitation. *Qualitative Health Research, 20*(2), 239–250.

Bodiam, C. (1999). The use of the COPM for the assessment of outcome on a neurorehabilitation unit. *British Journal of Occupational Therapy, 62*(3), 123–126.

Carswell, A., McColl, M. A., Baptiste, S., Law, M., Polatajko, H., & Pollock, N. (2004). The Canadian Occupational Performance Measure: A research and clinical literature review. *The Canadian Journal of Occupational Therapy, 71*(4), 210–222.

Chapparo, C., & Ranka, J. (2002). *PRPP research: Training manual CPE edition.* Darlington, New South Wales, Australia: The University of Sydney.

Christiansen, C., Baum, M. C., & Bass-Haugen, J. (2005). *Occupational therapy: Performance, participation, and well-being.* Thorofare, NJ: Slack.

Cott, C. A. (2004). Client-centred rehabilitation: Client perspectives. *Disability and Rehabilitation, 26*(24), 1411–1422.

Doig, E. J., Fleming, J., Cornwell, P., & Kuipers, P. (2009). Qualitative exploration of a client-centered, goal-directed approach to community-based occupational therapy for adults with traumatic brain injury. *American Journal of Occupational Therapy, 63*(5), 559–568.

Doig, E. J., Fleming, J., Cornwell, P., & Kuipers, P. (2010). Clinical utility of the combined use of the Canadian Occupational Performance Measure and the Goal Attainment Scale. *American Journal of Occupational Therapy, 64*(6), 904–914.

Doig, E. J., Fleming, J., Cornwell, P., & Kuipers, P. (2011). Comparing the experience of outpatient therapy in home and day hospital settings after traumatic brain injury: Patient, significant other and therapist perspectives. *Disability and Rehabilitation, 33*(13–14), 1203–1214.

Doig, E. J., Fleming, J., & Kuipers, P. (2008). Achieving optimal functional outcomes in community-based rehabilitation following acquired brain injury: A qualitative investigation of therapists' perspectives. *British Journal of Occupational Therapy, 71*(9), 360–370.

Doig, E. J., Fleming, J., Kuipers, P., Cornwell, P., & Khan, A. (2011). Goal-directed outpatient rehabilitation following TBI: A pilot study of programme effectiveness and comparison of outcomes in home and day hospital settings. *Brain Injury, 25*(11), 1114–1125.

Duncan, J. (1986). Disorganization of behaviour after frontal lobe damage. *Cognitive Neuropsychology, 3*, 271–290.

Elsworth, J. D., Marks, J. A., McGrath, J. R., & Wade, D. T. (1999). An audit of goal planning in rehabilitation. *Topics in Stroke Rehabilitation, 6*(2), 51–61.

Fischer, S., Gauggel, S., & Trexler, L. E. (2004). Awareness of activity limitations, goal setting and rehabilitation outcome in patients with brain injuries. *Brain Injury, 18*(6), 547–562.

Fleming, J., Strong, J., & Ashton, R. (1996). Self-awareness of deficits in adults with traumatic brain injury: How best to measure? *Brain Injury, 10*, 1–10.

Gagne, D. E., & Hoppes, S. (2003). Brief report – The effects of collaborative goal-focused occupational therapy on self-care skills: A pilot study. *American Journal of Occupational Therapy, 57*(2), 215–219.

Golledge, J. (1998). Distinguishing between occupation, purposeful activity and activity, park 1: Review and explanation. *British Journal of Occupational Therapy, 61*(3), 100–105.

Grieve, J., & Gnanasekaran, L. (Ed. 3). (2008). *Neuropsychology for occupational therapists: Cognition in occupational performance*. Oxford, U.K.: Blackwell.

Hinojosa, J., & Kramer, P. (1997). Fundamental concepts of occupational therapy: Occupation, purposeful activity, and function [Statement]. *American Journal of Occupational Therapy, 51*, 864–866.

Holliday, R. C., Cano, S., Freeman, J. A., & Playford, D. E. (2007). Should patients participate in clinical decision making? An optimized balance block design controlled study of goal setting in a rehabilitation unit. *Journal of Neurology, Neurosurgery and Psychiatry, 78*, 576–580.

Kiresuk, T. J., & Sherman, R. E. (1968). Goal attainment scaling: A general method for evaluating comprehensive community mental health programs. *Community Mental Health Journal, 4*, 443–453.

Kiresuk, T. J., Smith, A., & Cardillo, J. E. (1994). *Goal attainment scaling: Applications, theory and measurement*. Hillsdale, NJ: Lawrence Erlbaum Associates.

Kuipers, P., Carlson, G., Bailey, S., & Sharma, A. (2004). A preliminary exploration of goal-setting in community-based rehabilitation for people with brain impairment. *Brain Impairment, 5*(1), 30–41.

Kuipers, P., Foster, M., Carlson, G., & Moy, J. (2003). Classifying client goals in community-based ABI rehabilitation: A taxonomy for profiling service delivery and conceptualizing outcomes. *Disability and Rehabilitation, 25*(3), 154–162.

Lannin, N. (2003). Goal attainment scaling allows program evaluation of a home-based occupational therapy program. *Occupational Therapy in Health Care, 17*(1), 43–55.

Law, M., Baptiste, S., Carswell, A., McColl, M. A., Polatajko, H., & Pollock, N. (1998). *Canadian occupational performance measure manual*. Ottawa, Ontario, Canada: CAOT Publications.

Law, M., Cooper, B., Strong, S., Stewart, D., Rigby, P., & Letts, L. (1996). The person-environment-occupation model: A transactive approach to occupational performance. *Canadian Journal of Occupational Therapy, 63*(1), 9–23.

Law, M., Polatajko, H., Baptiste, W., & Townsend, E. (1997). Core concepts of occupational therapy. In E. Townsend (Ed.), *Enabling occupation: An occupational therapy perspective* (pp. 29–56). Ottawa, Ontario, Canada: Canadian Association of Occupational Therapists.

Leach, E., Cornwell, P., Fleming, J., & Haines, T. (2010). Patient centred goal-setting in a subacute rehabilitation setting. *Disability and Rehabilitation, 32*(2), 159–172.

Levack, W. M. M., Dean, S. G., Siegert, R. J., & McPherson, K. M. (2011). Navigating patient-centered goal setting in inpatient stroke rehabilitation: How clinicians control the process to meet perceived professional responsibilities. *Patient Education and Counseling, 85*(2), 206–213.

Levack, W. M. M., Taylor, K., Siegert, R. J., Dean, S. G., McPherson, K. M., & Weatherall, M. (2006). Is goal planning in rehabilitation effective? A systematic review. *Clinical Rehabilitation*, *20*(9), 739–755.

Levine, B., Robertson, I. H., Clare, L., Carter, G., Hong, J., Wilson, B. A., ... Stuss, D. T. (2000). Rehabilitation of executive functioning: An experimental–clinical validation of Goal Management Training. *Journal of the International Neuropsychological Society*, *6*, 299–312.

Locke, E. A., & Latham, G. P. (2002). Building a practically useful theory of goal setting and task motivation: A 35 year odyssey. *American Psychologist*, *57*, 705–717.

Malec, J. F. (1999). Goal attainment scaling in rehabilitation. *Neuropsychological Rehabilitation*, *9*(3/4), 253–275.

Mateer, C. A. (1999). The rehabilitation of executive disorders. In: Stuss, D. T., Winocur, G., Robertson, I. H., eds. *Cognitive Neurorehabilitation*. Cambridge, England: Cambridge University Press, pp. 314–332.

McGavin, H. (1998). Planning rehabilitation: A comparison of issues for parents and adolescents. *Physical and Occupational Therapy in Paediatrics*, *18*(1), 69–82.

McGrath, W. I., Meuller, M. M., Brown, C. B., Teitelman, J., & Watts, J. (2000). Caregivers of persons with Alzheimer's Disease: An exploratory study of occupational performance and respite. *Physical and Occupational Therapy in Geriatrics*, *18*, 51–69.

McPherson, K. M., Kayes, N., & Weatherall, M. (2009). A pilot study of self-regulation informed goal setting in people with traumatic brain injury. *Clinical Rehabilitation*, *23*, 296–309.

Miller, W. R., & Rollnick, S. (2002). *Motivational interviewing: Preparing people for change* (2nd ed.) New York, NY: The Guilford Press.

Miranti, V. S., & Heinemann, A. W. (2004). Systematic motivational counseling in rehabilitation settings. In W. Miles Cox & E. Klinger (Eds.), *Handbook of motivational counseling: Concepts, approaches and assessment* (pp. 301–318). West Sussex, England: John Wiley & Sons.

Ottenbacher, K. J., & Cusick, A. (1989). Goal attainment scaling as a method of clinical service evaluation. *American Journal of Occupational Therapy*, *44*(6), 519–525.

Ownsworth, T., Fleming, J., Shum, D., Kuipers, P., & Strong, J. (2008). Comparison of individual, group and combined intervention formats in a randomized controlled trial for facilitating goal attainment and improving psychosocial function following acquired brain injury. *Journal of Rehabilitation Medicine*, *40*, 81–88.

Pedretti, L. W., & Wade, I. E. (1996). Therapeutic modalities. In L. W. Pedretti (Ed.). *Occupational therapy: Practice skills for physical dysfunction* (4th ed., pp. 293–317). St Louis, MO: Mosby Incorporated.

Phipps, S., & Richardson, P. (2007). Occupational therapy outcomes for clients with traumatic brain injury and stroke using the Canadian Occupational Performance Measure. *The American Journal of Occupational Therapy*, *61*(3), 328–334.

Playford, D. E., Dawson, L., Limbert, V., Smith, M., Ward, C. D., & Wells, R. (2000). Goal-setting in rehabilitation: Report of a workshop to explore professionals' perceptions of goal-setting. *Clinical Rehabilitation*, *14*, 491–496.

Playford, D. E., Siegert, R., Levack, W., & Freeman, J. (2009). Areas of consensus and controversy about goal setting in rehabilitation: A conference report. *Clinical Rehabilitation*, *23*, 334–344.

Pollock, N. (1993). Client-centred assessment. *American Journal of Occupational Therapy*, *47*(4), 298–301.

Pollock, N., & Stewart, D. (1998). Occupational performance needs of school-aged children with physical disability in the community. *Physical and Occupational Therapy in Paediatrics*, *8*, 55–68.

Reed, K., & Sanderson, S. R. (1980). *Concepts in occupational therapy*. Baltimore, MD: Williams and Wilkins.

Roley, S. S., DeLany, J. V., Barrows, C. J., Brownrigg, S., Honaker, D., Sava, D. I., ... Youngstrom, M. J. (2008). Occupational therapy practice framework: Domain and process (2nd ed.). *American Journal of Occupational Therapy*, *62*(6), 625–683.

Rollnick, S., Miler, W. R., & Butler, C. C. (2008). *Motivational interviewing in health care: Helping patients change behavior*. New York, NY: The Guilford Press.

Schonberger, M., Humle, F., & Teasdale, T. W. (2006). The development of the therapeutic working alliance, patients' awareness and their compliance during the process of brain injury rehabilitation. *Brain Injury, 20*(4), 445–454.

Schwarzer, R. (1992). Self-efficacy in the adoption and maintenance of health behaviours: Theoretical approaches and a new model. In R. Schwarzer (Ed.), *Self-efficacy: Thought control of action* (1st ed., pp. 217–238). Washington, DC: Hemisphere Publishing Corporations.

Scobbie, L., Dixon, D., & Wyke, S. (2011). Goal setting and action planning in the rehabilitation setting: Development of a theoretically informed practice framework. *Clinical Rehabilitation, 25*, 468–482.

Sherer, M., Boake, C., Levin, E., Silver, B. V., Ringholz, G., & High, W. M. Jr. (1998). Characteristics of impaired awareness after traumatic brain injury. *Journal of the International Neuropsychological Society, 4*, 380–387.

Siegert, R. J., & Taylor, W. J. (2004). Theoretical aspects of goal-setting and motivation in rehabilitation. *Disability and Rehabilitation, 26*(1), 1–8.

Sivaraman Nair, K. P. (2003). Life goals: The concept and its relevance to rehabilitation. *Clinical Rehabilitation, 17*, 192–202.

Tennant, A. (2007). Goal attainment scaling: Current methodological challenges. *Disability and Rehabilitation, 29*, 1583–1588.

Toglia, J. P., & Kirk, U. (2000). Understanding awareness deficits following brain injury. *NeuroRehabilitation, 15*(1), 57–70.

Townsend, E. A., & Polatajko, H. J. (2007). *Enabling occupation II: Advancing an occupational therapy vision for health, well-being & justice through occupation.* Ottawa, Ontario, Canada: CAOT.

Trombly, C. A. (1995). Purposeful activity. In C. A. Trombly (Ed.), *Occupational therapy for physical dysfunction* (4th ed., pp. 237–253). Baltimore, MD: Williams and Wilkins.

Trombly, C. A., Radomski, M. V., & Davis, E. A. (1998). Achievement of self-identified goals by adults with traumatic brain injury: Phase I. *American Journal of Occupational Therapy, 52*(10), 810–818.

Trombly, C. A., Radomski, M. V., Trexel, C., & Burnet-Smith, S. E. (2002). Occupational therapy and achievement of self-identified goals by adults with acquired brain injury: Phase II. *American Journal of Occupational Therapy, 56*(5), 489–498.

Tryssenaar, J., Jones, E. J., & Lee, D. (1999). Occupational performance needs of a shelter population. *Canadian Journal of Occupational Therapy, 66*, 188–196.

Von Koch, L. V., Wottrich, A. W., & Widen-Holmqvist, W. L. (1998). Rehabilitation in the home versus the hospital: The importance of context. *Disability and Rehabilitation, 20*(10), 367–372.

Webb, P. M., & Glueckauf, R. L. (1994). The effects of direct involvement in goal setting on rehabilitation outcome for persons with traumatic brain injuries. *Rehabilitation Psychology, 39*(3), 179–188.

Wilson, B. A., Evans, J. J., & Keohane, C. (2002). Cognitive rehabilitation: A goal-planning approach. *Journal of Head Trauma Rehabilitation, 17*(6), 542–555.

Wressle, E., Eeg-Olofsson, A., Marcusson, J., & Henriksson, C. (2002). Improved client participation in the rehabilitation process using a client-centred goal formulation structure. *Journal of Rehabilitation Medicine, 34*, 5–11.

Wressle, E., Oberg, B., & Henriksson, C. (1999). The rehabilitation process for the geriatric stroke patient – An exploratory study of goal setting interventions. *Disability and Rehabilitation, 21*(2), 80–87.

11
Theory-Based Approach to Goal Setting

Lesley Scobbie and Diane Dixon

CONTENTS

11.1 Introduction

We begin this chapter with an overview of what theory is and what it can be used for. We suggest that theory is central to the development of a cumulative evidence base, especially in an area as complex as rehabilitation. However, it is possible to identify numerous theories relevant to rehabilitation in general and goal setting in particular. As a consequence, researchers and practitioners are faced with the problem of selecting a theory or theories suitable for their particular problem or question. Theory integration may offer a solution to this problem and we discuss recent work on theory integration in relation to goal setting within rehabilitation. We then go on to illustrate the process of theory selection and development by describing, in detail, a programme of work to develop a theory-based goal-setting professional practice framework. This practice framework focuses on stroke rehabilitation in a community setting but the development process is easily transferred across health conditions and settings.

11.2 What Is Theory and Why Is It Important in Rehabilitation?

We all have our own personal theories of how the world works and these theories guide and shape our behaviour, including professional practice. For example, a general practitioner is more likely to refer his or her patients to radiography for x-ray if he or she believes that degeneration of the spine typically plays a causal role in lower back pain, even though the evidence base indicates otherwise (Savigny, Watson, & Underwood, 2009; van den Bosch, Hollingworth, Kinmonth, & Dixon, 2004). These personal theories about the world are often implicit, that is, they are not shared and therefore are not open to scrutiny. Within research and practice, it is usual and useful to make theory explicit so it can be discussed, shared and evaluated.

Very simply then, theory can be considered to be a tool for thinking and doing. Theory provides an explicit and organized description of what is known about a particular phenomenon. Theory identifies and defines both the constituent parts of a system and the processes that relate one part to another. It can also specify the nature of interventions. As a consequence, theory enables us to predict, explain and change the world. It is fundamental to the development of a cumulative evidence base and to evidence-based practice.

11.3 Theory, Rehabilitation and the Concept of Disability

The relationship between theory and rehabilitation is a subject of much debate (Dunn & Elliott, 2008). It has been argued that an integrative theory of rehabilitation is lacking and that a unifying theory would confer benefit on the discipline as a whole, including the work of health professionals and researchers, and improve outcomes for patients (Siegert, McPherson, & Dean, 2005). However, it is also acknowledged that the development of a single unifying theory of rehabilitation poses many challenges, especially in regard to the wide scope required of such a theory. A somewhat boundless theory might risk violating the key requirements of a scientific theory, namely, that it (1) is composed of constructs that have logical consistency, (2) can generate hypotheses that can be empirically tested and (3) is parsimonious and operates within a clearly defined domain (Dekker, 2008). Others have suggested that rehabilitation requires two models, a model of illness and a model of the process of rehabilitation in the context of that model of illness (Wade, 2003). These discussions about theory and rehabilitation should not be taken to indicate that rehabilitation has not benefitted from the use of theory. Multiple theories have been used within rehabilitation but the focus has tended towards theories or models of disability, rather than on rehabilitation per se.

Multiple theories of disability are available, each of which is informed by how disability is conceptualized. Three conceptualizations of disability dominate the literature: impairment-based models (World Health Organization [WHO], 1980, 2001), social models (Oliver, 1990; Thomas, 2004) and behavioural models (Johnston, 1996). These disability concepts have been used to inform discipline-specific interventions. For example, an orthopaedic consultant would reduce disability associated with osteoarthritis of the hip through total hip replacement surgery, indicating the use of an impairment-based conceptualization of disability. In contrast, a social scientist might advocate for the adoption of equal opportunity legislation for people with disabilities or the redesigning of public transport to enable access by wheelchair users, indicating disability is conceptualized as a consequence of the structure of the social and physical environment. Conceptualizing disability as behaviour may initially seem rather strange. However, disability is typically measured in terms of the ability or inability of an individual to perform particular activities. For example, activities of daily living are measured by instruments such as the Barthel index (Mahoney & Barthel, 1965) and the Functional Independence Measure (Keith, Granger, Hamilton, & Sherwin, 1987). Activities of daily living are behaviours, for example, the ability to go up and down stairs, the ability to walk and the ability to wash your hair; stair climbing, walking and hair washing are discrete behaviours. As a consequence, these behaviours can be modelled by theories of behaviour drawn from psychology. It is the use of the concept of disability as behaviour that is the basis for the use of goal setting within rehabilitation because goals are an important construct within many theories of human behaviour. The use of behavioural theory within rehabilitation is increasingly recognized as an important theoretical tool to further our understanding of the factors that influence outcomes from rehabilitation and to inform intervention design and implementation (Siegert, Mcpherson, & Taylor, 2004; Siegert & Taylor, 2004; Wade, 2006).

11.4 Goal Setting and Rehabilitation

Goal setting is viewed as a core component of rehabilitation interventions (Levack et al., 2006; Scottish Intercollegiate Guidelines Network, 2010; Siegert & Taylor, 2004) and as a core skill of rehabilitation practitioners (Wade, 2000). The development of our understanding of how goals and goal setting operate within rehabilitation requires an appropriate theoretical framework. Locke and Latham's work on the effect of goal setting on performance within occupational settings represents the most comprehensive programme of work on goal setting to date (Locke & Latham, 2002). However, three features of Locke and Latham's approach to goal setting reduce its suitability as a model of goal setting within rehabilitation. First, its focus is to specifically increase task performance rather than goal achievement. Second, this focus does not require goals to be achievable. Third, goal importance is not defined in terms of patient relevance; rather, goal importance can be entirely external to the patient (Playford, Siegert, Levack, & Freeman, 2009). These limitations suggest other theories and models, which may be more relevant to application within a rehabilitation setting, should be considered.

The concept of a goal and goal setting occur in several other theories of behaviour. For example, goals can be found in social cognitive theory (Bandura, 2000), the health action process approach (Schwarzer, 1992), self-regulation theory (Carver & Scheier, 1981, 1982; Hart & Evans, 2006) and the common-sense self-regulation model (Leventhal, Leventhal, & Contrada, 1998). Further, other theories and models of motivation might also provide a theoretical framework within which goal setting in rehabilitation might be understood (Siegert & Taylor, 2004), for example, self-determination theory (Deci & Ryan, 1985). These social cognition models have often been used to understand health behaviours, such as diet and physical activity (Armitage & Conner, 2000), and outcomes from illness, including disability (Dixon, Johnston, Rowley, & Pollard, 2008; Johnston et al., 2007; Sniehotta, Scholz, & Schwarzer, 2006). Consequently, there is a growing evidence base for their utility in the relevant domain of health behaviour and with relevant (clinical) populations. Social cognition models have also been used to understand health professionals' behaviour and to design interventions to change health professionals' behaviour (Hrisos et al., 2008; Ivers et al., 2010). Thus, social cognition approaches may provide valuable theoretical insights into the role of goals and goal setting within rehabilitation from both patient and practitioner perspectives.

11.5 Identifying Appropriate Theoretical Frameworks for Goal Setting in Rehabilitation

As a result of the lack of a universal theory of rehabilitation and the availability of multiple theories of behaviour concerning the concept of a goal, the researcher or practitioner is faced with the difficult problem of deciding which theory to employ. Ideally, a systematic review of the evidence base should be undertaken to identify the model best suited to a particular problem. However, the predictive utility of a theory varies across behaviours, conditions and situations (Hagger, Chatzisarantis, & Biddle, 2002; Hagger & Orbell, 2003; Milne, Sheeran, & Orbell, 2000), and it is unlikely that any one theory will universally outperform all others. Rather, it is more likely that a review will indicate, at best, several theories that could be used, and unless the scope of the review is tightly focused, the choice of which theory to choose is likely to remain. Faced with the problem of identifying candidate theories for use in the development of a goal-setting practice framework for community rehabilitation in stroke, a recent literature review (by the present authors) focused on theories containing goal-setting concepts that had been used in a clinical context (Scobbie, Wyke, & Dixon, 2009). In this review, it was the explicit use of theory and the situation (clinical context), rather than the health condition (stroke), which was used to structure the review. This review identified 24 relevant studies that used 5 different theories, namely, social cognitive theory, goal-setting theory, health action process approach, proactive coping and the common-sense self-regulation model. Thus, even after a focused literature review, multiple potential theories remained.

Narrowing the scope of any literature review is dependent upon the availability of precise search terms. Unfortunately, there is no agreed standard terminology for goal setting in the rehabilitation literature. Goal setting has variously been described as goal planning, care planning, setting aims and objectives and action planning. Similarly, what constitutes goal setting, that is, what are its component parts, is unclear (Hurn, Kneebone, & Cropley, 2006; Levack et al., 2006; Playford et al., 2009; Wade, 1999). Further, there is not a universally accepted definition of goal setting in rehabilitation practice. The lack of a standard terminology hinders the development of a cumulative evidence base. It is difficult to structure a search strategy when different terms are used to describe the same underlying phenomenon, and it is especially difficult to determine if all relevant literature has been identified. Further, the content of goal-setting interventions is not always described in detail, making it difficult to ascertain precisely what has been delivered. Fortunately, recent efforts have begun to address these issues in an attempt to develop a consensus in relation to goal setting within neurological rehabilitation (Playford et al., 2009). It would benefit the development of a cumulative evidence base if the rehabilitation community could progress this work to develop clear and agreed definitions of goal setting and to specify the core content of goal setting within rehabilitation.

11.6 Integrating Goal Setting within a Wider Theoretical Framework for Rehabilitation

There is an emerging consensus within behavioural science that the application of a single theory may be limiting and that an approach that integrates across relevant theories may be better suited to understanding the complexity of human health-related behaviours (Hagger, 2009). Much of this work has focused on integrating elements from across different social cognition theories (Armitage, 2009; Gibbons, Houlihan, & Gerrard, 2009; Hagger & Chatzisarantis, 2009; Lippke & Plotnikoff, 2009; Ntoumanis, Edmunds, & Duda, 2009; Sniehotta, 2009), many of which share the same or similar constructs. For example, the concept of self-efficacy was originally developed by Bandura within the framework of social cognitive theory (Bandura, 1997), but it is also a fundamental component of Locke and Latham's work on the role of goals as drivers of performance (Locke & Latham, 2002) and the health action process approach (Schwarzer, 1992) and has been added to other theories to improve their predictive utility (Conner & Armitage, 1998; Hagger & Chatzisarantis, 2005; Prentice-Dunn & Rogers, 1986).

This overlap in content provides a useful basis for integration across social cognition theories. Consider the example earlier of a review that identified social cognitive theory, goal-setting theory, health action process approach, proactive coping and the common-sense self-regulation model as candidate theories for a goal-setting practice framework from community rehabilitation teams (Scobbie et al., 2009). Self-efficacy is a component part of the first four theories and on this basis any integrated theoretical framework should probably include the concept of self-efficacy.

Assuming that constructs that appear in multiple theories are more likely to have predictive utility across behaviours and situations, the process of comparing constructs within candidate theories should identify the key concepts for any integrative theoretical framework. That said, it is important to guard against what has been described as *cafeteria-style research* (Bandura, 2000, p. 299), whereby constructs from multiple similar theories are used to predict behaviour without regard to their original broader conceptual framework. This type of approach is more likely to result in fractionation of the evidence base rather than integration. A theoretical framework for rehabilitation should also consider inclusion of concepts that are theorized to have a causal role in behaviour. Some social cognition models have good predictive utility but may be less useful for the design of interventions to change behaviour because they are not causal models (Hardeman et al., 2002). Importantly, self-efficacy is theorized to be a causal construct and methods are available to increase self-efficacy (Bandura, 1997), for example, chronic disease self-management programmes employ techniques to increase self-efficacy as the means by which improvements in outcome are achieved (Bodenheimer, Lorig, Holman, & Grumbach, 2002; Marks, Allegrante, & Lorig, 2005). Self-efficacy would therefore appear to be a good candidate for inclusion in any integrated model of rehabilitation.

It could be argued that integrating across theories that share the same or very similar constructs should be quite straightforward. However, the process of rehabilitation, including goal setting, is complex and is likely to require a theoretical framework that is not limited to social cognition theories. This raises the question of whether goal and goal-setting theories from psychology can be integrated with broader models used in rehabilitation.

The International Classification of Functioning, Disability and Health (ICF) is a taxonomy of health outcomes developed by the World Health Organization (2001). It was designed to provide a common language to describe functioning, disability and health (WHO, 2002). For any given health condition, it identifies three health outcome domains – impairments (to body structures and functions), activity limitations and participation restrictions, each of which is clearly defined. It also indicates that contextual factors, in the form of personal and environmental factors, influence each health outcome and the relationships between them. The ICF is now widely used; a recent review of the ICF identified 672 papers that had used the ICF between 2001 and 2009, approximately a quarter of which reported the use of the ICF in clinical or rehabilitation contexts (Cerniauskaite et al., 2011).

However, the ICF was designed as a static taxonomy of health outcomes and has been criticized for neglecting the temporal nature of chronic health conditions (Wade & Halligan, 2003). Goals are a dynamic concept, as they relate to some future state; as a result, any integrative theory will need to be dynamic. That said, two features of the ICF enable its integration with social cognition theories. First, the ICF contains behavioural concepts. Activity limitations are behaviour, and behaviour is a component part of many participation restrictions. Second, social cognition theories can be used to operationalize the personal factors component of the contextual factors construct. The integration of social cognition models and the ICF transforms the ICF into a dynamic process model that identifies beliefs, including goals, as mediators of the relationship between the three health outcome domains. A schematic diagram of such an integrated model is shown in Figure 11.1. Empirical studies have shown that this integrated model is a better predictor of disability than either the ICF or psychological models alone in people awaiting joint

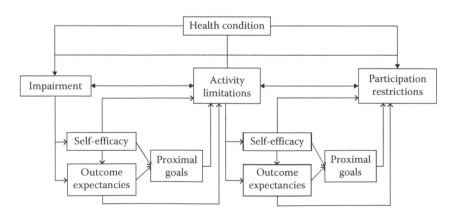

FIGURE 11.1
Integration of social cognitive theory into the ICF.

replacement surgery (Dixon et al., 2008) and in community samples (Dixon, Johnston, Elliott, & Hannaford, 2012).

Consider, for example, a 70-year-old man recovering from a stroke who has a drop foot (impairment). This might affect his confidence (self-efficacy) in his ability to walk in uncertain conditions, such as across rough terrain, or to walk quickly when needed. He might also anticipate that in these situations, he is at increased risk of falling (outcome expectancies) when he walks. He might, therefore, modify his goals of returning to playing golf and of being more active in general (activity limitations). His experience of activity limitations might then affect his involvement in valued social activities (participation restrictions), such as playing with his grandchildren, because he lacks confidence in his functional abilities and anticipates negative outcomes, such as being unable to prevent his grandchild running into the road.

This integrated model is, therefore, suitable for use in multidisciplinary settings because it is able to accommodate those constructs of most importance to both biomedicine (impairments) and social scientists (contextual factors). The model enables interventions at the level of impairment, activity limitations, participation restrictions, beliefs and the environment to be used to improve outcomes. Further, the inclusion of reciprocal relationships between the components of the model also accommodates interventions used by many rehabilitation professionals, for example, exercises (activity) to improve muscle strength (body structure and function).

11.7 Value of Theory to Practice and Patient Outcomes

Goal-setting practice continues to be largely atheoretical, with a *common-sense* approach to implementation rather than practice based on a sound theoretical rationale (Siegert & Taylor, 2004). It is of some concern that the evidence base to support the clinical efficacy of goal setting in rehabilitation is itself not robust (Siegert & Taylor, 2004; Wade, 2005). A recent, systematic review of the effectiveness of setting goals in rehabilitation settings concluded that there is some evidence that goal setting can improve patient adherence to rehabilitation; however, there was no consistent evidence to support its impact on patient outcomes. It was also noted that the quality of much of the evidence base was poor, for example, there was a lack of clarity about the purpose of goal setting which made it difficult to evaluate its effectiveness (Levack et al., 2006).

It has been accepted wisdom that interventions based on theory are likely to be more effective than those that are not (Albarracín et al., 2005; Downing, Jones, Cook, & Bellis, 2006). Whether this is the case for goal setting, interventions in rehabilitation cannot be examined because of the current lack of theoretically based interventions in the area. However, recent developments in behavioural science have begun to demonstrate that this is actually the case for interventions designed to change protective health behaviours. Meta-regression analyses of interventions to change physical activity and dietary behaviours have shown that those based on theory were more effective than those that were not (Michie, Abraham, Whittington, McAteer, & Gupta, 2009). These types of analyses are beginning to generate an evidence base in support of what was formerly simply a shared assumption that theory-based interventions are more effective.

Further, the value of theory has been recognized by the research community through published guidelines for the development of complex interventions (Craig et al., 2008).

These guidelines define best practice and identify a central role for theory, especially in the development and evaluation phases of complex interventions. Of particular importance is the ability of theory to guide and inform the modelling of processes and outcomes prior to a full scale evaluation of any intervention.

11.8 Theory to Practice: A Worked Example

Given the earlier discussion, the translation of theory into practice might seem a daunting prospect. In the next section of this chapter, we describe the development of a theory-based framework to guide goal-setting practice with people recovering from stroke in community rehabilitation settings. The focus of the framework was the practitioners delivering rehabilitation to stroke patients as part of a multidisciplinary team. The aim was to develop a theory-based practice framework to guide the delivery of goal setting so that practitioners would understand the rationale for goal setting and that practice would be optimized and standardized. We conclude the chapter with the recognition that carrying out systematic reviews and redesigning practice from scratch is probably impractical for most rehabilitation professionals and suggest ways in which theory can be used to evaluate and improve current practice.

11.9 Which Theories Should Inform Goal-Setting Practice in the Rehabilitation Setting?

Health professionals working in rehabilitation settings might find it difficult to name theories relevant to their goal-setting practice; this is probably because goal setting has been accepted as something that makes good clinical sense and therefore not in need of a strong theoretical rationale to support it (Siegert et al., 2004; Siegert & Taylor, 2004). However, the absence of a theoretical underpinning to goal-setting practice can lead to clinical uncertainties about what the key components of goal-setting interventions are, what terminology should be used to describe them, how they are likely to impact on patient outcomes and how to adjust the process if progress is not being made.

In addition to this theory–practice gap, there is a lack of evidence to support the impact of goal setting on patient outcomes in the rehabilitation setting. Sugavanam and colleagues (2013) systematically integrated and appraised the evidence for effects and experiences of goal setting in stroke rehabilitation. They concluded that no firm conclusions could be made on the effectiveness, feasibility and acceptability of goal setting in stroke rehabilitation and that further rigorous research was required to strengthen the evidence base. These findings concur with the findings of other studies examining the effectiveness of goal setting in the rehabilitation setting (Levack et al., 2006; Rosewilliam, Roskell, & Pandyan, 2011).

In view of the identified gaps in both evidence and theory, we have argued that goal setting is an important but complex intervention that should be developed and evaluated in a systematic way (Scobbie et al., 2009). The development of a theoretically informed goal-setting practice framework in which the key components and mechanisms of action are clearly defined should: (1) guide goal-setting practice in a structured and systematic way, providing health professionals with a shared understanding of *what* to do, *how* to go about doing it and *why* they are doing it in a particular way; (2) use terminology and concepts that are understood by the health-care team, patients and carers; and (3) clarify how patients (and carers) can best be involved in the process to optimize goal attainment in areas that reflect *their* priorities. Such a development would facilitate the systematic evaluation of a replicable goal-setting intervention, thus enabling the development of a cumulative evidence base.

The Medical Research Council (MRC) guidance for the development and evaluation of complex interventions (Craig et al., 2008) provides a framework to guide such development. This guidance emphasizes the importance of beginning the development process with the identification of a theoretical rationale to support the intervention. In line with the MRC recommendations, our first step in the development of a practice framework was to conduct a structured review of the rehabilitation and health-related self-management literature to identify those theories of behaviour change that offered the most potential to inform goal-setting practice in rehabilitation settings (Scobbie et al., 2009). We decided to focus on theories of behaviour change on the basis that the rehabilitation process primarily challenges people to change or adjust their behaviour at the level of impairment (e.g. forced use of an affected upper limb to improve motor control), activity (e.g. learning to get in and out of a bath using adaptive equipment) or participation (e.g. practising use of public transport to access the local library).

Our search identified three theories of behaviour change that were chosen on the basis of their capacity to inform goal-related rehabilitation or self-management interventions that had resulted in improved patient outcomes. The three theories were social cognitive theory (Bandura, 1997), health action process approach (Schwarzer, 1992) and goal-setting theory (Locke & Latham, 2002). Further review of these theories identified clear overlapping constructs within them, namely, self-efficacy, outcome expectancies, goal attributes, planning, appraisal and feedback.

Self-efficacy relates to how confident an individual is in their ability to achieve a desired goal in the presence of perceived barriers or facilitators (Bandura, 1997). Bandura (1997) argued that 'unless people believe they can achieve desired effects by their actions, they will have little incentive to act' (Bandura, 1997, p. 2). *Outcome expectancies* are beliefs about what the outcome of performing a particular goal-directed behaviour will be (Bandura, 2000, p. 306). Beliefs about self-efficacy and outcome expectancies operate together and are expected to exert their influence on health outcomes by improving motivation to set and pursue goals (Marks et al., 2005) and to increase resilience in the face of setbacks during goal pursuit (Schwarzer, Ziegelmann, Luszczynska, Scholz, & Lippke, 2008). Consider a person recovering from a stroke who believes they have the ability to dress themselves and that doing so will make them feel better. Social cognitive theory suggests they are more likely to be motivated to pursue that goal than someone who is not confident they can get dressed and believes that doing so will only use up energy they would rather have for other activities they think are more important.

Goal-setting theory has identified goal *specificity* and *difficulty* as the two primary *goal attributes* that will influence goal-related performance. The theory advocates that goals should be proximal and specific as opposed to vague *do your best*-type goals and should be difficult enough to challenge the person without taking them beyond the limits of their ability (Locke & Latham, 2002). The theory suggests that goals exert their influence by directing attention and effort, maximizing persistence and fostering problem solving in relation to the set goal (Locke & Latham, 2002). A goal such as *try to walk as much as you can* is less likely to be effective than a specific goal such as *aim to walk to the corner shop and back by the end of the month*. The specific goal creates a clear *benchmark* to focus attention on and measure performance against, both of which are important motivational influences.

Planning is about getting beyond the intention to do something, to actually doing it. There are two types of plans: action plans and coping plans. Action plans specify in behavioural terms exactly what has to be done, where it has to be done and when it has to be done. Coping plans encourage the person to think about barriers that may get in the way of carrying out the action plan and proactively think about strategies to overcome those barriers (Sniehotta et al., 2006).

Appraisal is the assessment of performance in carrying out the plan and gauging progress in relation to the goal. *Feedback* is the information provided to the actor (the person recovering from stroke in this case) on the basis of the appraisal of their performance (Locke & Latham, 2002). Appraisal and feedback perform several important functions. Where progress is being made, they motivate continued goal pursuit. If there is a problem with progress or circumstances have changed, they can prompt adjustments to goal-directed behaviour or disengagement from the goal (Maes & Karoly, 2005).

The clinical relevance of these theoretical constructs is clear; health professionals will recognize that confidence or self-efficacy, expectations about outcomes, specifying goals, making plans and giving feedback are all likely to impact on how patients engage in the goal-setting process. However, they are unlikely to have been considered or applied in a structured or standard way during usual goal-setting practice either within or between clinical settings. This probably goes some way to explaining why the practice of setting and achieving rehabilitation goals in the clinical setting is highly variable (Holliday, Antoun, & Playford, 2005; Levack et al., 2006; Playford et al., 2009) and often problematic (Borell, Daniels, & Winding, 2002; Parry, 2004).

11.10 How Can Theoretical Constructs Be Mapped onto the Goal-Setting Process?

Our next task was to consider how these theoretical constructs could inform clinical practice on a day-to-day basis. The MRC framework recommends Hardeman et al.'s causal modelling approach as one way of linking theory to health outcomes in complex interventions that are designed to promote behaviour change (Hardeman et al., 2005). A causal model can be thought of as a hypothetical process through which theory is used to identify the factors that determine behaviour change. We used the causal modelling approach to: (1) identify the factors likely to influence patients' motivation to pursue goals, (2) identify the behaviour(s) the goal should target and (3) consider the likely impact of a change in these behaviours on health outcomes.

The causal model also identifies the variables that are expected to mediate the relationship between the target behaviour and health outcomes. In other words, if a patient engages in the target behaviour, for example, practising climbing stairs, the causal model specifies how performing that behaviour will influence health outcomes, for example, improved functional outcomes. The causal modelling approach is useful for developing a practice framework because it identifies the points during the goal-setting process where health professionals can intervene with specific techniques to promote behaviour change.

The developed goal-setting causal model is outlined in Figure 11.2. It is important to consider what the practice implications of the causal model are – these can be summarized as follows:

- Self-efficacy, outcome expectancies, goal specificity and difficulty and planning will influence patients' goal-related behaviour.
- The behaviours targeted during the goal-setting process can be conceptualized in terms of the ICF functional levels of impairment, activity and participation.
- Successfully engaging in target behaviours is predicted to lead to incremental functional improvements at the level of impairment, activity or participation and enhanced self-efficacy.
- Health professionals can enhance patients' self-efficacy at intervention points by:
  - Setting plans that will optimize their chances of success (*mastery experience*)
  - Providing credible encouragement and positive feedback (*verbal persuasion*)
  - Highlighting other people in similar circumstances who have been able to achieve success (*vicarious experience*)
  - Helping their patients to correctly interpret their physical and/or emotional responses during tasks, for example, reassuring them it is natural to feel anxious the first time they try something new (*re-interpretation of physiological symptoms*)
- The cumulative effect of incremental functional improvements and enhanced self-efficacy is predicted to result in a measurable improvement in goal attainment and rehabilitation outcomes.

The causal model clearly identifies four intervention points where health professionals can act to influence and optimize behaviour change by: (1) facilitating the development of goal intentions, (2) identifying a specific goal to work on, (3) breaking this goal down into action plans with coping plans in place if barriers to action plan attainment are anticipated and (4) appraising performance and giving feedback. Strategies to enhance self-efficacy are included within all intervention points. It is also acknowledged within the causal model that goals and action plans may be assigned or self-set. The theoretical justification for this is found within goal-setting theory, which states that assigned goals do not reduce performance as long as the actor (in this case the patient) understands the rationale behind the goal and agrees that pursuing it is likely to result in a good outcome for them (Locke & Latham, 2002). Overall, the causal model makes an explicit link for health professionals between theory, practice and outcomes.

11.11 Developing a G-AP Framework for Clinical Practice

A multidisciplinary task group was set up within a community rehabilitation team in Scotland (*R*ehabilitation *a*t *C*ommunity and *H*ome (ReACH) Team) to explore how the goal-setting causal model could be applied in clinical practice (Scobbie, Dixon, & Wyke, 2011). The *workability* of each intervention point of the causal model was assessed by hypothetically applying it to case studies of patients currently seen by the team.

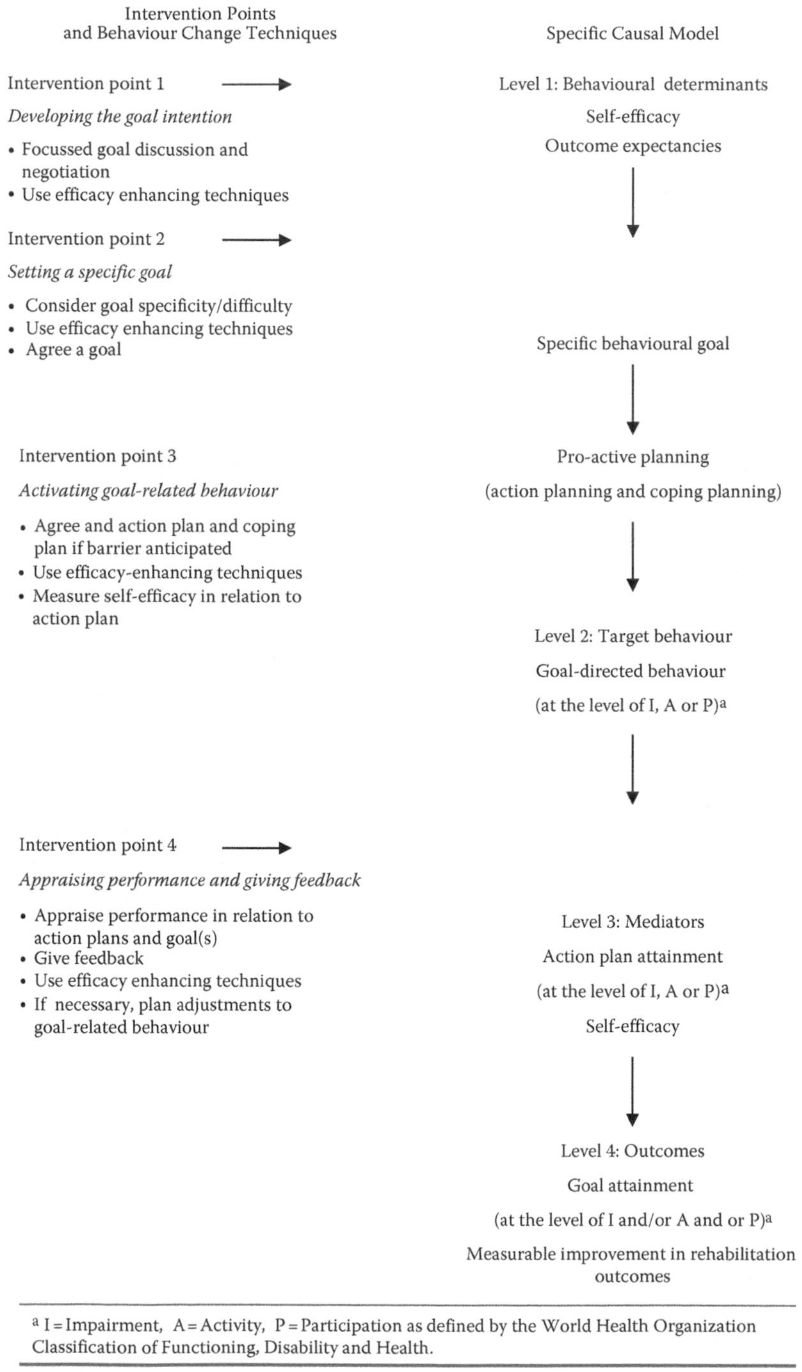

Intervention Points
and Behaviour Change Techniques

Specific Causal Model

Intervention point 1 ⟶

Developing the goal intention

- Focussed goal discussion and negotiation
- Use efficacy enhancing techniques

Level 1: Behavioural determinants

Self-efficacy

Outcome expectancies

Intervention point 2 ⟶

Setting a specific goal

- Consider goal specificity/difficulty
- Use efficacy enhancing techniques
- Agree a goal

Specific behavioural goal

Intervention point 3

Activating goal-related behaviour

- Agree and action plan and coping plan if barrier anticipated
- Use efficacy-enhancing techniques
- Measure self-efficacy in relation to action plan

Pro-active planning

(action planning and coping planning)

Level 2: Target behaviour

Goal-directed behaviour

(at the level of I, A or P)[a]

Intervention point 4 ⟶

Appraising performance and giving feedback

- Appraise performance in relation to action plans and goal(s)
- Give feedback
- Use efficacy enhancing techniques
- If necessary, plan adjustments to goal-related behaviour

Level 3: Mediators

Action plan attainment

(at the level of I, A or P)[a]

Self-efficacy

Level 4: Outcomes

Goal attainment

(at the level of I and/or A and or P)[a]

Measurable improvement in rehabilitation outcomes

---

[a] I = Impairment, A = Activity, P = Participation as defined by the World Health Organization Classification of Functioning, Disability and Health.

FIGURE 11.2

Goal-setting causal model with intervention points and behaviour change techniques. (From Scobbie, L. et al., *Clin. Rehabil.*, 25(5), 468, 2011.)

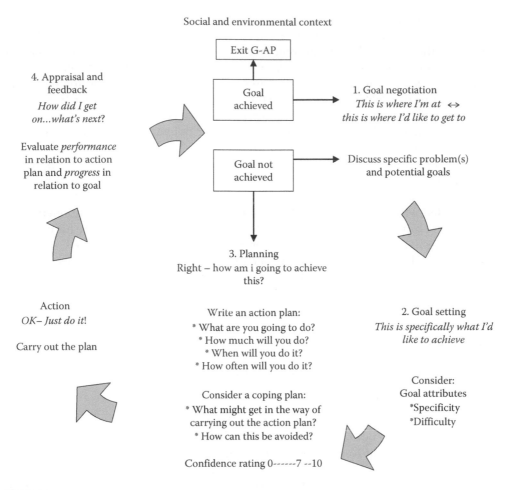

Social and environmental context

Exit G-AP

4. Appraisal and feedback
How did I get on...what's next?

Goal achieved

1. Goal negotiation
This is where I'm at ↔
this is where I'd like to get to

Evaluate *performance* in relation to action plan and *progress* in relation to goal

Goal not achieved

Discuss specific problem(s) and potential goals

3. Planning
Right – how am i going to achieve this?

Action
OK– Just do it!

Carry out the plan

Write an action plan:
* What are you going to do?
* How much will you do?
* When will you do it?
* How often will you do it?

Consider a coping plan:
* What might get in the way of carrying out the action plan?
* How can this be avoided?

Confidence rating 0------7 --10

2. Goal setting
This is specifically what I'd like to achieve

Consider:
Goal attributes
*Specificity
*Difficulty

FIGURE 11.3
G-AP framework. (From Scobbie, L. et al, *Clin. Rehabil.*, 25(5), 468, 2011.)

These discussions resulted in the linear goal-setting causal model being translated into a circular goal setting and action planning (G-AP) practice framework (see Figure 11.3).

In keeping with the causal model, the task group used the ICF (World Health Organization, 2001) alongside the G-AP framework to consider and set goals and action plans at the level of *impairment* (e.g. to improve breath control), *activity* (e.g. to dress independently) or *participation* (e.g. to use public transport to get to work) and to acknowledge the importance of considering contextual factors, that is, the patient's physical and social environment and relevant personal factors (such as coping styles) at each stage of the goal-setting process.

The G-AP framework was then iteratively applied to patients currently receiving rehabilitation services from task group members. The task group discussed the use of the G-AP framework with each patient in turn and reported on the *clinical usefulness* of each of the four intervention points and related behaviour change techniques specified in the causal model, the *feasibility* of implementing the components of the causal model and whether implementation of the causal model was *acceptable* to patients and their carers. These discussions resulted in further refinement of the G-AP framework and development of guidelines for its implementation in clinical practice.

The G-AP framework is designed to support health professionals, patients and carers through a collaborative G-AP process, acknowledging the experience and expertise that each brings to the process. This is important for two reasons. First, the theoretical constructs underpinning the framework, that is, self-efficacy, outcome expectancies, goal attributes, planning, appraisal and feedback, all need to be considered in relation to the patient and their life circumstances. How confident are the patients that they can achieve this goal? Do they believe it will result in a good outcome for them? Is the goal important to them? Will the goal challenge them without taking them beyond their potential? Are they confident they can carry out the action plans and coping plans? How do they think they are doing in relation to completing action plans and achieving their goal? What do they think the next step should be? If patients are not explicitly involved, the motivational potential of each stage of the G-AP process is at best compromised and at worst lost. Second, there is a strong value embedded within health-care policy in the United Kingdom that practitioners should work in partnership with patients and carers to create a shared responsibility for improving health outcomes (Department of Health, 2009; Scottish Executive, 2007). The G-AP framework creates an ideal opportunity for partnership working through the process of setting and working towards agreed goals within a specific time frame (Playford et al., 2009).

11.12 Four Stages of the G-AP Framework

11.12.1 Stage 1: Goal Negotiation

This stage focuses on developing goal intentions. First, patients are encouraged to consider their current situation – both things that are going well and not so well – and identify the main problems they want to address. Goals are more likely to be considered by patients if they have some confidence they can achieve them (self-efficacy), and they believe that achieving them will result in a positive outcome for them (positive outcome expectancies). Goal ideas can be suggested by the health professional and/or the patient (or carer) and discussed between them.

Outcome of this stage: The health professional and patient will agree on the general problem areas/goal(s) that will focus discussion in the next stage, for example, *I want to be able to talk better* or *I want to use my right arm more* or *I want to be able to get out of the house a bit more*.

11.12.2 Stage 2: Setting a Specific Goal

In this stage, the general goal is refined into a specific, challenging goal that will clarify for both the health professional and the patient what they are aiming for. Both should view the goal as important and worth pursuing. Setting a specific goal requires the health professional and patient to make an informed approximation about a future endpoint on the basis of the knowledge and expertise that each has at that particular time. As a consequence, this goal will be SMART*ish*, that is, *s*pecific, *m*easurable, *a*chievable, *r*elevant and *t*imed as it can be with the information currently available.

Outcome of this stage: The health professional and patient will agree on specific goal(s), for example, *I will be confident talking on the telephone to my friends* or *I will be able to use my right hand to sign my name* or *I will be able to take the dog for a walk to the local park on my own*.

11.12.3 Stage 3: Action Planning and Coping Planning

Action plans act as incremental *stepping stones* towards goal achievement, and coping plans prepare for barriers that might get in the way. Together, they work to activate and sustain goal-related behaviour. The action plan should detail, in behavioural terms, *what* has to be done, *when, where* and *how* often. It is an immediate plan that serves as a tangible focus in the here and now. Consequently, action plans do need to meet the *SMART* rule; they are *s*pecific (detail exactly what the patient has to do), *m*easurable (success of completion easily assessed), *a*chievable (represents the next incremental step, therefore should be highly achievable), *r*elevant (set in the current patient context) with a *t*ime frame (should be achievable in the immediate future; days not weeks).

A simple patient-report measure of self-efficacy using a 10-point visual analogue scale has been used to measure patient's confidence to successfully complete their action plans (0 = not at all confident; 10 = very confident). A lack of confidence (score less than 7) would suggest the plan should be modified or discussed further to optimize the chances of successful completion (Lorig, Holman, et al., 2006).

Outcome of this stage: The health professional and patient will agree the action plan that will create the next *stepping stone* to achieving a specific goal and, if necessary, a coping plan to deal with anticipated barriers. For example: Action plan: *Jane will complete her mouth and breathing exercises twice daily over the next week* (to work on the goal of being confident talking on the telephone to friends). Barrier: Jane is worried that she will not complete her exercises properly and will just give in. Coping plan: the speech and language therapist suggests that the rehabilitation assistant can visit the next day to supervise Jane practise her exercises and provide guidance if necessary. Jane agrees this is a good idea and rates her confidence to carry out the action plan as 7 on the self-report self-efficacy measure.

11.12.4 Stage 4: Appraisal and Feedback

At this stage, the health professional and patient appraise the outcome of the action plan and progress in relation to the goal. Health professionals have an opportunity to give feedback; verbal praising of success will act to enhance patient self-efficacy and motivation. Where the goal has not yet been achieved, but reasonable progress is being made through action plan attainment, new action plan(s) can be set. If action plans have not been successful and little or no progress is being made in relation to the goal, it might be necessary to rethink the action plans and/or coping plans or even to return to the goal negotiation phase and reconsider if the goal is worth pursuing.

Outcome of this stage: Progress will be collaboratively reviewed. Patient self-efficacy will be enhanced through positive feedback or support given where progress is lacking. Joint decisions are made about what should happen next.

11.13 Implementation and Evaluation of G-AP in Routine Clinical Practice

Having developed the G-AP framework using theory and practice-based methods, our next objective was to evaluate its implementation in everyday clinical practice from the perspective of patients and health professionals. We conducted a process evaluation of the

G-AP framework within the ReACH team in Scotland (Scobbie, McLean, Dixon, Duncan, & Wyke, 2013). Following team training, the framework was applied to people recovering from stroke over a 6-month period. The study focused only on people with stroke as goal setting is considered *best practice* with this patient group (Royal College of Physicians, 2008; Scottish Intercollegiate Guidelines Network, 2010). Additionally, we wanted to evaluate the multidisciplinary use of G-AP and the majority of stroke referrals to the ReACH team required multidisciplinary input.

The aim of the study was to investigate G-AP implementation and the practical experience of using G-AP, from the perspective of patients and health professionals, in routine clinical practice. Specifically, we were interested in whether G-AP was implemented as intended, the utility of the G-AP stages and patient and health professional views about its perceived benefits (if any).

Implementation of G-AP within the ReACH team was facilitated in three ways: (1) a G-AP protocol was illustrated on a visual flow chart to show how implementation of G-AP would fit within existing ReACH team goal-setting processes; (2) a G-AP patient-held record was developed to ensure that patients had information about their goals and action plans available to them in their own homes and (3) all team members participated in two training sessions, each lasting for 1 h, summarizing the G-AP framework and implementation protocol and use of the G-AP personal record (this training was in addition to the monthly updates team members had received on the stage-by-stage development of the framework).

The study involved two main methods of data collection: (1) *individual semi-structured interviews* with health professionals working within the ReACH team and with stroke patients receiving input from the service and (2) a detailed *audit examination* of the ReACH team service records of the stroke patients who participated in G-AP.

11.13.1 Was G-AP Implemented as Intended?

The case note analysis and discussion of implementation collected in patient and staff interviews revealed that goal negotiation, goal setting and action planning were largely implemented according to the protocol. However, there were inconsistencies noted in the implementation of the novel aspects of the framework, specifically coping planning, use of the visual analogue scale to measure self-efficacy and implementing appraisal and feedback on an *action plan-by-action plan* basis. Coping planning was viewed as a new and unfamiliar addition to practice which health professionals had not got into the habit of using. Health professionals tended to measure patients' confidence implicitly, for example, asking patients, 'do you think you'll be okay with that (action plan)?' rather than using the 0–10 self-efficacy scale. Reasons reported for non-use of the scale included forgetting to use it, not understanding its purpose and a belief it was laborious or could result in a negative emotional response if a patient rated their confidence as high then failed to complete an action plan. Health professionals also reported that the feasibility of implementing the appraisal and feedback stage could be compromised by time constraints.

11.13.2 Tools and Strategies to Facilitate G-AP Implementation

A variety of tools and strategies were used by health professionals to facilitate the goal negotiation and goal-setting stage of the process. Of particular importance was the use of Talking Mats® (Bornman & Murphy, 2006), a low-tech communication framework which uses symbols to facilitate communication. Health professionals referred to questions or *stock phrases* they would use to facilitate goal negotiation and goal setting, for example, *'think about what you would like to be able to do by (date)'* or *'what sort of things did you enjoy doing prior to having the stroke'* or *'think of something very specific to do with that particular activity you would like to work on.'* Giving patients a few examples of potential goals was sometimes used as a starting point and basis for discussion. Finally, the ICF was viewed as a useful framework to help health professionals and patients consider the full spectrum of potential goals at the level of impairment, activity and participation.

11.13.3 Clinical Usefulness/Acceptability of the G-AP Stages

Each of the G-AP stages made a useful contribution to the overall process; however, important insights were gained about implementation of G-AP in routine clinical practice. Firstly, goal negotiation and goal setting tended to be an iterative process merging into one rather than two separate stages. Secondly, the appraisal/feedback stage included a *support* and *decision-making* component. These findings have been used to inform development of the visual illustration of the G-AP framework (Scobbie et al., 2013). If self-appraisal led patients to believe they were successfully attaining action plans and on target for meeting their goals, it was encouraging. In these instances, health professionals' feedback acted to increase patient confidence (self-efficacy); the most commonly used self-efficacy enhancing technique was verbal praising of successes. However, if patients felt they were not attaining action plans or were not on target for meeting their goals, it could result in a negative emotional response. Health professionals tended to respond to this by providing support and reassurance.

Following appraisal and feedback, decisions were made about what to do next. Often, this resulted in either action plans being progressed to the next stage or deciding on a new goal on the basis that the previous goal had been achieved. In some cases, non-attainment of action plans led to a shared view that the goal was unachievable; this resulted in goal disengagement and renegotiation of an alternative goal. An important acceptability issue raised by health professionals was their concern that the appraisal and feedback stage made it explicit to patients if they were not making progress and that this could have a negative impact on their well-being. Different strategies used to manage this were reported including avoiding or not explicitly addressing goals that had not been achieved, reframing failure in a positive way or providing support and reassurance. Conversely, none of the patients voiced concerns about goal non-attainment or how it might impact on their well-being. Although failure to achieve action plans and goals was said to be disappointing, some patients said they used what they had learned from their experience to reassess their situation and to consider more realistic goals.

11.13.4 Health Professional and Patient Views about the Perceived Benefits of the Framework

Patients and health professionals reported that G-AP facilitated flexible patient/professional partnerships, attainment of unique patient goals and family member involvement in the process. Patients and health professionals described working together throughout the G-AP process; however, the nature of the partnership differed from patient to patient. Firstly, each had a different role to play. Patient accounts suggested their role was to tell health professionals about their priorities and preferences, give them feedback about what they felt they could and could not achieve and suggest goals that they would like to work on. Health professionals described their role in terms of guiding and encouraging patients through the G-AP process with a view to tailoring unrealistic or general goals into specific, achievable goals and providing education and information that would help patients make informed goal choices.

Secondly, the range of patient and staff views suggested that a G-AP continuum existed with *patient-led* at one end and *therapist-led* at the other. Patients who preferred health professionals to take the lead believed that they were the *experts*, someone who had experience dealing with other people in the same situation and so were better placed to suggest goals that would help them through their recovery process. Patients who were able to take the lead tended to have experience of setting goals in other life contexts (e.g. in their working lives) or had highly valued activities that they were very motivated to return to (e.g. returning to work). Regardless of who led the process, both groups described each stage of the process as collaborative with agreed goals and action plans reflecting patients' priorities and unique personal circumstances.

Patients judged the effectiveness of the G-AP framework on the basis of whether they were able to meet their goals and carry them out as planned. In describing how the G-AP process had helped them, patients talked about how identifying personal goals and action plans acted as an incentive, providing something to aim for. They also created a focus, with *steps* that made the process manageable for them. A repeated view was that achieving goals and action plans produced a sense of achievement and an important boost in confidence.

Health professionals tended not to focus on goal attainment when discussing the effectiveness of the G-AP framework; instead, they talked about the positive influence it had on their practice. In particular, they viewed their goal-setting practice to be more patient centred (with goals reflecting patients' priorities and personal circumstances rather than only their professional perspective), goal focused and efficient. Because goals and action plans acted as a benchmark against which progress could be gauged, it was easier for them to know if progress was being made or not and to identify when a change of plan was required. Health professionals felt that the G-AP process helped patients to have a greater sense of control and participation in the rehabilitation process. There was a commonly held view that using G-AP led patients to be more focused on their goals, which in turn had a positive impact on their motivation and adherence to a goal-directed behaviour.

Both patients and health professionals talked about *family member* involvement in the G-AP process. Patients gave examples of how family members had suggested goals and action plans and provided ongoing encouragement and support to optimize action plan attainment. In all examples given, the G-AP patient-held record had created the opportunity for family members to be involved as they had access to the record and could read for themselves the goals that were set and the kinds of action plans in place to facilitate meeting them. Health professionals acknowledged that family members could have an important role in facilitating the G-AP process, for example, suggesting goals, providing reassurance and encouragement, providing prompts to complete action plans (particularly if the patient had memory difficulties) and supervising patients carrying out their action plans.

11.14 Conclusion

The development of a framework to guide goal-setting practice in community-based stroke rehabilitation has been described. This process involved four main stages: a review of the literature to identify theories of behaviour change relevant to the goal-setting process, a causal modelling exercise to link theory to practice, convening of a clinical task group to develop the causal model into a G-AP practice framework and preliminary evaluation of the G-AP framework in one community rehabilitation team. The findings of the evaluation have informed development of the G-AP visual illustration and implementation protocol.

We are now in the process of conducting a process evaluation of the developed G-AP on a larger scale across diverse team settings. We aim to find out what patient, carer and therapist experiences can tell us about: (1) the acceptability of G-AP, (2) the important landmarks in stroke recovery and the contribution of G-AP (if any) to their achievement and (3) the feasibility of implementing G-AP according to protocol. This will inform the design of an effectiveness study in which the impact of G-AP on patient outcomes and professional practice will be compared to standard practice. An economic evaluation will be built into this study so a cost–benefit analysis can be completed.

The development of the G-AP framework was carried out whilst one of the authors (LS) was undertaking a part-time research fellowship and working clinically in the ReACH team. This meant that the project benefited from the time resources of LS, the academic resources of a university and the dynamic clinical–academic link between the ReACH team and the university. This level of resource is unlikely to be available to the majority of rehabilitation professionals. There is a question, therefore, of how the power of theory can be used to examine and perhaps improve usual clinical practice. However, it is possible to apply theory to everyday clinical practice. Rather than start with theory and build a practice framework or an intervention from theory, it is possible to start with current practice and apply theory to it.

Practitioners should begin a theory-based practice review by describing each component of their current practice and organizing this description so that it best represents the process of their rehabilitation practice from start to finish. Each component of current practice can then be compared to theory, for example, using any or some of the theories or models described in this book. This comparison could be carried out using a process of consensus within a rehabilitation team, whereby the team meets to discuss the relationship between theory and each component of their practice until a consensus agreement is achieved. In this way, each component of current practice can be labelled by one or more theoretical constructs. This information will provide the basis for understanding current practice and how it might be optimized.

Knowing which theoretical constructs current practice targets might enable the identification of opportunities to optimize that practice. For example, a theory-based review of practice might reveal simple techniques that are not currently being used, for example, assessing patient confidence in their ability to carry out an action plan prior to its implementation. Inclusion of such techniques may be simple and practicable within current resources. In contrast, the review might also reveal aspects of practice that appear inconsistent with current theoretical thinking. These practice components could be considered for review or removal from current practice, which might free up professional time to attend to those components that are theory-based. It may also be possible to review the order or sequence with which practice components are delivered, for example, are all action and coping plans thoroughly reviewed prior to progression to new action plans or goals? Again reordering practice components need not necessarily require additional resources to implement. Thus, a theory-based practice review offers rehabilitation teams the opportunity to use theory to understand and evaluate their current practice within the resource constraints experienced by practitioners.

References

Albarracín, D., Gillette, J. C., Earl, A. N., Glasman, L. R., Durantini, M. R., & Ho, M.-H. (2005). A test of major assumptions about behavior change: A comprehensive look at the effects of passive and active HIV-prevention interventions since the beginning of the epidemic. *Psychological Bulletin*, *131*(6), 856–897.

Armitage, C. J. (2009). Is there utility in the transtheoretical model? *British Journal of Health Psychology*, *14*, 195–210.

Armitage, C. J., & Conner, M. (2000). Social cognition models and health behaviour: A structured review. *Psychology & Health*, *15*(2), 173–189.

Bandura, A. (1997). *Self-efficacy: The exercise of control*. New York, NY: W.H. Freeman.

Bandura, A. (2000). Health promotion from the perspective of social cognitive theory. In P. Norman, C. Abraham, & M. Conner (Eds.), *Understanding and changing health behaviour: From health beliefs to self-regulation* (pp. 299–343). Amsterdam, the Netherlands: Harwood Academic Publishers.

Bodenheimer, T., Lorig, K., Holman, H., & Grumbach, K. (2002). Patient self-management of chronic disease in primary care. *The Journal of the American Medical Association*, *288*(19), 2469–2475.

Borell, L., Daniels, R., & Winding, K. (2002). Experiences of occupational therapists in stroke rehabilitation: Dilemmas of some occupational therapists in inpatient stroke rehabilitation. *Scandinavian Journal of Occupational Therapy*, *9*(4), 167–175.

Bornman, J., & Murphy, J. (2006). Using the ICF in goal setting: Clinical application using Talking Mats®. *Disability and Rehabilitation: Assistive Technology*, *1*(3), 145–154.

Carver, C. S., & Scheier, M. F. (Eds.). (1981). *Attention and self-regulation: A control theory approach*. New York, NY: Springer.

Carver, C. S., & Scheier, M. F. (1982). Control theory: A useful conceptual framework for personality–social, clinical, and health psychology. *Psychological Bulletin*, *92*(1), 111–135.

Cerniauskaite, M., Quintas, R., Boldt, C., Raggi, A., Cieza, A., Bickenbach, J. E., & Leonardi, M. (2011). Systematic literature review on ICF from 2001 to 2009: Its use, implementation and operationalisation. *Disability and Rehabilitation*, *33*(4), 281–309.

Conner, M., & Armitage, C. (1998). Extending the theory of planned behavior: A review and avenues for further research. *Journal of Applied Social Psychology*, *28*, 1429–1464.

Craig, P., Dieppe, P., Macintyre, S., Mitchie, S., Nazareth, I., & Petticrew, M. (2008). Developing and evaluating complex interventions: The new Medical Research Council guidance. *British Medical Journal*, *337*(7676), 979–983.

Deci, E., & Ryan, R. (1985). *Intrinsic motivation and self-determination in human behavior*. New York, NY: Plenum.

Dekker, J. (2008). Theories in behavioral medicine. *International Journal of Behavioral Medicine*, *15*(1), 1–3.

Department of Health. (2009). *Your health, your way – A guide to long term conditions and self care*. London, U.K.: The Stationary Office.

Dixon, D., Johnston, M., Elliott, A., & Hannaford, P. (2012). Testing integrated behavioural and biomedical models of activity and activity limitations in a population-based sample. *Disability and Rehabilitation*, *34*(14), 1157–1166.

Dixon, D., Johnston, M., Rowley, D., & Pollard, B. (2008). Using the ICF and psychological models of behavior to predict mobility limitations. *Rehabilitation Psychology*, *53*, 191–200.

Downing, J., Jones, L., Cook, P. A., & Bellis, M. A. (2006). *Prevention of sexually transmitted infections (STIs): A review of reviews into the effectiveness of non clinical interventions. Evidence briefing update*. London, U.K.: National Institute of Clinical Excellence.

Dunn, D. S., & Elliott, T. R. (2008). The place and promise of theory in rehabilitation psychology research. *Rehabilitation Psychology*, *53*(3), 254–267.

Gibbons, F. X., Houlihan, A. E., & Gerrard, M. (2009). Reason and reaction: The utility of a dual-focus, dual-processing perspective on promotion and prevention of adolescent health risk behaviour. *British Journal of Health Psychology*, *14*(2), 231–248.

Hagger, M. S. (2009). Theoretical integration in health psychology: Unifying ideas and complementary explanations. *British Journal of Health Psychology*, 14(2), 189–194.

Hagger, M. S., & Chatzisarantis, N. L. D. (2005). First- and higher-order models of attitudes, normative influence, and perceived behavioural control in the theory of planned behaviour. *British Journal of Social Psychology*, 44, 513–535.

Hagger, M. S., & Chatzisarantis, N. L. D. (2009). Integrating the theory of planned behaviour and self-determination theory in health behaviour: A meta-analysis. *British Journal of Health Psychology*, 14(2), 275–302.

Hagger, M. S., Chatzisarantis, N. L. D., & Biddle, S. J. H. (2002). A meta-analytic review of the theories of reasoned action and planned behavior in physical activity: Predictive validity and the v of additional variables. *Journal of Sport & Exercise Psychology*, 24(1), 3–32.

Hagger, M. S., & Orbell, S. (2003). A meta-analytic review of the common-sense model of illness representations. *Psychology & Health, 18(2),* 141–184

Hardeman, W., Johnston, M., Johnston, D. W., Bonetti, D., Wareham, N. J., & Kinmonth, A. L. (2002). Application of the theory of planned behaviour in behaviour change interventions: A systematic review. *Psychology & Health*, 17(2), 123–158.

Hardeman, W., Sutton, S., Griffin, S., Johnston, M., White, A., Wareham, N. J., & Kinmonth, A. L. (2005). A causal modelling approach to the development of theory-based behaviour change programmes for trial evaluation. *Health Education Research*, 20(6), 676–687.

Hart, T., & Evans, J. (2006). Self-regulation and goal theories in brain injury rehabilitation. *Journal of Head Trauma Rehabilitation*, 21(2), 142–155.

Holliday, R. C., Antoun, M., & Playford, E. D. (2005). A survey of goal-setting methods used in rehabilitation. *Neurorehabilitation and Neural Repair*, 19(3), 227–231.

Hrisos, S., Eccles, M., Johnston, M., Francis, J., Kaner, E. F. S., Steen, N., & Grimshaw, J. (2008). Developing the content of two behavioural interventions: Using theory-based interventions to promote GP management of upper respiratory tract infection without prescribing antibiotics #1. *BMC Health Services Research*, 8, 11.

Hurn, J., Kneebone, I., & Cropley, M. (2006). Goal setting as an outcome measure: A systematic review. *Clinical Rehabilitation*, 20(9), 756–772.

Ivers, N., Tu, K., Francis, J., Barnsley, J., Shah, B., Upshur, R., … Zwarenstein, M. (2010). Feedback GAP: Study protocol for a cluster-randomized trial of goal setting and action plans to increase the effectiveness of audit and feedback interventions in primary care. *Implementation Science*, 5(1), 98.

Johnston, M. (1996). Models of disability. *Physiotherapy Theory and Practice*, 12, 131–141.

Johnston, M., Bonetti, D., Joice, S., Pollard, B., Morrison, V., Francis, J. J., & MacWalter, R. (2007). Recovery from disability after stroke as a target for a behavioural intervention: Results of a randomised controlled trial. *Disability and Rehabilitation*, 29(14), 1117–1127.

Keith, R. A., Granger, C. V., Hamilton, B. B., & Sherwin, F. S. (1987). The functional independence measure: A new tool for rehabilitation. *Advances in Clinical Rehabilitation*, 1, 6–18.

Levack, W. M., Taylor, K., Siegert, R. J., Dean, S. G., McPherson, K. M., & Weatherall, M. (2006). Is goal planning in rehabilitation effective? A systematic review. *Clinical Rehabilitation*, 20(9), 739–755.

Leventhal, H., Leventhal, E. A., & Contrada, R. J. (1998). Self-regulation, health, and behavior: A perceptual-cognitive approach. *Psychology & Health*, 13(4), 717–733.

Lippke, S., & Plotnikoff, R. C. (2009). The protection motivation theory within the stages of the transtheoretical model – Stage-specific interplay of variables and prediction of exercise stage transitions. *British Journal of Health Psychology*, 14(2), 211–229.

Locke, E. A., & Latham, G. P. (2002). Building a practically useful theory of goal setting and task motivation: A 35-year odyssey. *American Psychologist*, 57(9), 705–717.

Lorig, K., Holman, H., Sobel. D., Laurent. D., Gonzalez, V., Minor, M. (2006) *Living a Healthy Life with Chronic Conditions*. Boulder, Co: Bull Publishing Company.

Maes, S., & Karoly, P. (2005). Self-regulation assessment and intervention in physical health and illness: A review. *Applied Psychology*, 54(2), 267–299.

Mahoney, F. I., & Barthel, D. (1965). Functional evaluation: The Barthel Index. *Maryland State Medical Journal*, *14*, 56–61.

Marks, R., Allegrante, J. P., & Lorig, K. (2005). A review and synthesis of research evidence for self-efficacy-enhancing interventions for reducing chronic disability: Implications for health education practice (Part II). *Health Promotion Practice*, *6*(2), 148–156.

Michie, S., Abraham, C., Whittington, C., McAteer, J., & Gupta, S. (2009). Effective techniques in healthy eating and physical activity interventions: A meta-regression. *Health Psychology*, *28*(6), 690–701.

Milne, S., Sheeran, P., & Orbell, S. (2000). Prediction and intervention in health-related behavior: A meta-analytic review of protection motivation theory. *Journal of Applied Social Psychology*, *30*(1), 106–143.

Ntoumanis, N., Edmunds, J., & Duda, J. L. (2009). Understanding the coping process from a self-determination theory perspective. *British Journal of Health Psychology*, *14*(2), 249–260.

Oliver, M. (Ed.). (1990). *The politics of disablement*. London, U.K.: Macmillan.

Parry, R. H. (2004). Communication during goal-setting in physiotherapy treatment sessions. *Clinical Rehabilitation*, *18*(6), 668–682.

Playford, E. D., Siegert, R., Levack, W., & Freeman, J. (2009). Areas of consensus and controversy about goal setting in rehabilitation: A conference report. *Clinical Rehabilitation*, *23*(4), 334–344.

Prentice-Dunn, S., & Rogers, R. W. (1986). Protection Motivation Theory and preventive health: Beyond the Health Belief Model. *Health Education Research*, *1*(3), 153–161.

Rosewilliam, S., Roskell, C. A., & Pandyan, A. D. (2011). A systematic review and synthesis of the quantitative and qualitative evidence behind patient-centred goal setting in stroke rehabilitation. *Clinical Rehabilitation*, *25*(6), 501–514.

Royal College of Physicians. (2008). *National clinical guidelines for stroke* (3rd ed.). London, U.K.: Royal College of Physicians.

Savigny, P., Watson, P., & Underwood, M. (2009). Early management of persistent non-specific low back pain: Summary of NICE guidance. *British Medical Journal*, *338*, 1441–1442.

Schwarzer, R. (1992). Self-efficacy in the adoption and maintenance of health behaviours: Theoretical approaches and a new model. In R. Schwarzer (Ed.), *Self-efficacy: Thought control of action* (pp. 217–245). Bristol, PA: Taylor & Francis.

Schwarzer, R., Ziegelmann, J. P., Luszczynska, A., Scholz, U., & Lippke, S. (2008). Social-cognitive predictors of physical exercise adherence: Three longitudinal studies in rehabilitation. *Health Psychology*, *27*(1), S54–S63.

Scobbie, L., Dixon, D., & Wyke, S. (2011). Goal setting and action planning in the rehabilitation setting: Development of a theoretically informed practice framework. *Clinical Rehabilitation*, *25*(5), 468–482.

Scobbie, L., McLean, D., Dixon, D., Duncan, E., & Wyke, S. (2013). Implementing a framework for goal setting in community based stroke rehabilitation: A process evaluation. *BMC Health Services Research*, *13*(1), 190.

Scobbie, L., Wyke, S., & Dixon, D. (2009). Identifying and applying psychological theory to setting and achieving rehabilitation goals. *Clinical Rehabilitation*, *23*(4), 321–333.

Scottish Executive. (2007). *Co-ordinated, integrated and fit for purpose. A delivery framework for adult rehabilitation in Scotland*. Edinburgh, Scotland: Scottish Executive.

Scottish Intercollegiate Guidelines Network. (2010). *Management of patients with stroke: Rehabilitation, prevention and management of complications, and discharge planning. A national clinical guideline*. Edinburgh, Scotland: Scottish Intercollegiate Guidelines Network.

Siegert, R. J., McPherson, K. M., & Dean, S. G. (2005). Theory development and a science of rehabilitation. *Disability and Rehabilitation*, *27*(24), 1493–1501.

Siegert, R. J., Mcpherson, K. M., & Taylor, W. J. (2004). Toward a cognitive-effective model of goal-setting in rehabilitation: Is self-regulation theory a key step? *Disability and Rehabilitation*, *26*(20), 1175–1183.

Siegert, R. J., & Taylor, W. J. (2004). Theoretical aspects of goal-setting and motivation in rehabilitation. *Disability and Rehabilitation*, *26*(1), 1–8.

Sniehotta, F. F. (2009). Towards a theory of intentional behaviour change: Plans, planning, and self-regulation. *British Journal of Health Psychology, 14,* 261–273.

Sniehotta, F. F., Scholz, U., & Schwarzer, R. (2006). Action plans and coping plans for physical exercise: A longitudinal intervention study in cardiac rehabilitation. *British Journal of Health Psychology, 11,* 23–37.

Sugavanam, T., Mead, G., Bulley, C., Donaghy, M., Van Wijke, F. (2013). The effects and experiences of goal setting in stroke rehabilitation a systematic review. *Disability and Rehabilitation,* 35(3), 117–190.

Thomas, C. (2004). How is disability understood? An examination of sociological approaches. *Disability & Society, 19*(6), 569–583.

van den Bosch, M. A. A. J., Hollingworth, W., Kinmonth, A. L., & Dixon, A. K. (2004). Evidence against the use of lumbar spine radiography for low back pain. *Clinical Radiology, 59*(1), 69–76.

Wade, D. T. (1999). Goal planning in stroke rehabilitation: Evidence. *Topics in Stroke Rehabilitation,* 6(2), 37–42.

Wade, D. T. (2000). Clinical governance and rehabilitation services. *Clinical Rehabilitation, 14*(1), 1–4.

Wade, D. T. (2003). Community rehabilitation, or rehabilitation in the community? *Disability and Rehabilitation, 25*(15), 875–881.

Wade, D. T. (2005). Describing rehabilitation interventions. *Clinical Rehabilitation, 19*(8), 811–818.

Wade, D. T. (2006). Belief in rehabilitation, the hidden power for change. In P. W. Halligan & M. Aylword (Eds.), *The power of belief: Psychosocial influence on illness, disability and medicine* (pp. 86–98). Oxford, U.K.: Oxford University Press.

Wade, D. T., & Halligan, P. (2003). New wine in old bottles: The WHO ICF as an explanatory model of human behaviour. *Clinical Rehabilitation, 17*(4), 349–354.

World Health Organization. (1980). *International classification of impairments, disabilities and handicaps.* Geneva, Switzerland: World Health Organization.

World Health Organization. (2001). *International classification of functioning, disability, and health.* Geneva, Switzerland: World Health Organization.

World Health Organization. (2002). *Towards a common language for functioning, disability and health: ICF.* Geneva, Switzerland: World Health Organization.

12

Goal Orientation and Goal Setting in German Medical Rehabilitation Research

Thorsten Meyer and Nadine J. Pohontsch

CONTENTS

12.1 Introduction

This chapter provides an introduction to research on goal setting and goal orientation within the German rehabilitation system. It is one of the peculiarities of German rehabilitation practice and rehabilitation research that it is hardly visible on an international level. This is presumably due to atypical approaches to rehabilitation that often do not conform to other countries' approaches or standards and result primarily in German language publications. Therefore, first of all we will describe the central features of the German rehabilitation system as well as outlining German rehabilitation research traditions that have evolved since the 1990s. This includes the introduction of a rehabilitation guideline related to goal setting. Thereafter, the results of German rehabilitation research will be presented and discussed.

12.2 Medical Rehabilitation in Germany

German health and social care is based on the Social Code (known as the *Sozialgesetzbuch*). This Social Code comprises 12 books, each established as social legislation and considered an independent Act of Parliament. Issues of health care and services can be found in

Social Code book V, issues of the statutory pension insurance can be found in Social Code book VI, and issues of accident insurance can be found in Social Code book VII. In 2001, Social Code book IX was added that integrated rules and regulations for the rehabilitation and participation of disabled people. The Social Code lays the foundation of a social insurance model built upon basic ideas which were developed during the 1870s within the rule of Chancellor Bismarck and which outlasted very different political systems and crises.

Rehabilitation is a service that can be delivered according to different code books. If the need for rehabilitation is due to an accident or illness directly related to work or education, accident insurance is in charge of all aspects of rehabilitation including acute treatments. If the need for rehabilitation is due to reduced or endangered working capacity, the statutory pension insurance is in charge. Its specific goal is to keep workers able to participate in the workforce as long as possible. Therefore, it is primarily concerned with health and social problems of people in the working age (at present, retirement starts at the age of 65, but this will slowly increase to the age of 67 in 2029) but also offers rehabilitation for children or teenagers with different types of severe or chronic diseases. Due to historical reasons, the statutory pension insurance also takes care of medical rehabilitation of cancer patients of all ages independent of their work ability. If both accident insurance and the statutory pension fund are not considered responsible for care of the rehabilitation needs of an insuree, then statutory health insurance is responsible for providing medical rehabilitation. This comprises primarily rehabilitation services for the elderly. The local social welfare office might take over the responsibility if no other insurance is in charge. Occupational rehabilitation without medical needs relates to Social Code book III that deals with promotion of employment.

Statutory pension insurance, statutory health insurance and accident insurance are the three most important legal institutions providing rehabilitation benefits in Germany. For example, the statutory pension insurance reported 1.669 million applications for medical rehabilitation benefits of which 1.062 million were granted and 996,000 rehabilitation measures were actually provided (Deutsche Rentenversicherung Bund, 2012) in 2010. Eighty-four percent of the cases were rehabilitation measures provided for adults within an inpatient setting, a further 12% were provided in an outpatient setting and another 3% were provided for children and teenagers in an inpatient setting. Most rehabilitation benefits related to musculoskeletal disorders (37%), oncological disorders (17%), mental disorders (14%), cardiac disorders (7%) and substance-related disorders (6%). Outpatient rehabilitation is in more than two out of three cases related to musculoskeletal disorders. In 2010, the statutory pension insurance spent about €5.38 billion for rehabilitation benefits. There are no comprehensive numbers on rehabilitation measures within the framework of the health insurances, but figures should be well below those of the statutory pension insurance. It has to be noted that close to 10% of the population is not insured according to the compulsory social insurances of the Social Code books, which is compulsory for employed persons up to a defined wage limit. These 10% mostly have private insurance where the services depend on the conditions of their respective contracts with insurance companies.

There are rehabilitation programmes for patients with myocardial infarction or coronary interventions, for hip or knee joint replacements, for cancer patients, for patients with arthritis, etc. In these and other specified indications, a patient is regularly obliged to undergo medical rehabilitation as part of a medical pathway. One characteristic of the German rehabilitation system is that these rehabilitation measures usually take place in rehabilitation clinics and mostly last for 3 weeks. Another characteristic of the German rehabilitation system is that the rehabilitation mostly takes place in inpatient institutions at rather remote places. This relates to the German *Kur* (health resorts, spa) tradition.*

In addition to these medical rehabilitation programmes within medical pathways, these institutions provide rehabilitation services that are not related to an acute medical event but are suited for persons with chronic diseases and a (risk of) decreased working capacity. Persons with chronic diseases, disabilities or at risk to experience a disability can apply for rehabilitation services. These rehabilitation services are usually provided over a time span of 3 weeks for most indications. This duration can be extended in individual (medically justified) cases. For further details on the German rehabilitation system, please refer to Vogel and Zdrahal-Urbanek (2004).

12.3 German Rehabilitation Research

Until the beginning of the 1990s in Germany, there was a yawning gap between resources spent for rehabilitation benefits and the small scale of research devoted to rehabilitation. In the wake of the work of a commission that made proposals for the future development of rehabilitation within the statutory pension insurances (Verband Deutscher Rentenversicherungsträger, 1992), rehabilitation research started to develop. With the rise of the era of assessment and accountability (Relman, 1988) and a political reform that led to a cut of rehabilitation services on a large scale in 1996, it became clear that rehabilitation needs to develop a sound evidence base for its practice and a strong foundation for quality improvement. The German Federal Ministry of Education and Research and the Federation of German Pension Insurances Institutes sponsored a joint rehabilitation research programme, *Rehabilitation Sciences*, for 6 years from 1998 to 2004.† A rehabilitation research infrastructure emerged, including rehabilitation research chairs at university level, especially within medical faculties, establishment of rehabilitation research departments within the statutory pension insurances, development of an unprecedented quality assurance programme, the foundation of a German Society on Rehabilitation Research in 2000 and different regional and national initiatives to support research by means of funding institutions, as well as setting up reference centres for training in research methodology. These initiatives were followed by further funding initiatives, especially within the wake of health services research development. To date, rehabilitation research has built up skills to compete with national research funds from other medical and social domains. There is a major conference addressing rehabilitation researchers and other professionals, the *Reha-Kolloquium*, which is jointly organized by a different regional statutory pension insurer each year and the national German statutory pension insurance. It has been established as a meeting point for German-speaking rehabilitation researchers, commissioners and rehabilitation clinicians. It has now evolved to become a regular meeting opportunity for more than 1500 rehabilitation professionals. Different scientific journals publishing

---

* A *Kur* uses place-bound remedies (e.g. springs, salines or altitude) to strengthen general health and differs markedly from medical rehabilitation although it can be provided within the same settings.
† One of the funded research networks of rehabilitation research programme, *Rehabilitation Sciences*, dealt with goal orientation in diagnostics, therapy and outcome assessment. Its results have been published in English (Jäckel, Bengel, & Herdt, 2006). Goal orientation was more of a general topic in this network; goal setting was not analysed in depth.

articles in German are devoted to rehabilitation issues, including *Die Rehabilitation**
and *Physikalische Medizin, Rehabilitationsmedizin, Kurortmedizin (Journal of Physical and
Rehabilitation Medicine)*,[†] both of which allow for scientific merits in terms of impact factors.

12.4 Goal Setting or Goal Orientation as Part of a General Rehabilitation Guideline

The German statutory pension insurance has published a general guideline on how rehabilitation should be conducted (Deutsche Rentenversicherung Bund, 2007). The determination of individual goals, both rehabilitation and treatment goals, is an essential component
of the rehabilitation process. The overarching goal of the German statutory pension insurance is to counter an imminent or already existing reduced capacity in working performance and to secure or reinstate (occupational) participation. Still, on an individual level,
the respective rehabilitation and treatment goals, related to the overarching goal of rehabilitation set by society, have to be selected on the grounds of a comprehensive diagnostic
process. This should usually take place in close partnership between the patient and the
rehabilitation team. It is a central task in the beginning of rehabilitation to set these goals.
Rehabilitation and treatment goals relate to different levels of specification. Rehabilitation
goals are usually termed on a more general level and relate to a holistic rehabilitation concept representing success of rehabilitation in general. Therapeutic goals are related to more
specific aspects, for example, on results of single therapies or interventions. They should be
more differentiated and specific compared to rehabilitation goals. For example, in a person
with long-term work absence due to disabling low back pain, a rehabilitation goal could
be to be able to work at least part-time in the former job at the end of the rehabilitation.
Therapeutic goals could be to adjust pain medication to the patient needs (medical treatment goal), to strengthen muscles of the trunk to enable a person to sit for longer periods or
to get heavy objects from a shelf (physiotherapy treatment goal) and to identify and practise
new movement-related sports that the patient is motivated to integrate into daily life (educational treatment goal). Goal setting should be understood as a process. Goals and their
priorities can change during the course of rehabilitation. This might be due to the results of
repeated diagnostics during the rehabilitation process and intermediate therapeutic results.

The general guideline on rehabilitation emphasizes the integration of the patient's view
into decision-making processes. They especially emphasize mutual goal setting. Mutual
goal setting is an important act to empower patients to actively engage in restoring their
health or coping with chronic illness and (impending) disability. Subjective concepts regarding health and illness as well as expectations towards rehabilitation have to be explored,
discussed and related to. The rehabilitation team has to react to inappropriate expectations
and try to alter those together with the patient. Rehabilitation and treatment goals have to
relate to the subjective perceptions of the patients and their individual and social resources.

---

* Official organ of the German Association for Rehabilitation, National Working Partnership for Rehabilitation
  and German Society for Rehabilitation Sciences.
† Official journal of the German Society of Physical Medicine and Rehabilitation, Association of Medical
  Rehabilitation Specialists, Austrian Society of Physical Medicine and Rehabilitation and Association of
  Austrian Medical Specialists on Physical Medicine and Rehabilitation; in association with the European Society
  of Physical and Rehabilitation Medicine (ESPRM), the International Society of Physical and Rehabilitation
  Medicine (ISPRM) and the European Union of Medical Specialists (UEMS) Physical and Rehabilitation
  Medicine (section and board).

Although most clinicians seem to acknowledge the usefulness of goal setting for successful rehabilitation (Dudeck et al., 2011), no consistent concepts or action strategies exist concerning the actual process of defining rehabilitation goals during the intake interview or at other points of the rehabilitation process. Different kinds of goal-setting strategies can be observed among rehabilitation services or even clinicians within a rehabilitation service. Some use open questions in a questionnaire to be filled out by the patient prior to rehabilitation admission, some guide their patients to draft rehabilitation goals according to the SMART model (Specific, Measurable, Assignable, Realistic and Time – related goals; Doran, 1981), some use checklists to be incorporated into the patient's training schedule, and others just note down goals in the individual patient's health record. The German statutory pension insurance puts a lot of emphasis on goal setting being essential for a (successful) rehabilitation process. However, it provides no guidelines for rehabilitation clinics to accomplish this task so far. A brochure (*Rehabilitation – What do I have to expect?**), distributed to prospective rehabilitation patients by the German statutory pension insurance, provides some information and guidance about rehabilitation goals. It advises patients to prepare for goal setting during the intake interview in the rehabilitation clinic. The brochure states different groups of rehabilitation goals: improvement of physical, mental or emotional capacity, clarification of vocational or social issues, improvement of disease management skills and lifestyle changes. Patients get instructions to think about possible tangible rehabilitation goals from each group, to write them down in the brochure and to rank their top three priorities. The brochure's use and benefits for goal setting and goal attainment in rehabilitation clinics have to our knowledge never been evaluated. However, there is an ongoing research project that evaluates a similar approach in a randomized controlled study (Buchholz, Glaser-Möller, & Kohlmann, 2012).

An ongoing project (results expected in 2014) sponsored by the Deutsche Rentenversicherung (http://forschung.deutsche-rentenversicherung.de/ForschPortal Web/contentAction.do?key=main_reha_ep_ab-ziel) aims at reviewing national and international studies about goal setting in medical rehabilitation and collecting existing approaches to goal setting used in German rehabilitation clinics. The final output of this project shall be a manual outlining a consistent, practical and scientifically sound strategy for goal setting in medical rehabilitation in Germany (*Arbeitsbuch Reha-Zielvereinbarung in der medizinischen Rehabilitation*).

12.5 Goal Setting or Goal Orientation as a Topic of German Rehabilitation Research

In 1994, a seminal paper on goal orientation was published by Vogel, Tuschhoff, and Zillessen. It presented the results of a working group on process quality in rehabilitation. The authors made a strong plea for an integration of individual goal setting into rehabilitation processes. The first author, Heiner Vogel, is a psychologist with a psychotherapeutic background, a field where individual goal setting is a regular part of the treatment process. In the paper, there was a strong call to understand goal setting as an essential, independent treatment phase. They laid emphasis on the following: (1) goals to be the result of a cooperative dialogue between therapists and rehabilitation patients and the patient

---

* Rehabilitation – Was erwartet mich dort? (Deutsche Rentenversicherung Bund, 2008).

TABLE 12.1

Examples of Therapeutic Goals for Orthopaedic/Rheumatic Patients

Somatic	Psychosocial
Pain reduction (area)	Anxiety reduction (psychological level)
Stabilization (area)	Depression reduction (psychological level)
Improvement of the mobility of the spine (area)	Improvement of occupational integration (social level)

Functional	Educational
Improvement of ability to perform personal hygiene	Improvement of information about illness
Improvement of ability to climb stairs	Mastering techniques and strategies to reduce risk behaviour (e.g. smoking, alcohol, nutrition, leisure)
Improvement of ability to use public transport	Mastering stress-management techniques and strategies

Source: Translated and modified from Verband Deutscher Rentenversicherungsträger (Ed.), *Das Qualitätssiche-rungsprogramm der gesetzlichen Rentenversicherung in der medizinischen Rehabilitation. Instrumente und Verfahren*, DRV-Schriften, 18, VDR, Frankfurt am Main, Germany, 2000.

being able to accept the defined goals, (2) rehabilitation goals to be appropriate to the individual situation and being in a proper hierarchy, (3) goals having been made transparent and having been defined to be measureable, (4) goals to be realistic and reachable and (5) goals to have a long-term perspective.

Subsequently, goal setting was introduced as one aspect of rehabilitation quality in the quality assurance programme of the statutory pension insurances. Questions concerning goal setting and rehabilitation planning were included in the regular patient survey on satisfaction and treatment success. Here, a random sample of about 1/6 of all rehabilitation patients under the auspices of the statutory pension insurance is surveyed (ongoing monitoring of about 20 patients per month in each institution) 6–8 weeks after their inpatient rehabilitation stay. This survey was developed in the mid-1990s, started around 1997, modified in 2008 and is still in use. Goal orientation has also been integrated as a quality indicator in a peer-review approach to quality assurance. Another part of these quality assurance initiatives was the development of treatment goals on the level of general medical indications (Protz, Gerdes, Maier-Riehle, & Jäckel, 1998; Verband Deutscher Rentenversicherungsträger, 2000), for example, cardiac rehabilitation or orthopaedic rehabilitation. The authors distinguished somatic, functional, psychosocial and educational goals. Within these domains, different indication-specific treatment goals were made explicit. Examples of goals for orthopaedic/rheumatic disorders are shown in Table 12.1. These goals are not necessarily identical with individual treatment goals but direct attention towards the decision about possible individual treatment goals. For quality assurance and research purposes, these goals provide support in selecting appropriate outcome domains or indicators.

12.6 Goal Setting as a Problem Domain in Quality Assurance

From the beginning, the quality assurance programmes found aspects of goal setting to be deficient. Patients rated their satisfaction with *goals and rehabilitation planning* repeatedly worse than other satisfaction domains (Beckmann, Pallenberg, & Klosterhuis, 2000; Berking, Dreesen, & Jacobi, 2004; Dorenburg, Huck-Langner, Nischan, & Winnefeld, 2001; Meyer, Pohontsch, Maurischat, & Raspe, 2008; Meyer, Pohontsch, Maurischat, & Raspe, 2009a).

There were indications for substantial differences in the patients' appraisal of goal setting between clinics (Widera & Klosterhuis, 2007). Also, in the peer-review process, the goal-setting items were rated worse compared to other quality domains (Baumgarten & Klosterhuis, 2007; Farin et al., 2003). Therefore, the statutory pension insurance funded a study with the aim to explore reasons for this phenomenon. A mixed-methods study was set up by the first author and his working group. First, we aimed to model the patients' ratings of *goals and rehabilitation planning*, a subscale of the patient questionnaire in quality assurance, statistically. Then we set up a league table of inpatient rehabilitation institutions and identified the upper and lower 10% of the institutions with regard to patients' ratings of goals and rehabilitation planning after case-mix adjustment for person characteristics. Two rehabilitation institutions of the upper and two of the lower end of the distribution (one with musculoskeletal patients and one with cardiologic patients, respectively) were contacted. We conducted guided qualitative interviews with 10 patients in each institution. In addition, we confronted the rehabilitation teams with the results of the study and their discussions served as further reference for this study.

Interestingly, in a systematic qualitative comparison of the clinics rated well above or below average with regard to satisfaction with rehabilitation goals and planning, we found that differences between rehabilitation clinics could not primarily be accounted for by superficial differences in goal and rehabilitation planning. Rather, clinics rated high above average provided an atmosphere that made the patients feel more respected and valued as a person. There was a higher degree of devotion towards the patient (e.g. talks besides the regular therapies, being known by name and being talked to on the hallway). Also, the continuity experienced by the patients was another important distinguishing category. For example, clinics rated high above average were characterized by continuity of doctor–patient and/or therapist–patient relationships, while the reports of patients from the clinics rated much below average gave evidence of no or disrupted relationships. On the positive side, clinicians were viewed to act concertedly, that is, they follow a common philosophy. On the negative side, there were strong indications of heterogeneity of clinicians' approaches from the perspective of the patients. Thirdly, in the institutions rated below average, deficient organizational characteristics were reported from the patients' point of view. These included insufficient staff numbers, time overlaps of therapies or priority of ward rounds to therapies.

The results of the qualitative analysis phase related to the statistical analyses where satisfaction ratings of the patients were associated with different aspects of patient orientation. Important predictors of satisfaction with goal orientation and planning were whether the patients reported that recommendations on how to deal with their chronic illnesses and/or disabilities at home, at the work place and during leisure time were given to them, as well as satisfaction with medical doctors and satisfaction with the accommodation facilities. In summary, this study paved the way for the idea that problems in goal setting were not of procedural or technical origin but inextricably related to the broader concept of patient orientation (Meyer, Pohontsch, Maurischat, et al., 2009a; Meyer, Pohontsch, & Raspe, 2009b).

12.7 Goals from the Patients' and Physicians'/Therapists' Perspective

Another field of interest in German rehabilitation research is related to differences and communalities between patients' and physicians' or therapists' treatment goals (Bergelt, Welk, & Koch, 2000; Brandes & Niehues, 2012; Dörner & Muthny, 2006; Glattacker,

Farin, & Jäckel, 2006; Höder, Josenhans, & Arlt, 2006; Nagl & Farin-Glattacker, 2011; Rietz, Höder, Josenhans, & Arlt, 2001; Weis, Moser, & Bartsch, 2002). All studies reported on substantial differences between patients' and physicians' or therapists' perceptions of treatment goals both at a group and individual patient level. For example, Bergelt et al. (2000) reported that individual agreement between physicians and patients with an onco-logical disease at the level of therapeutic goal domains (e.g. physical capacity, nutrition/body weight, pain, daily activities, social life, working capacity) documented after admission of the patient including an intake interview was astonishingly low. A maximum of agreement in a pre-specified list of goals of a little above 50% was found in the domain of physical capacity; a little above 40% regarding nutrition/weight maintenance, psychological strain and working capacity; only 30% of agreement regarding pain and coping with consequences of treatment; and less than 20% regarding social life, information and education, daily living and issues dealing with life planning. Differences in the number and type of treatment goals chosen by physicians and patients can indicate different priorities in rehabilitation goals. Here, information and education, daily living, social life, issues dealing with life planning and pain were important domains for patients but received much less priority from physicians. Höder et al. (2006) showed that physicians and phys-iotherapists select fewer types of rehabilitation goals, that is, they have a more restricted perspective on rehabilitation goals compared to patients. Patients preferred a higher num-ber of goals from the domains of activities and participation as well as personal factors, to use terms from the World Health Organization's (2001) International Classification of Functioning, Disability and Health (ICF), whereas physicians and therapists emphasized goals related to impairments of body functions. Brandes and Niehues (2012) reported that female patients with endometriosis reported considerably fewer rehabilitation goals before rehabilitation than documented by the physicians during the admission talk. There was also only limited agreement between the patients' pre-rehabilitation goals and those documented in the discharge report. Goals also differed considerably according to the ICF dimensions. Using a checklist approach, Glattacker et al. (2006) found that patients reported a higher number of goals compared to physicians or therapists. A recent study by Farin & Fleitz (2009) found that only 57% of patients with musculoskeletal disorders reported that rehabilitation goals had been set or agreed on. The respective proportions were 67% in patients with a cardiac disease and 62% in patients with a neurological disease.

These studies rely on questionnaire or checklist approaches to identify treatment goals. Qualitative studies, in comparison, identify a fundamental problem to do with how patients are able to talk about their rehabilitation goals (Meyer et al., 2008; Meyer, Pohontsch, & Raspe, 2009b). There have been patients in every clinic under study who claimed to have no rehabilitation goal at all even after having attended their intake interview and having been in the clinic for about 2 weeks. These patients made it necessary, in the qualitative studies, to go beyond the notion of goals in terms of explicitly developed or selected ideas about a future state and to make use of the notion of expectations. The distinction here between *goals* and *expectations* is that the latter do not have to be developed or selected or stated explicitly. In qualitative research, their presence can be inferred by analysis of surprises or disappointments with the rehabilitation experience. Still, pinpointing these expectations during the qualitative interviews can be difficult. Often, patients in these studies referred to very general expectations, for example, to improve one's health, or that one is somehow better off afterwards. These results (which are based on interviews made about 2 weeks after the start of rehabilitation) indicated that the integration of treatment goals into rehabilitation practice is far from being substantial. Interestingly, another quali-tative study by Quatmann et al. (2011) reported that physicians tend to avoid the term *goals* while talking with patients. They also found that patients would not distinguish different terms like goals, wishes, expectations or demands. However, Dudeck et al. (2011) reported that patients were quite able to state rehabilitation goals by means of a questionnaire with an open-ended response format.

12.8 Goal Orientation and Outcome Assessment

The problem of the existence of a wide range of multiple endpoints in the evaluation of rehabilitation has been tackled in a research project using an outcome instrument widespread in German rehabilitation research, the Indikatoren des Reha-Status (IRES) – literally, *indicators of rehabilitation status* (Gerdes, 1998). Not every indicator is important for every rehabilitation patient. For example, there are usually a number of indicators where patients start off with positive values that have no chance of getting substantially better during rehabilitation. It is argued that these dimensions reduce the true effects of rehabilitation when they are integrated into the evaluation of rehabilitation, that is, they dilute possible large effects in patients to whom this indicator represents an important problem area. The Zielorientierte Ergebnismessung or *ZOE* approach (literally *goal-oriented outcome assessment*) tries to overcome this problem by defining a patient profile at the beginning of the evaluation in terms of the individual rehabilitation goals for each patient. That means patients are asked to select a number of goals important to them. Only these goals are included in the subsequent evaluation. In contrast to goal-attainment scaling, the selection of the goals may be more standardized, and the effect is based not on a rating of goal attainment or a direct appraisal of change but on calculation of pre–post differences only for those domains that were identified as a goal in these patients. In a study comprising seven institutions including patients with musculoskeletal, cardiac or psychosomatic indications, it was shown that effect sizes with the ZOE approach are substantially larger than the conventional approach. The conventional approach takes into account all patient data, that is, independent of whether the respective dimension represents an individual goal for the patient. The higher the number of patients who do not see a certain dimension (e.g. sleep quality) as a personal goal, the more attenuated the effect sizes should be. Although the *ZOE* approach proved useful for tackling an important problem in rehabilitation research, it has also been subjected to substantial criticism (Zwingmann, 2003). For example, it is especially prone to the effects of regression to the mean and cannot take into account changes in the goals or goal structure of a patient during the process of rehabilitation, which can be a goal of rehabilitation in itself. Consequently, it has not become part of routine clinical practice or outcome research.

A study by Weis et al. (2002) reported results on goal-attainment scaling in comparison with pre–post assessment of outcome. It was a controlled, observational study with 1-year follow-up after rehabilitation in female patients with non-metastatic breast cancer. Here, a comparison was made between patients with and without rehabilitation (i.e. *usual care*). It could be shown that results of pre–post assessments and goal-attainment scaling were only weakly related with each other. However, the relationships were found within similar domains, that is, improvement in psychological functioning was related to improvement in psychological issues in goal-attainment scaling. This means that inclusion of personal goals into outcome assessment may change the interpretation of effects of rehabilitation interventions. At the same time, they do not represent totally different information but should be related to the same underlying change processes.

12.9 Goal Setting and Rehabilitation Outcome

There are inconsistent results regarding the association between characteristics of goal setting and rehabilitation outcomes, which are all based on observational studies. Höder et al. (2006) could not find a relationship between the degree of agreement on rehabilitation goals between physicians and patients and the degree of goal attainment or the course of rehabilitation in patients with orthopaedic disease. A similar result has been reported by Glattacker et al. (2006) in patients with oncological diseases. However, in an early study on determinants of psychological therapy goals in cardiac and orthopaedic patients by Farin, Follert, and Jäckel (2002), a positive relationship could be found between a higher degree of agreement between physicians and patients and positive outcome of rehabilitation.

In a prospective, multi-centre cohort study by Schochat and Neuner (2007), the relationship between therapy goals (immediate rehabilitation goals) and the long-term goal of avoiding early retirement was analysed. Two thousand rehabilitation patients, primarily with musculoskeletal indications, were followed up for 5 years and were contacted each year. Improvement of mobility and pain reduction (as immediate rehabilitation goals) were the two most valid predictors of work status 5 years after rehabilitation, in addition to (younger) age and (higher) level of education.

12.10 Approaches to Integrate Goal Orientation into Rehabilitation

Dudeck et al. (2011) developed and evaluated a training module to support shared goal setting. It could be shown that four out of five of the participating therapists reported asking patients about their goals. However, only about half of the surveyed therapists (including physicians) reported integration of patients into rehabilitation goal setting. It became evident that goal setting has increasing relevance and acceptance among clinicians. They see the use of shared goal setting in improved motivation and compliance, better rehabilitation outcome, empowerment of the patients and improved transparency of processes. Possible steps for improvement of goal setting in rehabilitation included discussions about goals during different time points of rehabilitation; implementation of participation in the goal-setting process, that is, shared goal setting; documentation of stipulated goals; sensitivity towards changes of goals during rehabilitation; explanation of therapies in relation to goal achievement; preparation of patients with regard to measures to be taken after the rehabilitation phase to keep up goal achievement; exchange of individual goals within the rehabilitation team; better integration of non-medical therapists into goal-setting process; and integration of goal orientation into rehabilitation concepts.

While the study by Dudeck et al. (2011) provided evidence for increased acceptance of goal orientation in rehabilitation, only a few studies have tackled the problem of how to best integrate goal setting and further goal orientation into rehabilitation practice. A recent study by Buchholz et al. (2012) reported on the use of a simple, structured but open-ended questionnaire sent to the patients before admission to a rehabilitation unit. In this study, 2782 patients with musculoskeletal, oncological or psychosomatic diseases were asked *What do I want to achieve in rehabilitation?* along with instructions to stimulate different lines of thought and possible outcome domains. The researchers reported that about 62%

of the patients had the filled-in questionnaire available at the admission meeting and that it was a useful starting point for the clinicians to talk about rehabilitation goals. Forty-five percent of clinicians found the questionnaire to be useful for treatment planning and in the overall rehabilitation process.

In a pilot study involving this chapter's authors and colleagues (Pohontsch, Deck, Höder, Schönrock-Nabulsi, & Meyer, 2009), patients were introduced to the idea of goal setting before admission to rehabilitation. Here, oncology patients were invited to a special *rehabilitation information day* on a Saturday before their scheduled admission. Besides getting an introduction into the surroundings and accommodations of the rehabilitation clinic, patients were informed about rehabilitation goals and their importance for the rehabilitation process. They took time to elaborate on their rehabilitation goals with the support of other rehabilitation patients and a professional instructor and learned techniques to discuss their individual goals with the physician during the intake interview. Evaluation at the end of the day showed that patients judged the information given as helpful and felt sufficiently prepared to discuss their goals with the physician. After rehabilitation, patients who attended the *rehabilitation information day* reported slightly more often that all therapists knew about their rehabilitation goals. No further effects (e.g. influence of personal goals on therapy planning, attainment of rehabilitation goals) could be found. All participants reported that attending the *rehabilitation information day* helped them to focus on their personal goals and to discuss them during the intake interview.

12.11 Conclusion

Goal orientation is an essential aspect of the German rehabilitation system. It has become evident that the focus of goal setting in rehabilitation research is intrinsically related to the quality assurance activities that have substantially impacted the field of rehabilitation in Germany. The studies cited earlier demonstrate that the challenge to integrate goal orientation into every step of the rehabilitation process has not yet been fully met. Although results of studies that demonstrate a positive influence of goal setting on rehabilitation outcomes in Germany are equivocal, much research has been done in the field of rehabilitation goals, (mutual) goal setting and goal attainment. This research on goal setting in rehabilitation is primarily oriented towards practical problems and still lacks an explicit theoretical foundation. The German rehabilitation system suffers the same lack of agreement on terminology which is emerging in the English-speaking research field (Playford, Siegert, Levack, & Freemann, 2009; Scobbie, Wyke, & Dixon, 2009). The only substantial agreement in sight is to distinguish (rather medium- or long-term) rehabilitation goals from treatment goals that are part of the intervention phase, that is, admission to a rehabilitation institution (Korsukéwitz, 2008). The German rehabilitation system also has no standard approach regarding how to best agree on rehabilitation and treatment goals with individual rehabilitation patients. Nevertheless, the importance of mutual goal setting and goal orientation in the rehabilitation setting is currently undisputed.

The studies cited earlier show very different results on the relevance of goals to patients depending on the type of goal assessment. While results of the use of goal checklists or open-ended questionnaires were optimistic about patients having (specific) rehabilitation goals, qualitative enquiries resulted in more pessimistic appraisals. German rehabilitation research has started to tackle general methodological issues related to outcome assessment with reference to individual patient goals, the *goal-oriented outcome assessment* being one of these approaches deserving further consideration.

While the importance of rehabilitation goals is increasingly accepted by rehabilitation therapists, most effort has been devoted to analysing the type of goals that patients and physician or therapists have and how goal setting takes place – although it is not known what happens behind closed doors in intake interview concerning the definition of goals (Dudeck et al., 2011). The most important challenge to research in this field is how to implement goal orientation into the process of rehabilitation and to analyse respective effects of different measures taken. It has also been recognized that approaches to implementation of goal setting or goal orientation in rehabilitation has not necessarily resulted in better rehabilitation outcomes. Still, goal setting and goal orientation should not only be appraised in terms of their contribution to effectiveness. They can be thought of as a valuable means to improve patient orientation in rehabilitation in its own right, that is, independent of effectiveness considerations. In fact, German Code book IX which lays the foundation of rehabilitation states two overarching goals of rehabilitation: self-determination and participation. Mutual goal setting and goal orientation could be valuable means to foster self-determination in rehabilitation.

References

Baumgarten, E., Klosterhuis, H. (2007). Aktuelles aus der Reha-Qualitätssicherung: Peer Review-Verfahren ausgewertet – bessere Reha-Qualität, aber deutliche Unterschiede zwischen Reha-Einrichtungen. *RVaktuell* 54(5), 152–154.

Beckmann, U., Pallenberg, C., & Klosterhuis, H. (2000). Berichte zur Qualitätssicherung. Informationen der BfA für die Rehabilitationseinrichtungen im Rahmen des Qualitätssicherungsprogramms. *Angestelltenversicherung*, 3, 1–11.

Bergelt, C., Welk, H., & Koch, U. (2000). Erwartungen, Befürchtungen und Therapieziele von Patienten zu Beginn einer onkologischen Rehabilitationsmaßnahme. *Rehabilitation*, 39, 338–349.

Berking, M., Dreesen, J., & Jacobi, C. (2004). Was wollen Patienten wann und wo erreichen? Die Veränderungen von Therapiezielen während und nach einer stationären Verhaltenstherapie. *Verhaltenstherapie*, 14, 245–252.

Brandes, I., & Niehues, C. (2012). Welche Zusammenhänge bestehen zwischen den von Patienten selbst beschriebenen und den im ärztlichen Entlassbericht dokumentierten Reha-Zielen? Am Beispiel von Endometriose-Patientinnen in einer Reha-Klinik. *DRV Schriften*, 98, 137–138.

Buchholz, I., Glaser-Möller, N., & Kohlmann, T. (2012). Die Erfassung von Reha-Zielen vor Antritt der medizinischen Rehabilitation – "Schicksal" und Nutzen eines vorab versandten Fragebogens. *DRV-Schriften*, 98, 135–136.

Deutsche Rentenversicherung Bund. (2007). *Rahmenkonzept zur medizinischen Rehabilitation in der gesetzlichen Rentenversicherung*. Berlin, Germany: Deutsche Rentenversicherung Bund.

Deutsche Rentenversicherung Bund. (2008). *Rehabilitation – Was erwartet mich dort?* Berlin, Germany: Deutsche Rentenversicherung Bund.

Deutsche Rentenversicherung Bund. (2012). Reha-Bericht 2012. *Die medizinische und berufliche Rehabilitation der Rentenversicherung im Licht der Statistik*. Berlin, Germany: Deutsche Rentenversicherung Bund.

Doran, G. T. (1981). There's a S.M.A.R.T. way to write management's goals and objectives. *Management Review*, 70(11), 35–36.

Dorenburg, U., Huck-Langner, K., Nischan, P., & Winnefeld, M. (2001). Kontinuierliche, klinikvergleichende Patientenbefragung im Reha-Qualitätssicherungsprogramm der Rentenversicherung: Konzept, Methodik, Erfahrungen. In W. Satzinger, A. Trojan, & P. Kellermann-Mühlhoff (Eds.), *Patientenbefragungen in Krankenhäusern* (pp. 361–369). St. Augustin, Germany: Asgard.

Dörner, U., & Muthny, F. A. (2006). Ziele in der kardiologischen Rehabilitation aus Sicht von Patienten und Ärzten – Passt das zusammen? *Prävention und Rehabilitation, 18*, 131–139.

Dudeck, A., Glattacker, M., Gustke, M., Dibbelt, S., Greitemann, B., & Jäckel, W. H. (2011). Reha-Zielvereinbarungen – gegenwärtige Praxis in der stationären medizinischen Rehabilitation. *Rehabilitation, 50*, 316–330.

Farin, E. & Fleitz, A. (2009) The development of an ICF-oriented, adaptive physician assessment instrument of mobility, self-care, and domestic life. *International Journal of Rehabilitation Research 32*, 98–107.

Farin, E., Carl, C., Lichtenberg, S., Jäckel, W. H., Maier-Riehle, B., & Rütten-Köppel, E. (2003). Die Bewertung des Rehabilitationsprozesses mittels des Peer-Review-Verfahrens: Methodische Prüfung und Ergebnisse der Erhebungsrunde 2000/2001 in den somatischen Indikationsbereichen. *Rehabilitation, 42*, 323–334.

Farin, E., Follert, P., & Jäckel, W. H. (2002). Die Therapiezielfestlegung bei Patienten mit psychischen Belastungen in der orthopädischen und kardiologischen Rehabilitation. *Rehabilitation, 41*, 389–400.

Gerdes, N. (1998). Rehabilitationseffekte bei "zielorientierter Ergebnismessung". Ergebnisse der IRES-ZOE-Studie 1996/97. *Deutsche Rentenversicherung, Heft 3–4*, 217–237.

Glattacker, M., Farin, E., & Jäckel, W. H. (2006). Rehabilitationsziele aus Patienten und Arztsicht in der onkologischen Rehabilitation – Wie hoch ist die Kongruenz und welchen Einfluss hat dies auf das Outcome? *DRV-Schriften, 64*, 414–415.

Höder, J., Josenhans, J., & Arlt, A. C. (2006). Ziele von Patienten, Ärzten und Therapeuten in der stationären Rehabilitation von Rückenschmerzpatienten. *DRV-Schriften, 64*, 363–364.

Jäckel, W. H., Bengel, J., & Herdt, J. (Eds.). (2006). *Research in rehabilitation. Results from a research network in Southwest Germany*. Stuttgart, Germany: Schattauer.

Korsukéwitz, C. (2008). Medizinische Rehabilitation – Den Patienten dort abholen, wo er steht. *Deutsches Ärzteblatt, 105*, A-2312.

Meyer, T., Pohontsch, N., Maurischat, C., & Raspe, H. (2008). *Patientenzufriedenheit und Zielorientierung in der Rehabilitation*. Lage, Germany: Jacobs.

Meyer, T., Pohontsch, N., Maurischat, C., & Raspe, H. (2009a) Warum beurteilen Rehabilitanden die Rehaplanung und Zielorientierung weniger positiv als andere Aspekte der medizinischen Rehabilitation? *Physikalische Medizin, Rehabilitationsmedizin, Kurortmedizin, 19*, 85–92.

Meyer, T., Pohontsch, N., & Raspe, H. (2009b). Zielfestlegungen in der stationären medizinischen Rehabilitation – die Herausforderung bleibt. *Rehabilitation, 48*, 128–134.

Nagl, M., & Farin-Glattacker, E. (2011). Patientenseitige Gesundheitsbewertungen und arztseitige Zielfestlegungen in der Rehabilitation: Übereinstimmung oder Diskrepanz? *DRV-Schriften, 93*, 147–148.

Playford, E. D., Siegert, R., Levack, W., & Freemann, J. (2009). Areas of consensus and controversy about goal setting in rehabilitation: A conference report. *Clinical Rehabilitation, 23*(4), 334–344.

Pohontsch, N., Deck, R., Höder, J., Schönrock-Nabulsi, P., & Meyer, T. (2009). Der Rehabilitanden-Informationstag – Ein rehabilitandenzentriertes Programm zur Zielorientierung der medizinischen Rehabilitation. *DRV Schriften, 83*, 60–61.

Protz, W., Gerdes, N., Maier-Riehle, B., & Jäckel, W. H. (1998). Therapieziele in der medizinischen Rehabilitation. *Rehabilitation, 37*, 24–29.

Quatmann, M., Dibbelt, S., Dudeck, A., Glattacker, M., Greitemann, B., & Jäckel, W. H. (2011). Zielvereinbarung in der Rehabilitation: Verständnis und Handhabung des Begriffs "Reha-Ziele" bei Ärzten und Patienten. *DRV-Schriften, 93*, 161–163.

Relman, A. S. (1988). Assessment and accountability. The third revolution in medical care. *The New England Journal of Medicine, 319*, 1220–1222.

Rietz, I., Höder, J., Josenhans, J., & Arlt, A. C. (2001). *Ziele von Patienten, Ärzten und Therapeuten in der stationären Rehabilitation von Rückenschmerzen.* Lübeck, Germany: Verein zur Förderung der Rehabilitationsforschung der LVA SH (vffr).

Schochat, T., & Neuner, R. (2007). *Prädiktive Validierung von Therapiezielen am Frühberentungsrisiko 3–5 Jahre nach der Rehabilitation. Abschlussbericht.* Retrieved 4 March 2012, from http://forschung. deutsche-rentenversicherung.de/ForschPortalWeb/rehaDoc.pdf?rehaid=21A7D8D1CC61C8 F0C1256E99004071C3.

Scobbie, L., Wyke, S., & Dixon, D. (2009). Identifying and applying psychological theory to setting and achieving rehabilitation goals. *Clinical Rehabilitation, 23,* 321–333.

Verband Deutscher Rentenversicherungsträger (Ed.). (1992). *Bericht der Reha-Kommission – Empfehlungen zur Weiterentwicklung der medizinischen Rehabilitation in der gesetzlichen Rentenversicherung.* Frankfurt am Main, Germany: VDR.

Verband Deutscher Rentenversicherungsträger (Ed.). (2000). *Das Qualitätssicherungsprogramm der gesetzlichen Rentenversicherung in der medizinischen Rehabilitation. Instrumente und Verfahren.* DRV-Schriften, 18. Frankfurt am Main, Germany: VDR.

Vogel, H., Tuschhoff, T., & Zillessen, E. (1994). Die Definition von Rehabilitationszielen als Herausforderung für die Qualitätssicherung. *Dtsch Rentenversicher, 49,* 751–765.

Vogel, H., & Zdrahal-Urbanek, J. (2004). Rehabilitation in Germany: New challenges of a structured social security scheme. *International Journal of Rehabilitation Research, 27,* 93–98.

Weis, J., Moser, M. T., & Bartsch, H. H. (2002). *Zielorientierte Evaluation stationärer onkologischer Rehabilitationsmaßnahmen (ZESOR-Studie). Abschlussbericht.* Retrieved 4 March 2012, from http://forschung.deutsche-rentenversicherung.de/ForschPortalWeb/rehaDoc.pdf?rehaid=5f 5eb3b5f78bf136c1256e9b002f82b6.

Widera T, Klosterhuis H. (2007). Patientenorientierung in der Praxis – 10 Jahre Rehabilitanden- befragung im Rahmen der Reha-Qualitätssicherung der Rentenversicherung. *RVaktuell* 54(6), 177–182.

World Health Organization. (2001). *International Classification of Functioning, Disability and Health.* Geneva, Switzerland: WHO.

Zwingmann, C. (2003). Zielorientierte Ergebnismessung (ZOE) mit dem IRES-Patientenfragebogen: Eine kritische Zwischenbilanz. *Rehabilitation, 42,* 226–235.

Section III

Specific Applications

13

Goal Setting in Social Competence Treatment after Brain Injury

Lenore A. Hawley and Jody K. Newman

CONTENTS

13.1 Introduction

Social competence impairments are among the most common and potentially devastating sequelae of brain injury, often disrupting relationships with family, friends, co-workers and others in the community. The effect of brain injury on an individual's cognitive, behavioural and emotional abilities has been well documented (Ben-Yishay et al., 1985; Malec, Smigielski, DePompolo, & Thompson, 1993; McDonald, Tate, et al., 2008; Prigatano, Fordyce, & Zeiner, 1994; Thomsen, 1984; Ylvisaker & Feeney, 2001). After a brain injury, impaired social functioning is often the main obstacle to successful relationships, employment and social confidence and may lead to social anxiety, frustration and avoidance of social situations, loneliness and depression (Gordon & Hibbard, 2005; McDonald, Tate, et al., 2008; Oddy & Humphrey, 1980). Additionally, social interactions with individuals following traumatic brain injury (TBI) have been described as effortful and unrewarding (Galski, Tomkins, & Johnston, 1998).

Social competence encompasses the cognitive, emotional and communication skills needed to interact successfully, as well as the ability to determine how to apply those skills in a variety of social situations (Bellack, Mueser, Gingerich, & Agresta, 2004; Hawley & Newman, 2010; McDonald, Tate, et al., 2008; Welsh & Bierman, 1998). Individuals with TBI may have difficulty with a wide range of social competence skills such as starting, sustaining or ending conversations; staying focused on a social interaction; respecting and setting social boundaries; taking turns; initiating social activities; interacting assertively;

resolving conflicts; initiating appropriate topics; and social problem solving. Being socially competent requires some of the very skills that are frequently impaired after TBI including initiation, awareness, sustained attention, social perception, problem solving, language, speech and emotional regulation. The ability to communicate one's thoughts and needs, to listen to and support others and to develop social and vocational relationships is critical to being an active member of society (Hawley & Newman, 2010). Due to the array of deficits common to this population, the ability to formulate and address one's social competence goals following brain injury can be difficult.

In this chapter, we will define social competence, provide a brief history of goal setting within social competence treatment and present a model of goal setting within an evidence-based social competence group treatment programme for individuals with brain injury. There are multiple terms used to describe social competence and related behaviours, including social skills, social communication skills, interpersonal skills, psychosocial skills and pragmatic language skills. The term social competence appears to best describe the broad array of skills and behaviours needed to interact successfully.

13.2 History of Goal Setting in Social Competence Treatment

Social competence has been formally studied since the early 1920s and was initially described simply as the successful interaction between an individual and his or her specific environment (Knapp, 2001). The study of social competence accelerated in the 1950s and 1960s when researchers discovered a relationship between social competence and mental health in children (Dodge, Asher, & Parkhurst, 1989). Subsequent definitions incorporated the concepts of social problem solving, specific cognitive and behavioural processes and judgements regarding one's overall social ability (Knapp, 2001; Pelegrini, 1985; Rubin & Rose-Krasnor, 1992; Warnes, Sheridan, Geske, & Warnes, 2005). Goldfried and D'Zurilla (1969) described social competence as a judgement someone makes about how another person is performing in a social situation and noted that assessment of social competence needs to take place in context. Today, there are a variety of definitions of social competence, most incorporating cognitive, affective and behavioural components and emphasizing judgement, problem solving and contextual relevance. Wentzel (1991) noted that to be socially competent requires the self-regulatory capabilities of planning and goal setting.

Social skills are a major component of social competence and have been defined as 'goal-directed, learned behaviours that allow one to interact and function effectively in a variety of social contexts' (Sheridan & Walker, 1999, p. 687). Protocols for social skills treatment have been described for adults and children with various diagnoses including depression, anxiety, autism spectrum disorders, learning disabilities, developmental disabilities, addiction, juvenile delinquency and schizophrenia. Social skills treatment is rooted in behavioural and social learning theory (Bandura, 1969, 1977; Skinner, 1938, 1953), and strategies related to these theories are described as key components of social skills treatment. These strategies include modelling, shaping, feedback, reinforcement, cueing, social problem solving, generalization and goal setting. Goal setting is often seen as the core upon which social skills treatment is based. As Rose (1998) noted in discussing social skills group treatment, 'the structure provided by goals gives both members and the group therapists a sense of direction' (p. 153).

Social skills treatment has traditionally taken place in group settings, capitalizing on the natural social environment of the group and the ability of the group to provide feedback, reinforcement and modelling. Group treatment may employ a psycho-educational skills-training approach or may involve group psychotherapy, emphasizing group moderators of change including universality, altruism, group cohesiveness and interpersonal learning (Yalom & Leszcz, 2005). Thus, goal setting in social skills treatment may involve individual goals as well as interactive goals for the group as a whole (Bellack et al., 2004; Rose, 1977). The timing of goal setting in group treatment is crucial. Rose (1998) cautioned that not all group members will be prepared to set goals at the same time and that premature goal setting can result in energy spent proceeding toward a goal that is not realistic or relevant for the individual.

Goal setting in social skills treatment is frequently described as a collaborative process. Liberman and Kopelowicz (2002) noted that few outcomes are as valuable or empowering to an individual as meeting one's own personal goals. The individual is encouraged to take the lead role, with input from the therapist, family and other group members (Bellack et al., 2004; Liberman et al., 1986; Rose, 1998). Goals provide a structure around which social skills group sessions are organized, providing a sense of direction for the group process, as well as a method to evaluate outcomes (Bellack et al., 2004; Rose, 1998). Bellack et al. noted that when individual clients' goals are kept central in the treatment process, group members are more active and engaged. Various models have been described for developing goal setting within social skills groups. For example, Liberman et al. outlining a social skills model for individuals with schizophrenia described the goal-setting process as beginning with identifying the individual's assets and deficits, pinpointing behaviours as functional goals, breaking goals into measureable steps and cueing others (family, friends, etc.) to reinforce goal behaviours. Bellack and colleagues added that the therapist can meet individually with each group member prior to the group to assess what the individual's goals were before the onset of their illness or condition, as well as what goals the individual may be interested in addressing in the group, and to ensure that goals are meaningful and relevant to the individual's daily life.

Many of the social competence approaches and strategies developed and implemented in the fields of mental health and special education have been adapted for individuals with brain injury. For example, the use of group treatment, the influence of behavioural and social learning theory, the need for contextual relevance and an emphasis on client-lead, goal-oriented treatment have been used extensively with individuals following brain injury (Ben-Yishay et al., 1985; Deaton, 1991; Hawley & Newman, 2008; Kuipers, Carlson, Bailey, & Sharma, 2004; Malec et al., 1993; McDonald, Bornhofen, et al., 2008; Ownsworth, McFarland, & Young, 2000; Prigatano et al., 1994; Rath, Simon, Langenbahn, Sherr, & Diller, 2003; Thomsen, 1984; Walker, Onus, Doyle, Clare, & McCarthy, 2005; Ylvisaker & Feeney, 1998).

Specific interventions designed to improve the social functioning of individuals with brain injury have generally focused on one or more of the following areas: (1) social skills and behaviours, (2) emotional perception and (3) the ability to attribute beliefs and intentions in others – a cognitive function called *mentalizing* in the theory of mind (Aboulafia-Brakha, Christe, Martory, & Annoni, 2011; Driscoll, Dal Monte, & Grafman, 2010; McDonald, Tate, et al., 2008; Stronach & Turkstra, 2008; Ylvisaker & Feeney, 1998). In this chapter, we have focused on goal setting within social competence treatment that addresses social skills and behaviours.

13.3 Goal Setting in Social Competence Treatment for Individuals with Traumatic Brain Injury

Goal setting requires self-awareness, self-regulation and executive functioning (Bergquist & Jacket, 1993; Walker et al., 2005; Ylvisaker & Feeney, 1998). Impairments in self-awareness and self-regulation are common sequelae of brain injury and have been associated with poor psychosocial functioning as well as difficulty in formulating and monitoring performance on goals, as well as problem solving and persisting toward goal achievement (Bergquist & Jacket, 1993; Malec, 1999; Ownsworth et al., 2000; Ylvisaker & Feeney, 1998). Stuss and Benson (1986) noted that disorders of self-awareness result from disruption of the executive control system, affecting anticipation, planning, goal selection, initiation, execution and self-regulation. Executive functioning has been defined as the set of abilities that allow a person to carry out goal-directed behaviours (Lezak, Howieson, & Loring, 2004). Positive outcomes following brain injury have been found to occur in individuals who recognize their deficits, set realistic goals for themselves and are active participants in their rehabilitation (Bergquist & Jacket, 1993; Deaton, 1986; Ownsworth et al., 2000).

Several authors have described the goal-setting process and given examples of specific social skills goals for individuals with brain injury. Malec et al. (1993) studied the effects of a comprehensive brain injury neurorehabilitation programme consisting of six treatment groups targeting six different areas of treatment, including social skills. The social skills group treatment involved the participants taking an active role in the process of setting individual goals and additionally used goal attainment scaling (Kiresuk, Smith, & Cardillo, 1994) as a means for monitoring progress on those goals. McGann, Werven, and Douglas (1997) described a brain injury social competence group treatment which also involved the participant, working together with the group facilitator, to select communication goals.

Several concepts and strategies have been consistent throughout goal setting in social skills treatment following brain injury. The value of patient and family involvement in the formulation and selection of rehabilitation goals has been described by many authors (Hawley & Newman, 2008; Kuipers et al., 2004; Levack, Siegert, Dean, & McPherson, 2009; Malec et al., 1993; Ownsworth et al., 2000; Walker et al., 2005; Ylvisaker & Feeney, 1998). This type of collaboration may result in the development of a broader range of goals which are personally and contextually relevant, realistic and more likely to generalize to various situations. Active engagement in the goal-setting process may enhance the self-awareness of an individual with a brain injury (Braden et al., 2010; Hawley & Newman, 2010; Kuipers et al., 2004). Common goal areas generally addressed in social skills treatment following brain injury include the following: greetings, introducing oneself, listening, conversational skills, topic selection, asking questions, interpreting non-verbal feedback, starting conversations and keeping them going, assertiveness, social boundaries, conflict resolution, controlling emotions during social interactions and development of opportunities to socialize (Hawley & Newman, 2008; McDonald, Bornhofen, et al., 2008; Ownsworth et al., 2000; Rath et al., 2003; Walker et al., 2005). Several brain injury research studies have investigated the efficacy of social skills interventions (Dahlberg, Cusick, & Hawley, 2007; Helffenstein & Wechsler, 1982; Malec et al., 1993; McDonald, Tate, et al., 2008; Walker et al., 2005; Wiseman-Hakes, Stewart, Wassertnan, & Schuller, 1998). A number of these emphasize the importance of goal setting in the treatment process.

13.4 Model for Goal Setting within a Social Competence Intervention for Individuals with Brain Injury

Group interactive structured treatment (GIST) is an evidence-based social competence programme designed to address social skills problems faced by people with brain injuries (Hawley & Newman, 2008). GIST uses a structured cognitive behavioural group therapy model addressing the underlying cognitive, communicative and emotional impairments interfering with social competence after brain injury. This dual-disciplinary intervention draws upon the theoretical areas of holistic neurorehabilitation, group therapy and cognitive behavioural therapy. Sessions take place once per week over 13 weeks and involve six to eight group participants and two group therapists. Each week, key points from the previous session are reviewed, and then a new topic is introduced, followed by interactive group practice of strategies and skills. The session topics include the following: self-assessment and goal setting, starting conversations, keeping conversations going, giving and receiving feedback, assertiveness, social problem solving, social confidence through positive self-talk, social boundaries and conflict resolution.

The GIST developers have applied this group model over the past 20 years for individuals with mild, moderate and severe brain injury, including active duty military and veterans. A randomized control trial, funded by the National Institute on Disability and Rehabilitation Research and conducted at Craig Hospital (in Denver, Colorado, United States), demonstrated the efficacy of this programme (Dahlberg et al., 2007). Within GIST's structured group therapy sessions, active mediators from cognitive behavioural therapy are used to promote behavioural change. These include observation, verbal persuasion, feedback, cognitive restructuring, cueing, modelling, social reinforcement, goal setting and homework. The group process offers the opportunity for development of universality, altruism and a sense of group cohesion which can lead to increased self-awareness and behaviour change. Specific social competence skills are discussed, modelled and practised in small and large interactive groups. Group members receive a session-by-session workbook with weekly homework, providing an opportunity for repetition and practice in the real world, as well as feedback and reinforcement from available support persons. Generalization is targeted through the involvement of family or significant others, weekly homework, practice across environments, video feedback and social problem solving. Family or significant others have the opportunity to participate in three support person sessions, allowing them to learn about the group as well as learning strategies to assist group members in reaching individual treatment goals (Hawley & Newman, 2010).

Self-assessment and individual goal setting are key elements of the GIST programme and provide an individualized path through the treatment process. The self-assessment and goal-setting process span three sessions, allowing the opportunity for feedback from family and friends regarding social skills strengths and challenges and eventual goal development. Self-assessment is the first step to setting realistic and relevant goals. In the GIST programme, self-assessment begins within the second session of the group, as group members complete a written self-assessment of their social competence strengths and challenges. Through group discussion, each participant receives feedback from other group members and then takes the self-assessment home for additional input from family or friends. Based on this feedback, each individual may make revisions to goals and then finalizes two or three social competence goals to address over the course of the group.

The group therapists guide this process, as needed, to assure that the goals are measureable, realistic and relevant for the individual.

There are a number of factors that affect goal choices, such as the age of the individual, level of self-awareness, family situation and whether the individual is employed. Another significant factor, within the context in which the GIST programme has been implemented, is whether the individual is civilian or military. Examples of goal areas commonly chosen by civilian group members include the following: keeping conversations going, thinking of topics to talk about, making friends, finding places to socialize, being assertive and controlling emotions. Goal areas commonly chosen by military and veteran group members include the following: controlling emotions, parenting assertively (rather than aggressively), being patient in social interactions, socializing more and re-developing the desire to socialize with others (Hawley & Newman, 2010).

After the goals are finalized, they are written on a goal form which is placed in the front of the individual's workbook. Group members are asked to share the finalized goals with family and friends or others (i.e. employers, teachers) so that goal-directed behaviours can be reinforced. It is also suggested that a copy of the goals be posted somewhere in the individual's home where he or she will see it frequently. The goals are written behaviourally so that the individual can assess when movement has been made toward the goal. Some examples of common goals include the following:

- I will get out of the house and socialize with others at least once per week.
- I will initiate a fun activity with my son once per week.
- I will ask questions during conversations with my wife.
- I will ask for clarification when I do not understand instructions at work.

At the beginning of each session, after the previous week's homework is reviewed, the group members share progress on their social competence goals and problem solve any obstacles. Group members often exhibit extraordinary insight and altruism in their desire to help each other through this process. The homework assignments are frequently geared toward assessing progress on individual social competence goals and gathering feedback on goal behaviours from others. The group therapists model this by providing positive feedback on even the smallest steps toward goal achievement and encouraging persistence.

The GIST programme uses a modified version of goal attainment scaling (Kiresuk et al., 1994) as a means to track goal progress. Goal behaviours are placed on a five-point scale, with the current behaviour scaled at a Level 2, allowing for an increase or decrease in behaviour. Level 4 indicates the level that the individual believes he or she could realistically attain during the group sessions, with Level 5 indicating progress beyond the group member's expectations. (For more information on goal attainment scaling, see Chapters 7 and 8 in this book.)

At the end of the 13-week group session, goals are reassessed and the individual receives feedback and reinforcement from the group members and therapists. Group members begin to discuss how they might continue to work on their social competence goals if needed or set new social goals for themselves. In addition, the group therapists develop individual written recommendations for each group member. Based on this collection of feedback and recommendations, group members discuss potential new strategies and goals. There are two follow-up sessions, usually scheduled for 1 and 2 months after the group has ended. This is a time when group members can come back together, reconnect, share goal progress and problem-solve solutions to any obstacles they have encountered. If someone has completed a goal, new social goals may be developed with input from the group.

13.4.1 Case Study

John is a 25-year old veteran of the US Army having served in the conflicts in Iraq and Afghanistan. He sustained a documented mild TBI 1 year ago and was also later diagnosed with post-traumatic stress disorder by the military physician. He reports that he was exposed to at least two other blast injuries which were not documented. After returning to the United States, John received psychological and cognitive therapy and was subsequently discharged from the army. Since discharge, several of his symptoms persisted including a lack of desire to socialize with others, difficulty controlling his emotions with his family, difficulty maintaining the topic during conversations and difficulty initiating conversations especially with civilians.

John joined a GIST social competence group in his community along with seven other army veterans. During the initial session of the group, John and the other group members shared information about themselves and discussed the key ingredients of social competence. During the second session, the group discussed skills required for good communication and also completed a social skills self-assessment. John noted the following social skills strengths and challenges:

13.4.2 Strengths

1. I have a wife and two kids who love me.
2. I have a variety of interests and topics that I can discuss.
3. Eye contact is easy for me.

13.4.3 Challenges

1. I do not want to socialize with people outside of my family.
2. I get angry at my wife and kids at least once a day and end up yelling.
3. When I am in a conversation, I can't seem to stay on the topic – I jump from one topic to another and forget where I started.

The homework assignment that week was to take the self-assessment form home and ask for input and feedback from a family member or close friend. John's wife reviewed the information with him and agreed with his strengths and challenges. She noted an additional strength is his desire to be a good father. She also noted that he specifically needed to interact more often with civilians. The following week in the group, John and the other group members shared their self-assessments and the feedback they had received from family. The group members then gave each other input and, based on all of the feedback received, developed social competence goals.

With guidance from the GIST group therapists, John's final social skills goals written in measurable terms were the following:

1. I will interact with civilians in social settings at least once a week.
2. I will manage my anger when interacting with my kids (i.e. I will not yell at my kids more than once a week).
3. I will stay on topic during conversations with my wife 75% of the time.

John was then asked to write down these goals on the goal form at the front of his workbook. At the suggestion of the therapists, John wrote his goals in a format that would be easy for him to remember:

1. Get out and talk to civilians every week.
2. Control my anger with family (Don't yell).
3. Stay on the topic.

The development of John's individual goals was instrumental in identifying key strategies for success. The strategies that proved to be most helpful for John included the following: (1) the group process (universality, support and alliance among the group members and social problem solving); (2) the development of positive self-talk strategies addressing social confidence, ability to stay focused and control of emotions; and (3) learning assertive communication skills for managing his interactions with family.

John was consistent in attending all of the sessions over the 13-week group session and his wife continued to give feedback and support throughout the group. John returned for a follow-up session 3 months after the group ended. At that time, he reported that his relationship with his children had improved and that he was able to interact with his children without yelling (yelling less than twice per month). He and his wife described that he was interacting with civilian friends at home or in the community, at least once per week. John and his wife agreed that he seemed more focused in conversations and stayed on the topic of conversation most of the time. They were encouraged to continue working on these goals and to develop new social skills goals as needed, using the same goal-setting process and strategies.

13.5 Conclusion

In this chapter, we have provided an overview of goal setting within social competence treatment. Additionally, we described the application of goal-setting methods within social competence treatment to the field of brain injury rehabilitation. Finally, we provided a model for goal setting within an evidence-based social competence intervention for individuals with brain injury. More work needs to be done in this area to acquire additional evidence regarding the individual factors that affect goal setting and goal attainment in social competence treatment following brain injury.

References

Aboulafia-Brakha, T., Christe, B., Martory, M. D., & Annoni, J. M. (2011). Theory of mind tasks and executive functions: A systematic review of group studies in neurology. *Journal of Neuropsychology, 5*(1), 39–55.

Bandura, A. (1969). *Principles of behavior modification.* New York, NY: Holt, Rinehart & Winston.

Bandura, A. (1977). *Social learning theory.* Englewood Cliffs, NJ: Prentice Hall.

Bellack, A., Mueser, K., Gingerich, S., & Agresta, J. (2004). *Social skills training for schizophrenia: A step-by-step guide.* New York, NY: Guilford Press.

Ben-Yishay, Y., Rattok, J., Lakin, P., Piasetsky, E. B., Ross, B., Silver, S., ... Ezrachi, O. (1985). Neuropsychologic rehabilitation: Quest for a holistic approach. *Seminars in Neurology, 5,* 252–259.

Bergquist, T., & Jacket, M. (1993). Awareness and goal setting with the traumatically brain injured. *Brain Injury, 7*(3), 275–282.

Braden, C., Hawley, L., Newman, J., Morey, C., Gerber, D., & Harrison-Felix, C. (2010). Social communication skills group treatment: A feasibility study for persons with traumatic brain injury and comorbid conditions. *Brain Injury, 24*(11), 1298–1310.

Dahlberg, C., Cusick, C., & Hawley, L. (2007). Treatment efficacy of social communication skills training after traumatic brain injury: A randomized treatment and deferred treatment controlled trial. *Archives of Physical Medicine and Rehabilitation, 88,* 1561–1573.

Deaton, A. (1986). Denial in the aftermath of traumatic head injury: It's manifestations, measurements, and treatment *Rehabilitation Psychology, 31*(4), 231–240.

Deaton, A. (1991). Group interventions for cognitive rehabilitation: Increasing the challenges. In J. Kreutzer & P. Wehman (Eds.), *Cognitive rehabilitation for persons with traumatic brain injury* (pp. 191–200). Baltimore, MD: Paul H. Brookes.

Dodge, K., Asher, S., & Parkhurst, J. (1989). Social life as a goal-coordination task. In C. Ames and R. Ames (Eds.), *Research on motivation in education* (pp. 107–135). San Diego, CA: Academic Press.

Driscoll, D., Dal Monte, O., & Grafman, J. (2010). A need for improved training for the remediation of impairments in social functioning following brain injury. *Journal of Neurotrauma, 28,* 319–326.

Galski, T., Tomkins, C., & Johnston, M. (1998). Competence in discourse as a measure of social integration and quality of life in persons with traumatic brain injury. *Brain Injury, 12,* 769–782.

Goldfried, M., & D'Zurilla, T. (1969). A behavioral analytic model for assessing competence. In C. Spielberger (Ed.), *Current topics in clinical and community psychology* (Vol. 1, pp. 151–196). New York, NY: Academic Press.

Gordon, W., & Hibbard, M. (2005). Cognitive rehabilitation. In J. Silver, T. McAllister, & S. Yudofsky (Eds.), *Textbook of traumatic brain injury* (pp. 655–660). Washington, DC: American Psychiatric Publishing.

Hawley, L., & Newman, J. (2008). *Group interactive structured treatment-GIST: For social competence* (Rev. ed.) (Previously titled Social skills and traumatic brain injury: A workbook for group treatment; 2006). Denver, CO: Authors.

Hawley, L., & Newman, J. (2010). Group interactive structured treatment (GIST): A social competence intervention for individuals with brain injury. *Brain Injury, 24*(11), 1292–1297.

Helffenstein, D., & Weshsler, F. (1982). The use of interpersonal process recall (IPR) in the remediation of interpersonal and communication skill deficits in the newly brain-injured. *Clinical Neuropsychology, 4,* 139–142.

Kiresuk, T., Smith, A., & Cardillo, J. (Eds.). (1994). *Goal attainment scaling: Applications, theory, and measurement.* Hillsdale, NJ: Lawrence Erlbaum Associates.

Knapp, K. (2001). *Social competence of children: Definitions and assessment.* Retrieved from https://www.msu.edu/~dwong/StudentWorkArchive/CEP900F01-RIP/Knapp-SocialCompetence.htm. Accessed on 26 March, 2014.

Kuipers, P., Carlson, G., Bailey, S., & Sharma, A. (2004). A preliminary exploration of goal-setting in community-based rehabilitation for people with brain impairment. *Brain Impairment, 5*(1), 30–41.

Levack, W. M. M., Siegert, R. J., Dean, S. G., & McPherson, K. M. (2009). Goal planning for adults with acquired brain injury: How clinicians talk about involving family. *Brain Injury, 23,* 192–202.

Lezak, M. D., Howieson, D. B., & Loring, D. W. (2004). *Neuropsychological assessment* (4th ed.). New York, NY: Oxford University Press.

Liberman, R., & Kopelowicz, A. (2002). Teaching persons with severe mental disabilities to be their own case managers. *Psychiatric Services, 53*(11), 1377–1379.

Liberman, R. P., Mueser, K. T., Wallace, C. J., Jacobs, H. E., Eckman, T., & Massel, H. K. (1986). Training skills in the psychiatrically disabled. *Schizophrenia Bulletin, 12*(4), 631–647.

Malec, J. (1999). Goal attainment scaling in rehabilitation. *Neuropsychological Rehabilitation: An international Journal, 9*(3-4), 253–275.

Malec, J. F., Smigielski, J. S., DePompolo, R. W., & Thompson, J. M. (1993). Outcome evaluation and prediction in a comprehensive-integrated post-acute outpatient brain injury rehabilitation programme. *Brain Injury, 7*(1), 15–29.

McDonald, S., Bornhofen, C., Togher, L., Flanagan, S., Gertler, P., & Bowen, R. (2008). *Improving first impressions: A step-by-step social skills program.* Sydney, New South Wales, Australia: University of New South Wales.

McDonald, S., Tate, R., Togher, L., Bornhofen, C., Long, E., Gertler, P., & Bowen, R. (2008). Social skills treatment for people with severe, chronic acquired brain injuries: A multicenter trial. *Archives of Physical Medicine and Rehabilitation, 89*(9), 1648–1659.

McGann, W., Werven, G., & Douglas, M. (1997). Social competence and head injury: A practical approach. *Brain Injury, 11*, 621–628.

Oddy, M., & Humphrey, M. (1980). Social recovery during the year following severe head injury. *Journal of Neurology, Neurosurgery and Psychiatry, 43*, 798–802.

Ownsworth, T., McFarland, K., & Young, R. (2000). Self-awareness and psychosocial functioning following acquired brain injury: An evaluation of a group support programme. *Neuropsychological Rehabilitation, 10*(5), 465–484.

Pelegrini, D. (1985). Social cognition and competence in middle childhood. *Child Development, 56*(1), 253–264.

Prigatano, G., Fordyce, D., & Zeiner, H. (1994). Neuropsychological rehabilitation after closed head injury in young adults. *Journal of Neurology, Neurosurgery, and Psychiatry, 47*, 505–513.

Rath, J. F., Simon, D., Langenbahn, D. M., Sherr, R. L., & Diller, L. (2003). Group treatment of problem-solving deficits in outpatients with traumatic brain injury: A randomised outcome study. *Neuropsychological Rehabilitation, 13*(4), 461–488.

Rose, S. D. (1977). *Group therapy: A behavioral approach.* Englewood Cliffs, NJ: Prentice Hall.

Rose, S. D. (1998). *Group therapy with troubled youth: A cognitive-behavioral interactive approach.* Thousand Oaks, CA: Sage Publications.

Rubin, K., & Rose-Krasnor, L. (1992). Interpersonal problem solving and social competence in children. In V. B. Van Hasselt & M. Hersen (Eds.), *Handbook of social development: A lifespan perspective* (pp. 283–323). New York, NY: Plenum Press.

Sheridan, S., & Walker, D. (1999). Social skills in context: Considerations for assessment, intervention and generalization. In C. R. Reynolds & T. B. Gutkin (Eds.), *The handbook of school psychology* (3rd ed., pp. 687–708). New York, NY: Wiley.

Skinner, B. F. (1938). *The behavior of organisms: An experimental analysis.* New York, NY: Appleton-Century-Crofts.

Skinner, B. F. (1953). *Science and human behavior.* New York, NY: Macmillan.

Stronach, S., & Turkstra, L. (2008). Theory of mind and use of cognitive state terms by adolescents with traumatic brain injury. *Aphasiology, 22*(10), 1054–1070.

Stuss, D., & Benson, D. (1986). *The frontal lobes.* New York, NY: Raven Press.

Thomsen, I. (1984). Late outcome of very severe blunt head trauma: A 10–15 year second follow-up. *Journal of Neurology, Neurosurgery, and Psychiatry, 47*, 260–268.

Walker, A. J., Onus, M., Doyle, M., Clare, J., & McCarthy, K. (2005). Cognitive rehabilitation after severe traumatic brain injury: A pilot programme of goal planning and outdoor adventure course participation. *Brain Injury, 19*(14), 1237–1241.

Warnes, E., Sheridan, S., Geske, J., & Warnes, W. (2005). A contextual approach to the assessment of social skills: Identifying meaningful behaviors for social competence. *Psychology in the Schools, 42*(2), 173–187.

Welsh, J. A., & Bierman, K. L. (1998). *Gale encyclopedia of childhood and adolescence.* Detroit, MI: Gale Research.

Wentzel, K. (1991). Relations between social competence and academic achievement in early adolescence. *Child Development, 62*, 1066–1078.

Wiseman-Hakes, C., Stewart, M. L., Wassertnan, R., & Schuller, R. (1998). Peer group training of pragmatic skills in adolescents with acquired brain injury. *Journal of Head Trauma Rehabilitation, 13*(6), 23–38.

Yalom, I., & Leszcz, M. (2005). *The theory and practice of group psychotherapy* (5th ed.). New York, NY: Basic Books.

Ylvisaker, M., & Feeney, T. (1998). *Collaborative brain injury interventions.* San Diego, CA: Singular Publishing Group.

Ylvisaker, M., & Feeney, T. (2001). What I really want is a girlfriend: Meaningful social interaction after traumatic brain injury. *Brain Injury Source, 5*(3), 12–17.

14

Self-Management for People with Chronic Conditions

Fiona Jones

CONTENTS

14.1 Introduction

The concept of self-management is not necessarily new, and successful strategies used by individuals living with long-term conditions to manage their daily lives have been described and studied for decades (Taylor & Bury, 2007). Self-management in the context of healthcare has largely been associated with separate programmes organized and provided in addition to other care. Promotion of active self-management through rehabilitation has not previously received much attention. It is timely to review current evidence relating to self-management and how it could be utilized within rehabilitation.

The recent growth of interest in self-management programmes amongst policymakers in health has been attributed to the prospect of more people living into older age with a chronic condition and the concern associated with meeting their needs (Newman, Steed, & Mulligan, 2009). Policymakers and researchers have highlighted the need for a reorientation away from acute interventions towards more self-care models. Patient involvement in their health is commonly referred to in healthcare policy and is closely linked to self-management, which is defined by Barlow and colleagues as referring to 'an individual's ability to manage the symptoms, treatment, physical and psychosocial consequences and life style changes inherent with living with a chronic disease' (Barlow, Sturt, & Hearnshaw, 2002). Self-management as a concept is considered multidimensional and complex and can involve a broad range of attitudes, behaviours and skills directed at managing life with a chronic disease (Lawn & Schoo, 2010).

The basic premise of many self-management programmes is enabling individuals to take greater control of their health and everyday lives. Methods often include group work or individual programmes using different behaviour change methods, facilitated by lay people or healthcare professionals (Coulter & Ellins, 2006). Research has shown that self-management programmes can be more effective than educational programmes on a number of health outcomes, thought to be largely due to the behaviour change aspect including goal setting (de Silva, 2011). However, self-management programmes have been criticized by some authors, who liken them to more of a professional compliance model with the balance of therapeutic relationship weighted heavily towards the professional (Kendall, Ehrlich, Sunderland, Muenchberger, & Rushton, 2011). This could be counterproductive to enabling choice and control about managing life with a long-term condition, and some research shows that need for healthcare can increase after attendance at a self-management programme (Coulter & Ellins, 2006).

Self-management is a concept which has been defined in different ways. Some definitions link it closely to managing health, whereas other definitions place a greater emphasis on community participation and individual control. As with rehabilitation, it can be thought of as a complex intervention with many interacting components. The *active ingredient* is thought to be behaviour change, but the skills required by professionals or lay people to support self-management are often poorly defined (Hardeman & Mitchie, 2009).

Supporting an individual to manage life with a complex chronic condition or disability may need a number of different approaches. There may be little benefit associated with attending a generic group-based self-management programme and more benefit from a responsive, individualized intervention that can be integrated into rehabilitation. Whilst research on self-management programmes has been developing, the link to rehabilitation has not been clearly made, despite sharing many of the same principles such as goal setting, problem-solving and enabling activity. The question of whether it is more effective for individuals to attend a distinct self-management programme or learn the principles of self-management through rehabilitation has not been tested nor has the cost effectiveness of different models for delivery of self-management been explored.

Along with questions about the content and delivery of self-management programmes comes the question about the best time to introduce self-management principles. A recent paper by Taylor, Todman, and Broomfield (2011) proposed a cyclical and dynamic model of adjustment after stroke, which was strongly influenced by social context and individual differences such as beliefs about one's past and future self (Taylor et al., 2011). Having an understanding of an individual's beliefs about their self-identity and the degree of discontinuity experienced may influence how and when to introduce interventions to encourage and support self-management. This may take a different form depending on the nature of the condition, for example, whether it is a progressive or relatively static condition or disability.

Individuals will also interact with professionals at different stages of their recovery and adjustment depending on whether the condition is progressive or a single incident such as stroke. The messages given by professionals at times of particular stress or change could be highly influential in forming beliefs about autonomy and self-management

(Coulter & Ellins, 2006; Hardeman & Mitchie, 2009). In fact the beliefs and attitudes of professionals have been found to determine the direction and philosophy of rehabilitation (Jones & Lennon, 2009; Lake & Staiger, 2010). In addition, the organizational context of a rehabilitation team, the time available and outcomes used could all have an influence on the choices made by professionals and the level of input given to supporting self-management.

The degree of social support and how family and friends interact and support an individual's self-management could also be critical to success with self-management. Mastery of new tasks, problem-solving and self-discovery are all thought to be critical components of active self-management, so interactions from caregivers could have the potential to both support and hamper these processes (Lorig & Holman, 2003). In spite of targeted intervention for caregivers, there has been little investigation of the role of caregivers in self-management and goal setting (Evans, Hendricks, Haselkorn, Bishop, & Baldwin, 1992; Mackenzie et al., 2007).

Critics of self-management programmes have warned of the potential for them to become structured towards the needs of professionals and the organization rather than focusing on individual responses and learning styles (Lawn & Schoo, 2010). Careful exploration of the overlap between theories supporting self-management programmes and goal setting is required. It would be helpful to understand more fully some of the factors which influence successful goal attainment and how these experiences are then utilized to inform future behaviours. The interactions of professionals could have a positive effect to support the attribution of success to an individual's own effort and skills, thus informing future behaviour. Further research on self-management programmes used within rehabilitation or outside of the clinical setting also have the potential to add to theory development.

Overall, evidence to support self-management programmes is generally positive, but the outcomes chosen to measure success may not fully reveal the more iterative, cyclical process involving in learning to take control and feeling more confident to self-manage. Changes may be more linked to self-identity and confidence and these outcomes are underrepresented in rehabilitation.

There is scope for more work to unpick the links between programme outcomes and meaningful areas of change for an individual. This chapter will explore self-management by discussing three interrelated areas. The first section will examine theories which have informed the most common self-management programmes with a main focus on social cognitive theory and self-efficacy principles. The second section will explore the evidence relating to self-management programmes, including research which relates to long-term conditions, but also reviewing an emerging body of evidence on self-management programmes for people after stroke. Finally, the third section will explore and discuss the practical implications of self-management programmes in the context of individual needs, professionals working in rehabilitation and finally the service and organization. Practical examples will be used to illustrate some of the ways in which self-management programmes can be used alongside rehabilitation or embedded into rehabilitation practice.

14.2 Theoretical Influences on Self-Management

Overall, most definitions of self-management suggest a focus on individuals taking control after a health event or when living with a disability. The way in which individuals strive for control over their lives is thought to permeate almost everything they do, and the ability to influence an outcome can foster a greater sense of preparedness (Bandura, 1995).

The beliefs that an individual holds with regard to their sense of self-identity could also influence the level of effort and connectedness to future efforts and change. In addition, the way in which an illness or threat to health is perceived by an individual could also relate to apparent causes and level of control over events and inform subsequent courses of action. Memories of our own illnesses and in others can contribute to a knowledge base that can inform potential coping strategies (Levanthal et al., 1997). Having to contend with the changes involved in living with a chronic disease or disability and navigating a different sense of self can involve different meanings of disability at different time points and settings (Bury, 2005).

There is an increasing recognition of the importance of understanding individual's beliefs about their health, and many self-management programmes now incorporate strategies based on behaviour change and behaviour change theories (de Silva, 2011; Lawn & Schoo, 2010). Several theories have been used as a framework to inform and develop self-management programmes which enables them to be better described, replicated and tested (Hardeman et al., 2005). The theories also allow for specific aspects of behaviour to be targeted and measured. There is not an actual *theory of self-management*, but one of the most common and influential concepts to inform self-management programmes is that of self-efficacy, which has been incorporated in some instances as both a mediator and possible outcome of value (Jones & Riazi, 2011). Other theories which have informed the development of programmes include self-regulation theory, transtheoretical change theory and the stress coping model. The following section provides an overview of social cognition theory and self-efficacy, including discussion of how it has influenced the content and delivery of self-management programmes. This is followed by a briefer discussion of other theories that have been applied to self-management strategies.

14.2.1 Self-Efficacy and Social Cognitive Theory

Bandura described self-efficacy as 'the level of confidence a person has in their ability to perform certain behaviours' but stresses that this includes organizing and executing the course of action (Bandura, 1997). Self-efficacy beliefs have been suggested to have the potential to not only influence what an individual chooses to do but importantly how much effort they put towards the task and how long they will persevere in the event of failures or difficulties (Bandura, 1997). Self-efficacy principles have been used as a central tenet of many self-management programmes, often as a structure for exploring key skills involved in living with a health problem, for example, coping, problem-solving and goal setting (Newman et al., 2009).

A key empirical distinction made by Bandura with regard to the differences in beliefs about the action (e.g. locus of control) and beliefs about whether an individual can produce the course of action (self-efficacy) resonates with many of the principles of self-management in that it is not just what a person states they *intend* to do but it is what they *actually* go on to do that is important. This relates closely to the perceived confidence required to make a change, try out a new task and not be put off when it might fail the first time.

Individuals with strong self-efficacy tend to select more challenging goals and approach difficult tasks as challenges to overcome, rather than as threats to avoid. In the face of failure, such individuals are more likely to heighten and sustain their efforts, quickly recover their sense of efficacy and even attribute failure to insufficient effort or deficient knowledge and skills that can be acquired (Bandura, 1994).

Self-efficacy is a principle construct within social cognition theory, which replaced the earlier social learning theory, extending the theory to emphasize more of a collective agency underpinning learning and social development (Bandura, 1995). Social cognitive theory offers an important consideration in the delivery of self-management programmes in that it acknowledges that individuals are not only the product of their own beliefs but are also informed by beliefs shared with those around them, for example, social contacts and healthcare professionals. Self-managing relies in part on an individual acting for themselves, often by using processes such as self-monitoring, assimilating past knowledge and utilizing cognitive processes such as self-incentives to produce desired change (Bandura, 1989). The effectiveness of these actions is also likely to be influenced by an individual's knowledge about their condition and also the social environment and interactions with others.

Social cognition theory has thus provided the knowledge to guide translational principles of programmes by converting the theoretical principles into operational models. There are numbers of self-management programmes that have found that enhancing self-efficacy makes a change in performance and successful outcome more likely (de Silva, 2011; Newman, Steed, & Mulligan, 2004). Understanding the sources of information used by individuals to form self-efficacy beliefs has also been a guiding principle of many programmes. Self-efficacy beliefs are said to be constructed from four principle sources of information: (1) mastery experiences, (2) modelling, (3) social persuasion and (4) physiological and emotional states (Bandura, 1997). Self-management programmes often incorporate strategies which address these four sources.

14.2.1.1 Mastery Experiences

Mastery experiences are said to be the most powerful source of self-efficacy information and relate entirely to experiences of success in a particular task or skill. Personal successes can build a robust sense of self-efficacy made more influential when attributed to the individual's own efforts and persistence. The way in which successes and failures in tasks are perceived and cognitively appraised will determine the extent to which self-efficacy can be altered. The accomplishment of a small goal through independent effort may persuade an individual that they have the necessary skill to go beyond their current level and extend their performance (Jones, Mandy, & Partridge, 2008). Mastery experiences can be targeted in rehabilitation through a variety of methods (Johnston et al., 2007; Kendall et al., 2007; Watkins et al., 2007). But the critical factor is not only the success alone but the ability to judge the success and develop a greater sense of self-knowledge and determination to influence future performance. Therefore, successful self-management may only be achieved if an individual can use the mastery experiences to create the tools and strategies to organize and produce effective actions to manage life with a disability or change in health. Programmes which are aimed at helping people understand *how* they made the changes and achieved the goals coupled with social validation of personal efficacy may offer a more effective method of raising self-efficacy and self-management skills.

Example: Many programmes use a method of monitoring progress through action plans or *to-do* lists, with individuals being encouraged to note any changes and achievements (however small) as reinforcement of mastery experiences.

14.2.1.2 Modelling

Modelling may serve as another tool for promoting self-efficacy. Vicarious experience is gained through the comparison and modelling of others, and it can be beneficial to observe someone perceived to be similar (a model) successfully performing a task. By social comparison with a person facing similar difficulties, an individual can form a judgement about their own capabilities. The persuasion that can be gained by observing others' mastery experiences can typically raise self-efficacy beliefs, that is, *if they can do it, I too should have the capabilities* (Bandura, 1997). Self-management programmes have used this principle in many ways, such as through peer support groups and through approaches such as the UK Expert Patients Programme (Phillips, 2010). Although it is thought that vicarious experiences may have less impact than personal mastery, they could override the impact of direct experience. If a person with low self-efficacy observes failure of a task in another person, it may act as a reinforcement of lack of personal capability, confirming beliefs and predictions about whether change or management of a task is possible. Modelling may be incorporated into self-management programmes in various ways, and it has been suggested there may be greater benefit from seeing others that have used effort and coping skills to make a change gradually overtime, rather than quick personal mastery experiences (Bandura, 1997).

Example: Some programmes use peer support or buddy schemes, in which individuals with greater experience of living with a long-term condition offer support and advice to someone newly diagnosed. Modelling is also achieved through group work and books describing people experiences and strategies to self-manage.

14.2.1.3 Social Persuasion

Social persuasion can strengthen self-efficacy beliefs by encouraging individuals that they do possess the skills to complete a particular task. Persuasion may be used to sustain effort when struggling with a difficult task, especially when expressed by significant others showing faith rather than doubts. Self-management programmes make use of this source again through peer support groups and also encouragement and feedback about performance from healthcare professionals (Lake & Staiger, 2010). If individuals are facing new and challenging tasks (e.g. after first stroke), they are likely to rely more on feedback from a credible and knowledgeable source (such as a health professional). However, over time, this may create conflict for the individual if the beliefs expressed by others do not match the individual's lived experience. Another consideration is that people may be more likely to believe those who have faced the same challenges and have had similar experiences of coping and developing successful strategies (Bury, Newbold, & Taylor, 2005).

Example: Many group programmes are led by lay people with experience of long-term condition self-management or healthcare professionals, who provide a source of information and support for participants. Persuasion can be achieved through encouragement from group leaders, friends, family and supporters who notice and reinforce achievements and efforts of individuals to self-manage.

14.2.1.4 Physiological and Emotional States

Physiological and emotional states can help individuals judge their own capability. Feedback from somatic and physical information can affect self-efficacy through cognitive appraisal of the extent of the sources, providing reasons for successes or difficulties. For example, anxiety during a new task may be perceived as positive and indicative of the degree of challenge involved or negative and a reflection on personal failings.

Mood states can also influence how events are appraised; a person with low self-efficacy and despondency about their performance may be less likely to sustain effort and set goals. Conversely, a more buoyant mood state can facilitate motivation, effort and more positive responses to setbacks (Bandura, 1997). There is a critical function for cognitive appraisal of these different states, and application of self-management principles will be far more challenging in individuals who have difficulties in recognizing symptoms and limited insight into their potential to set goals and solve problems (Taylor et al., 2011).

Example: Physiological states can be related to an individual feeling less anxious or feeling that a task requires less effort. Reflection on how easy a task has become compared to an earlier time is often used as a strategy by trainers to enhancing motivation. Self-management programmes also frequently include education sessions for participants to learn to correctly interpret physiological signs such as breathlessness or muscle ache as positive evidence of their individual effort (rather than negative signs of their inability to succeed).

14.2.2 Other Theories of Note

Other theories such as *self-regulation theory* have informed self-management programmes through introducing the view of the individual as an active problem solver. This theory emphasizes the role of both cognitive and emotional responses towards self-management behaviours. The way in which an individual perceives a health threat will determine their responses and subsequent coping action. However, these actions do not only take place in a vacuum but are also responsive to contextual influences such as cultural and institutional factors. Intrapersonal and interpersonal factors can mediate problem-solving processes having a direct effect on behavioural outcomes (Levanthal et al., 1997). This theory supports the concept that changing illness perceptions may lead to positive changes in active coping strategies and self-management.

The *transtheoretical change model* highlights the stages of acceptance and adjustment required to make a change in behaviour and has been used to determine the timing of interventions. Programmes based on this theory often incorporate *motivational interviewing*, a method used to help individuals explore and resolve any barriers to behaviour change. Motivational interviewing originally started from a central principle of empathy and reflective listening. Underpinning the transtheoretical change model and the use of motivational interviewing is the notion that interventions may be more successful if matched to each individual's level of readiness for change. This however relies on having accurate definition of stages of readiness, and the theory has been heavily criticized in this regard (Treasure & Maissi, 2007). It has also been suggested that areas such as fear and anxiety, which require specific targeting at different stages, are not easily specified (Newman et al., 2009).

The *stress coping model* has also been used to inform self-management programmes (Lazurus, 1990). This model focuses on the strategies people use to overcome the challenges and stresses of living with a chronic disease. Programmes usually incorporate the use of cognitive behavioural techniques to encourage individuals to develop more positive and active coping strategies. An example can be taken from cardiac rehabilitation, where self-management programmes involve individuals learning to perceive feelings of breathlessness and raised heart rate as a positive and necessary step towards fitness, as opposed to a negative experience indicative of a possible medical complication (Ewart, 1992).

14.3 How Does Theory Inform Self-Management Interventions?

Self-management programmes like many rehabilitation interventions are complex and include a number of components which may act dependently or independently of one another (Medical Research Council Health Services and Public Health Research Board, 2000). Some programmes have been developed without a clear understanding of the mechanisms through which behaviour change may occur and therefore make it difficult to fully understand the active ingredients and thus to inform future practice. The need to carefully link theory, development and evaluation, particularly in the early stage of design, has been emphasized (Hardeman et al., 2005). In response to this limitation, Hardeman and colleagues have described some general methods of mapping objectives, intervention, strategies and outcomes and highlight that published studies rarely include a justification of the theory selected. They have illustrated a causal model with a case study involving a primary care–based programme aimed at increasing physical activity (Hardeman et al., 2005). When developing this programme, these authors considered questions about which intervention techniques might be most effective at supporting increases in physical activity and how the efficacy of these interventions could best be tested. A generic causal model was then modified and a new model developed for the specific programme. Epidemiological evidence helped define the health outcome, target group, target behaviours and objective measures. Psychology informed the causal model and defined behavioural determinant, intervention points, techniques to support behaviour change and measure of behaviour change. This process provided a clearer understanding of the links between behaviour, health outcomes, measures and interventions. If self-management programmes are to be used more extensively as recommended in the health policy, the complexity of design, delivery and implementation needs careful consideration (Barlow et al., 2002; Hardeman et al., 2005; Schreurs, Colland, Kuijer, de Ridder, & van Elderen, 2003).

The content of many self-management programmes is varied but in general involves practical and interactive components. An appreciation of the theoretical influences that guide the delivery and content of self-management programmes will also enable an awareness of skills required by lay tutors and professionals and identification of the variables and outcomes to be defined and tested using the relevant measures. Common components of self-management programmes are summarized in Table 14.1.

An understanding of theory is critical in the development and testing phases of new programmes but also needs to inform practical implementation and sustainability over time. In addition, well-developed programmes need to take into account social and contextual issues which may influence effectiveness. There is an overall aim in much health policy in the developing world for self-management programmes to become the main method for increasing patient involvement, choice and control over their health (Imison et al., 2011). But it could be counterintuitive to deliver programmes in clinical settings by healthcare professionals when the aim is to promote autonomy and control over health.

One qualitative study exploring the perspective of providers of self-management programmes illustrated a sense of burden felt by many about delivering such programmes and disbelief about its effectiveness (Johnston, Liddy, & Ives, 2011). It is also the case that many programmes only deliver parts of the recommended approach and this is commonly just the education component of self-management (Johnston et al., 2011). This is despite a consistent finding that education approaches alone are not usually as successful in improving

TABLE 14.1

Common Components of Self-Management Programmes

Self-Management Component	Action or Task by Tutor
Problem-solving	An individual is supported to define the problem as they see it and to work out possible strategies. If a group-based programme is used, participants may be given ideas by others that have experienced a similar problem.
Self-discovery (and taking risks)	An individual is encouraged to try things out and work out ways around a particular issue. Tutors and peers may be critical in encouraging a person to have a try on their own or with appropriate support.
Goal setting	The starting point may be *a thing I want to do*. The individual is supported to work out the steps or particular skills required to achieve the goal and enable a feeling of success (mastery).
Resource utilization	This involves making use of what other resources may be available to sustain participation or enable further progress. It could include accessing local self-help groups, seeking expert advice if a problem emerges or using friends or family to support access to services or activities.
Decision making	An individual is encouraged to be more involved in their own daily life especially issues relating to health. To weigh up the pros and cons of a particular action, it is important that the individual, not the tutor, chooses the ultimate strategy or action.
Taking action	An individual is supported to produce action in any form; this may be used as a way of challenging unhelpful beliefs, e.g. that exercise may lead to a second stroke. They may be encouraged to record specific activities of action and discuss progress with their group or tutor.
Collaboration	This involves working together with the tutor to decide together on a course of action or preferred direction in relation to health. There is a sharing of expertise, a shift from traditional thinking whereby the professional is perceived to be the expert.
Reflection on progress	Reflecting on progress can encourage an individual to make the link between their own efforts and progress made. This is a useful strategy to use to help an individual recognize the ways in which they have made a positive change and what has helped or hindered in pursuit of this change.
Knowledge	Living with a disability or chronic disease can involve a continuous process of learning from new experiences, particularly when the condition can fluctuate and change over time, such as multiple sclerosis. Increased knowledge about a condition, symptoms and treatment is an important aspect of self-management but should represent a more active process of learning than just gaining knowledge. A key skill is being able to gather, to process and to evaluate the information.

The content of this table has been influenced by the work of Lorig and Holman (2003) and Newman et al. (2009).

outcomes for people with chronic illness (Gibson, Powell, Wilson, Abramson, Haywood, Bauman, & Roberts, 2002; Jovicic, Holroyd-Leduc, & Straus, 2006). Self-management can thus be interpreted and programmes delivered in different ways and as such have attracted as many critics as proponents.

Some authors have questioned whether it is appropriate to have one model or rigid protocol to support self-management and queried the limitations of having a *one-size-fits-all* approach, particularly with more complex disability. Whilst there is clearly a need for programmes to provide greater transparency and rigour in their use of theory to inform development, structure and delivery of interventions, a self-management programme will not be suitable for all. There are concerns about making the focus about living with chronic disease or disability to be solely about health, despite the fact that many individuals use social networks and other informal sources as their main forms of support (Kendall & Rogers, 2007). A critique of the UK Expert Patients Programme, drawing on qualitative studies, found a paradox between the proactive, organized approaches taken in group work almost reinforcing medical paradigms and the peer support and acknowledgement of the subjective experience of living with a chronic disease (Wilson, Kendall, & Brooks, 2007).

14.4 Self-Management and Goal Setting

It may be helpful to make the distinction between self-management *programmes* and self-management *principles*. Many individuals with a new disability, such as stroke, will start their recovery period in an ultra-medical environment and continue to receive intensive rehabilitation for up to 6 months. Self-management skills such as self-discovery, goal setting and problem-solving may be undermined particularly in inpatient rehabilitation settings (Jones et al., 2007; Levack, Dean, Siegert, & McPherson, 2011), yet a main aim of rehabilitation is to promote independence and control. It may be beneficial, therefore, to utilize some of the theories underpinning self-management programmes to develop specific strategies and interventions to integrate into rehabilitation practice. One way in which there could be greater harmony between rehabilitation and self-management programmes is by examining methods of goal setting.

Goal setting has been described as a principal component within self-management programmes, but the process involved or the theory behind goal setting is rarely described. Studies on self-management programmes often purport to utilize *collaborative goal setting*, stating that involving the patient in their goal setting can increase self-efficacy. However, the precise methods and skills required to achieve this are unclear (Langford, Sawyer, Gioimo, Brownson, & O'Toole, 2007).

Programmes which focus on the outcome of individuals developing specific and realistic goals may also be using methods which potentially challenge choice and control. A delicate balance may be required by professionals to provide support to individuals to develop their goals and self-management strategies but not run the risk of individuals feeling abandoned to manage alone or conversely be directed to goals and strategies which are not of equal value to that expressed by the professional. A study exploring how self-management programmes shaped patient perceptions of their care suggested that professionals do not always possess the communication skills required to avoid individuals feeling their views are being overridden (Kielman et al., 2010). A recent systematic review and synthesis of evidence behind goal setting suggests that despite a policy and service ambition of person-centred goal setting in practice, this is hard to achieve (Rosewilliam, Roskell, & Pandyn, 2011).

In general, there is agreement from most proponents of self-management that programmes should always involve supporting individuals towards *taking action*: whether mobilizing support or finding a new way of doing something, the action is on the part of the individual or together with a tutor (de Silva, 2011; Department of Health, 2006). If self-management is to be integrated more readily into rehabilitation, we need to consider ways of individuals discovering their own strengths and difficulties, experimenting and trying out different strategies and activities; inevitably, this requires an element of risk-taking. If the goals or activities are not achieved, then ways to support individuals to learn to set their targets slightly differently or devise an alternative target are required (Creer & Holroyd, 1997). In this way, there is a stronger link back to some of the theoretical assumptions underpinning self-management such as strengthening self-efficacy through mastery experiences.

This brief overview of the theory supporting self-management provides many areas of consideration for practice in rehabilitation, not least how to enhance and sustain individual's self-efficacy and sense of autonomy over their health but also to retain a focus on important personal goals and managing any worries. By having a greater understanding of theories, rehabilitation could be more directed towards supporting self-management and potentially avoid some of the negative aspects experienced by individuals such as a sense of abandonment when discharged from treatment (Cott, Wiles, & Devitt, 2008). The following section provides an overview of the evidence base relating to different self-management programmes and explores the varied methods of delivery. An illustration of how an individualized self-management programme for stroke could be embedded into rehabilitation is also discussed.

14.5 Current Research Base of Self-Management Programmes

The development of self-management programmes has followed a trend towards individuals having a greater responsibility for their health. Underpinning this development is the need to move away from didactic methods of teaching management of chronic illness to a more interactive problem-solving approach that focuses on coping and goal setting. The wide diversity of programmes that have been developed and in some cases fully implemented into healthcare makes it hard to identify the key messages regarding what works best and for whom.

There is reasonable evidence to support condition-specific programmes in areas such as diabetes and asthma but less for other conditions such as arthritis (Challis et al., 2010). This is suggested to be a reflection on the complexities associated with living with arthritis, whereby the set of skills necessary for successful self-management has not been clearly defined. Self-management programmes for people with even more complex disabilities such as multiple sclerosis, stroke and traumatic brain injury are starting to emerge, but there are considerable challenges in getting to a stage whereby the programme has been thoroughly tested and implemented into practice (de Silva, 2011).

Seminal research to develop a lay-led group intervention by Lorig and colleagues known as the Chronic Disease Self-Management (CDSM) programme has informed many subsequent programmes (Lorig et al., 1999). An example of this is the Expert Patient Programme, which is now delivered in some parts of the United Kingdom (Department of Health, 2001). The precursor of these generic chronic disease programmes was more condition-specific programmes in areas such as arthritis, which often take the form of a 6–8-week programme facilitated by a lay tutor. Research has shown that the CDSM programme does lead to moderate short-term improvements in some health outcomes, self-efficacy and use of health services (Lorig, Sobel, Ritter, Laurent, & Hobbs, 2001). However, the longer-term effects of such programmes are unclear, and follow-up studies have failed to demonstrate sustained improvement between intervention and control groups (Newbold, Taylor, & Bury, 2006).

A national evaluation of the UK Expert Patients Programme, including a randomized trial of 629 patients, does not seem to support early assertions that such interventions lead to any marked improvements in health status and/or efficiency savings (Kennedy et al., 2007).

However, previous evaluations have found several benefits of the programme, and results from a qualitative study and process evaluation showed that participants enjoyed the social support, practical exchange of ideas and reduced social isolation, and generally, satisfaction was quite high amongst attendees (Kennedy, Rogers, & Gately, 2005).

The use of self-management programmes as an integral part of chronic disease management is likely to remain high, as is the prevalence of people with long-term conditions and disability. One of the drivers for the growth of self-management programmes is the rising costs associated with care, and this was one of the main reasons for involving volunteers in the delivery genetic group-based programmes (Lorig, 1986). However, there is conflicting evidence of the effect that self-management programmes have on the costs associated with health and social care. In a review of over 600 studies relating to self-management initiatives, it was found that although programmes can alter the pattern of healthcare usage, many studies have not proven that greater self-care leads to reduced resource use (de Silva, 2011). However, the applicability of the findings of many reviews may be limited as the interventions are so diverse, and it can be unclear which intervention has been successful and for what outcome (Newman et al., 2004). Several questions remain about these national programmes to support self-management, not least the lack of uptake from different ethnic communities, and there have been particular difficulties engaging people from these groups (Coulter & Ellins, 2006). In addition, there are concerns that participators in self-management groups tend to be younger, female, middle class, better educated and, importantly, at a stage of readiness to participate in sharing their experiences and learning something new (Corben & Rosen, 2005).

Overall, the evidence strongly supports the conclusion that proactively supporting self-management and that focusing on behaviour change can have a positive impact on health outcomes (Coulter & Ellins, 2006; de Silva, 2011). However, there needs to be more ways of integrating the evidence into practice and recognition that self-management is not necessarily a panacea for chronic disease management (Bury et al., 2005). If self-management is viewed more of a continuum of support, then there is also a need to explore alternative ways of integrating common principles into rehabilitation. Reviews summarizing findings regarding the optimum mode of delivery of self-management programmes have so far been inconclusive. Group programmes offer the possibility of more peer support and learning and in some conditions have shown more favourable results than individual programmes (Mulligan & Newman, 2007). A study exploring the experiences of individuals with stroke, multiple sclerosis and spinal cord injury again supported the beneficial effects of group support, but because of the long-standing and unpredictable nature of some conditions such as multiple sclerosis, participants felt they would benefit from a more flexible approach to delivery and possible refresher courses to maintain behaviour changes (Hirsche, Williams, Jones, & Manns, 2011).

There also continues to be a debate about whether self-management programmes should be delivered by healthcare professionals or lay leaders. The benefits of healthcare professionals are that they may have more current knowledge about alternative treatments and skills to assist with disease-specific aspects of management. But there may be limitations with programmes delivered by healthcare professionals whose background is strongly biomedical. Critics have warned that there may be a tendency for these programmes to be focused too much on compliance using education approaches, and strategies such as collaborative goal setting and problem solving may only be incorporated at a tokenistic level (Johnston et al., 2011; Wilson et al., 2007).

It is not clear whether individuals with more complex disability such as stroke would find benefit from a generic group-based intervention such as the CDSM programme, but the evidence to support any one type of programme is extremely limited. Previous research on self-management has often excluded people with complex disability such as stroke (Cadilhac et al., 2011). Some researchers have tried to refine the CDSM programmes for stroke with varying results. Huijbregts, Myers, Streiner, and Teasell (2008) and Kendall et al. (2007) showed some beneficial effects of their programmes modified for stroke, with a reduction in early decline in activities of daily living, and family and personal roles, and some improvements in balance and reintegration to daily life in intervention groups (Huijbregts et al., 2008; Kendall et al., 2007). However, the benefits were not stable over a prolonged period of time. Both of these programmes stated they were based on self-efficacy principles, but the way in which learning and self-management skills were facilitated was unclear. Attrition, unlike other programmes, was relatively low, particularly in the study by Huijbregts and colleagues, which may have been to do with the timing of interventions relative to individuals' stages of readiness to engage in such programmes. A recent phase II trial carried out in Australia found that a group-based stroke-specific self-management was both safe and feasible, with some favourable effects on mood. This study adds to the evidence that self-management programmes are feasible to modify to a broader population including individuals with cognitive, language and more severe physical impairments (Cadilhac et al., 2011). Participants also found the content to be more relevant than a generic chronic disease programme.

These interventions and others may benefit from iterative modelling of causal relationships such as those suggested by Hardeman and described earlier (Hardeman et al., 2005). The target outcomes such as quality of life are multidimensional, and self-efficacy is often perceived to be both a measure and a mediator through which behavioural change will occur.

The majority of self-management research within stroke has focused on group-based programmes, but there are some examples of more individualized interventions which could be delivered either separately or integrated into rehabilitation and care. Johnston et al. (2007) used a workbook approach for people after stroke, designed to influence control cognition (perceived control) based on a similar intervention used for individuals post heart attack (Johnston et al., 2007). This included tasks and activities to support knowledge, goal setting and problem-solving skills relevant to stroke. The intervention group showed a significant change in recovery from disability and confidence, but failed to impact on the target variables, perceived control and distress. This programme was limited by attrition and a large proportion of participants failed to complete the workbook tasks.

The Bridges stroke self-management programme is also an individualized programme for stroke survivors which uses a patient-held workbook, based on social cognitive theory and self-efficacy principles (Jones, Mandy, & Partridge, 2009a). Stroke practitioners use one-to-one sessions to support individuals to set goals, record progress and plan future activities. These strategies are supported by the use of a stroke workbook to facilitate a personal record of self-management strategies such as independent activity, future goals and targets. The workbook is used as a personal record of goals and progress after stroke and is not kept by the professional. It has been developed together with an advisory group of stroke survivors and avoids technical terms, including vignettes, activities, ideas and solutions from other individuals for successful self-management.

Preliminary results from a series of case studies showed significant changes in self-efficacy after supported use of the workbook for a period of 4 weeks (Jones et al., 2009). A further pilot randomised controlled trial testing Bridges as an additional intervention and showed favourable changes in quality of life in the intervention group (McKenna, Jones, Glenfield, & Lennon, 2011). Qualitative results exploring the feasibility and acceptability with patients, carers and clinicians suggested the programme facilitated more person-centred goal setting and helped participants manage their own progress. However, in this study, Bridges was delivered as an additional intervention to usual stroke rehabilitation which has cost and time implications. Further studies are now underway to test the feasibility of integrating the programme into rehabilitation through a cluster trial.

Although some programmes are already being adopted by stroke rehabilitation teams, there are a similar range of questions which beset the development and implementation of many self-management programmes. One issue relates to the skills required by professionals for them to be able to incorporate self-management principles into their practice, when their natural tendency may be more towards an educational didactic approach. The communication skills and focus of the therapeutic relationship could have a potent effect on the effectiveness of supporting self-management, and principles may not be matched by practice as highlighted by a number of authors (Lake & Staiger, 2010; Langford et al., 2007; Lawn, McMillan, & Pulvirenti, 2011).

14.6 What Is the Way Forward with Self-Management Research?

Overall, there are some favourable results with regard to self-management programmes for people with long-term conditions, but the results between different conditions are inconsistent. There are several issues that continue to prevent any firm conclusions about the evidence being made. These are summarized in the following:

- Many programmes use a group-based format, but this fails to attract people from hard to reach groups, for example, those with severe disability; more creative methods of self-management are needed, for example, telephone, on-line support and peer and buddy support schemes.

- Programmes often fail to identify the theoretical influences and specific behaviour change strategies. A causal modelling approach is missing from most programmes.

- Individualized interventions are often more reliant on the skills of healthcare professionals; whilst this can be positive in managing disease-specific issues, it may be counterproductive in supporting autonomy and control over decisions.

- Goal setting is a common aspect of self-management programmes, but is rarely described in any detail, and heavily influenced by SMART approaches. This may reduce the opportunity of individuals' aspirational goals to be recognized and for the outcome to be directed towards *realistic* tasks as defined by the tutor/professional. There is very little reference to goal setting theories which could underpin the activities used.

- Professionally led programmes will be dependent to a degree on the skills of the professional. There has been minimal documentation or discussion of the training and core skill set required for health professionals to deliver these programmes.

- Many group-based programmes are delivered over a fixed time period, and a more flexible approach may be useful. People with complex needs and changing disabilities may need help and support to manage at different time points in their life span.

There are clearly a number of limitations in the current evidence base for self-management programmes, and a healthy debate has arisen on the current ambition in much of health-care policy to have more programmes as part of healthcare management. Self-management invokes a sense in many of an *organized model of support*, and there is increasing evidence and arguments to support more informal self-help networks, which are not part of any healthcare programme (Kendall & Rogers, 2007). There is also recognition of the potential of more flexible, tailored approaches to self-management which may have greater possibilities for people with more complex rehabilitation needs.

The next section focuses on the more practical implication of self-management as part of rehabilitation and particular issues for teams and professionals when considering introducing a self-management programme or principles into their practice.

14.7 Self-Management and Rehabilitation

14.7.1 Considering Individual Needs First

Individuals with a new or progressive disability that access rehabilitation will all have very different background experiences and methods of learning accumulated through their lives. Understanding an individual's personal narrative, for example, their aspirations, worries, past successes and limitations, can assist with planning towards self-management. There are several authors who have highlighted the importance of acknowledging a person's sense of change in identity particularly after a sudden onset and change in circumstances, for example, after stroke or spinal cord injury (Ellis-Hill, Payne, & Ward, 2008; Rittman, Boylstein, Hinojosa, Hinojosa, & Haun, 2007). The sense of discontinuity which can be experienced by some individuals, coupled with emotional issues such as post-stroke depression, is not an ideal background to expect self-determination and active problem-solving (Taylor et al., 2011).

The value and opportunities for reflecting on the meaning of self-management for each individual could be limited within a more organized group-based approach. A study which explored individuals with respiratory disease and their perceptions of self-management found that although they were aware of the shift towards more self-responsibility for their health, this approach did not necessarily feel new (Kielman et al., 2010). Many of them had been using self-care practices before and had gained significant levels of knowledge before attending self-management programmes. This highlights the importance of exploring individual strategies of self-management before embarking on more organized forms of support. It has been pointed out by several authors that many individuals will not want to conform to what's perceived to be a good *self-manager* (Bury et al., 2005; Kendall et al., 2011; Lawn et al., 2011). There will also be times when an individual requires minimum support and other times when there is a need for more complex forms of support. Studies have shown that individuals can also feel a sense of abandonment when being strongly encouraged to self-manage and can experience times when they have reached the boundaries of their individual knowledge and need expert care provided by healthcare professionals (Kielman et al., 2010; Lawn & Schoo, 2010).

An individual's perceived confidence or self-efficacy has been strongly linked to mood and functional performance of people with stroke, multiple sclerosis and other long-term conditions, and there could be value in introducing more targeted ways of enhancing self-efficacy without the need for a structured self-management programme (Dixon, Thornton, & Young, 2007; Ewart, 1992; Holman & Lorig, 1992; Jones & Riazi, 2011). Encouraging reflection on progress and attribution of change to individual efforts has shown some promise as a method of supporting self-efficacy (Audulv, Asplund, & Norbergh, 2010; Jones et al., 2009). One study amongst people with chronic illness showed those that attributed responsibility to a combination of internal and external factors were flexible in their self-management and less reliant on one form of support (Audulv et al., 2010). They could also adhere to more standardized or multifaceted forms of support and alternate between them according to the situation. This highlights the importance of programmes which take account of individual learning styles and attributions and the need to be aware of how different individuals will respond to self-management principles or programmes. Rehabilitation which follows a philosophy which is largely guided and controlled by the professional may be at odds with enhancing self-efficacy and supporting an individual to formulate flexible responses to any challenges or difficulties (Robinson-Smith & Pizzi, 2003; Sabari, Meisler, & Silver, 2000).

In addition to exploring an individual's responses to their condition and opportunities to self-manage, there is also a need to consider the impact of family and other social networks. Authors have highlighted the association of self-management to health and the medical paradigms, which neglects the potential value of some of the more informal mechanisms of support. The effects of social isolation and the value of maintaining social networks have been well documented in relation to people with long-term conditions (Boden-Albala, Litwak, Elkind, Rundek, & Sacco, 2005; Salter, Hellings, Foley, & Teasell, 2008; Vassilev et al., 2011). Social networks could play a more important role in an individual's management of their long-term condition, particularly for those who do not traditionally seek access or maintain links with organized forms of healthcare (Ch'Ng, French, & Mclean, 2008; Vassilev et al., 2011). Individuals may feel more at ease accepting interventions to promote adjustment or accept lifestyle changes in non-clinical settings.

14.7.2 Family Involvement and Social Networks

The interaction between social support and psychological wellbeing has been clearly shown in many studies (Boden-Albala et al., 2005; Luger, Cotter, & Sherman, 2009). There are also links between social support and the ability to adjust to a chronic illness, not just for the individual but also caregivers (Adriaansen, Van Leeuwen, Visser-Meily, van den Bos, & Post, 2011). There is scope for further exploration of the role of informal social networks to provide a kind of *buffer* to the challenges and stresses associated with self-management. People who have more reliable and secure social networks tend to have a stronger sense of life satisfaction, and this is not necessarily associated with the severity of the condition. This also raises the importance of securing longer-term support for individuals and their family, beyond the fixed period of self-management training. The unique benefit offered by informal peer support groups has been highlighted by individuals recovering after stroke, particularly after the initial acute stages of rehabilitation. The enjoyment felt by being with others who understand can help to normalize experiences as well as being a source of practical tips and advice about self-management (Ch'Ng et al., 2008).

There have been some efforts to translate the positive effects of social support into the design and delivery of self-management programmes. Direct evidence of the efficacy of more family-focused self-management programmes is limited, but this could depend on whether the primary end point is seen to be the individual with the chronic condition or their carer and whether the intervention is aimed at functional or psychosocial changes.

A study which aimed to increase social support and self-efficacy amongst stroke survivors and their families showed no influence on outcomes related to the stroke participants' disability measured by the Barthel index (Glass et al., 2004). The authors questioned whether the findings were due in part to the characteristics of the cohort as it included individuals with psychological impairments and those with a relatively mild physical disability. These questions only serve to highlight the challenges of designing and implementing self-management programmes for people who have such a multifaceted and varied disability as stroke and having dual-purpose programmes which include caregivers that provide an additional complexity. Nonetheless, self-management relies on the successful integration of strategies into everyday life, and here, the role of the carer seems critical (Mackenzie et al., 2007).

Self-help groups, whilst sharing some of the benefits of organized self-management programmes, operate with a range of values including support and friendship. It has also been suggested that they can provide a safe haven for people with more stigmatized conditions and a place for recognition and support (Kendall & Rogers, 2007). There have been attempts to integrate strategies such as informal story telling into self-management education and to address some of the criticisms associated with the rigid structure in many programmes. A programme based on the sharing of personal stories in minority ethnic groups with diabetes led to better attendance and personal enablement than a nurse-led group; however, there was no impact on clinical outcomes (Greenhalgh et al., 2011). The lack of clinical efficacy could be explained by many factors including the possibility that the focus was only on the individual with diabetes and not the wider family and social network. The authors also highlighted that the relatively unstructured story telling did not necessarily relate to goal setting and care planning aimed at improving diabetic health and outcomes. In addition, groups may have failed to cover some of the key learning domains which define self-management such as goal setting, action planning, using community resources and collaborative decision making. Nonetheless, informal self-help groups may impact on outcomes other than those clinically determined, such as self-esteem and confidence.

Social networks can play an important role in self-management in people with long-term conditions and disability, by shifting the emphasis from healthcare to more of a shared responsibility. A realist synthesis of social networks and CDSM showed the huge variation in potential networks which can occur in a consistent or entirely reflexive way within communities. These networks may both support and undermine self-management and there is little known about the processes involved. A greater understanding of the influence of social networks may also be more appropriate for engaging people from more hard to reach groups, such as those in socially and economically deprived areas (Vassilev et al., 2011). Structured and unstructured social networks and support could add to a more holistic model of self-management which is inclusive of different forms of support.

14.7.3 Knowledge, Attitudes and Practices of Practitioners towards Self-Management

In order to optimize the use of self-management programmes or principles, a number of issues have been discussed in relation to the individual with a chronic disease or disability, but the attitudes, skills and training needs of healthcare professionals have been a relatively ignored area in self-management research. This is a concern as the growth of self-management programmes continues and is not only an issue for healthcare professionals but also raises questions regarding the skills and attributes required by lay tutors.

One area of concern is the issue that self-management programmes are not necessarily led by personal need but rather tend to centre on areas of activity that are prioritized by the professional (Kendall & Rogers, 2007; Wilson et al., 2007). There are a number of examples of practices which are largely focused on professionally led practices, which could be serving to foster dependency rather than promote autonomy and control (McKevitt et al., 2011). Implicit in many discussions on self-management is the shared assumption that self-management will lead to better quality of life and that healthcare professionals as educated experts are in an ideal position to promote self-management (Kendall et al., 2007). However, *good compliance* may act as a barrier to a more reflexive style of self-management and could reinforce the assumption that what the professionals value are most important. If compliance with prescribed self-management practices is considered a measure of successful outcome, then this also conflicts with more contemporary approaches to self-management, advocated in some health policy, which promotes the role of autonomous individuals rather than passive recipients of medical advice (Wilson et al., 2007). There can also be discrepancies between how self-determination and compliance are conceptualized by healthcare professionals. For example, Maclean explored the concept of motivation amongst stroke professionals and found it was commonly used as a way of labelling individuals they worked with in their practice (Maclean, Pound, Wolfe, & Rudd, 2002). The criteria used by practitioners to determine a *motivated patient* were sometimes blurred, and individuals were often expected to be proactive as long as their behaviour did not manifest itself in non-adherence to therapy (Maclean et al., 2002).

A new and progressive disability often creates a personal and unique event for each individual. In order to facilitate effective self-management, the importance of developing a therapeutic relationship which is based on trust, mutual respect, shared decision making and good communication should not be underestimated. This is vital if self-management is to be part of a *guided process* in which professionals use enhanced communication to respond to individual reactions and support the process of goal setting and self-discovery. Ellis-Hill has highlighted the importance of the shared discourse between the therapist and patient, to facilitate self-discovery, goal setting and problem-solving on behalf of the patient (Ellis-Hill et al., 2008). The healthcare professional acts in collaboration as a coach, rather than an expert, and there is an emphasis on shared planning and decision making. Using this model, the balance of power between professionals and patients is recognized and involves more planning *with*, not *for*, individuals and a focus on self-management which fits in with individual needs and lives (Corben & Rosen, 2005). This could create a tension between the professional and individual when the goals and aspirations are not one and the same.

A model of shared decision making by Zoffman and colleagues highlights the importance of co-created person-centred knowledge, communication and mutual reflection (Zoffman, Harder, & Kirkevold, 2008). They suggested that a key issue for the therapeutic relationship is bringing the patients' perspective and difficulties to the foreground and enabling shared decision making by mutual situational refection; this can help to close the gap between personal experience and general clinical evidence. However, there is a need for professionals to move away from a disease-focused approach to more of a life–disease approach and challenging individuals to adopt a more independent reflection as a way of clarifying their approaches to decision making and self-management. This may require a critical change to the ways in which healthcare professionals interact and communicate with individuals.

Overall, some learning strategies that actively involve individuals and include planned follow-up can be effective (Smith et al., 2008). But there are limitations to education provision alone, and this may be due to the way in which information is given which often does not take into account individual learning styles and use methods which promote active involvement and problem-solving. If rehabilitation is to embrace a self-management approach, then interactions between the healthcare professional and individual need to emphasize a sharing of expertise, changing from the more didactic provision of information (Newman et al., 2004). In spite of an overall ambition in health policy to move away from professionals being seen as experts, the ways in which rehabilitation is organized may make this difficult to achieve. There can be a lack of flexibility and opportunity to deliver services which allow time for individuals to learn the skills of self-management particularly when the time frame and criteria for rehabilitation are fixed as is the case in many inpatient rehabilitation settings.

14.7.4 Service and Organization

The role played by both formal and informal self-help groups can be a vital aspect of a more collective approach to self-management (Ch'Ng et al., 2008). However, these groups can be difficult to access by individuals with restricted mobility or communication impairments or minority and ethnic groups (Davidson, How, Worral, Hickson, & Togher, 2008). In general, the organization and delivery of self-management programmes have given little recognition to the role of social context and the collective value of a group of people with similar experiences coming together for support. Additionally, follow-up support after acute care is often not clearly defined and can provide an impression of extension to rehabilitation instead of supporting individuals to engage with their communities to make full use of community resources.

In considering the organizational and contextual issues surrounding self-management, there is a gap in our understanding about the provider's perspective, although there are a number of perceived barriers amongst healthcare professionals to successful implementation within usual practice. These barriers include lack of time, concerns over sustainability and cultural relevance of some self-management programmes (Jones & Lennon, 2009; Lake & Staiger, 2010). In addition, the attitudes and beliefs of practitioners with regard to the credibility and confidence about self-management could impact on the sustainability of key principles. There is the concern that if professionals do not integrate the key aspects of behaviour change using methods which show sensitivity to individual needs, learning and social circumstances, then they will revert to delivering basic educational interventions. The elements most at risk can be the interactions perceived to be more time consuming such as active problem-solving, shared decision making and goal setting.

Rehabilitation may need to consider a whole system change, whereby professionals have the skills and services and have the flexibility to offer access to different types of self-management support (Kielman et al., 2010). The fixed period of rehabilitation that is offered by many organizations may not provide the flexibility to support self-management over time. The timing of rehabilitation may not coincide with the right time for an individual to learn new strategies to self-manage. In addition, the very nature of accessing a specialist in rehabilitation may promote a reliance on professional support, particularly if delivered in a clinical setting. Teams and services will need to examine ways of promoting autonomy and control earlier during rehabilitation, if self-management is not to come as a shock to individuals once discharged.

The success of rehabilitation is measured in different ways, and teams are monitored according to different outcomes. If self-management is promoted as part of rehabilitation, then the ways in which change is captured and recorded will also need to be re-evaluated. Self-management is multifaceted and one outcome measure will not be sufficient to record change, but there could be value in measuring some of the factors associated with successful self-management such as levels of self-activity or confidence. Rehabilitation teams considering doing more to promote self-management should also consider what model of support is best for their patient groups, and a mix of group and individualized interventions may be most appropriate. There also needs to be careful consideration of how to utilize people with experience of self-management of different conditions to work alongside and advise professional teams.

14.8 Conclusion

A report published by the Kings Fund in 2005 reviewed evidence on self-management programmes but with a focus on patient perspectives. This included qualitative interviews to explore individuals' experiences of living with a long-term condition (Corben & Rosen, 2005). The report draws attention to several key issues which still have resonance now in relation to this chapter:

1. That people's ability to self-manage changes over time
2. That participation in self-management programmes is influenced by many factors, including time since diagnosis, severity of the disease, age, social support and level of education
3. That there is a need for good, ongoing, flexible relationships between professionals and patients
4. That professionals should be planning with, not for, their patients and offer a clear signposting towards support services, community resources and assistive devices and equipment

The current guidance in much of health policy is that self-management should be the top priority for commissioners and providers of healthcare (Imison et al., 2011). There is also an emphasis on the need to move away from acute and episodic care and towards prevention and self-management. This is a consistent theme across the developed world which underlines the need to develop a more systematic and proactive management of individuals with long-term conditions.

Rehabilitation could offer a real opportunity to add on or integrate principles of self-management, and evidence suggests that one of the most effective ways is through focusing on behaviour change and supporting self-efficacy (de Silva, 2011). A formal organized programme may not be the right approach for all, and a more flexible integrated approach may be more appropriate, particularly for individuals with complex disability. It is also important to recognize that self-management programmes are not necessarily an alternative to specialized and timely rehabilitation interventions.

This chapter has raised a number of issues which could be used personally, professionally or more generally within a rehabilitation service and include the following:

- There are many challenges and ethical issues associated with self-management. These include the importance of acknowledging power within the therapeutic relationship, in order to achieve shared decision making and mutual refection on priorities to take control.

- There needs to be sensitivity about the timing of self-management programmes and consideration of individuals' learning needs and priorities. There may be times when support and guidance are needed from an expert especially during periods of anxiety and change in health status, for example, in fluctuating conditions such as multiple sclerosis.

- The skills required by professionals to support self-management may be different to those commonly used within rehabilitation. Professionals may need to adapt current strategies to those that address behaviour change according to different individual needs.

- An understanding of the relevance of self-management to individuals is important in order to address perceived barriers. This may include a wide range of beliefs including those influencing decisions about heath and the level of desire for control.

- Self-management will not be appropriate for everyone, and there should not be a *one-size-fits-all* approach. In particular, programmes are under-researched in complex conditions such as stroke and traumatic brain injury. Clinical trials rarely include individuals with cognitive and communication problems or those with severe disability.

- Organized self-management programmes should not take the place of informal self-help and social networks. They could be seen to complement each other instead of being mutually exclusive.

Overall, self-management offers great promise to support individuals to take greater control of their lives when living with a chronic condition or disability. Further research is needed on the efficacy of different programmes but also to explore the barriers and attitudes of individuals and professionals to self-management and how self-management principles can be integrated into rehabilitation practice. Goal setting and self-management are not separate processes and are linked by both theory and practice and may offer efficient ways of promoting autonomy control and greater confidence through rehabilitation.

References

Adriaansen, J.J.E., Van Leeuwen, C.M.C., Visser-Meily, J.M.A., van den Bos, G.A.M., Post, M.W.M., (2011). Course of social support and relationships between social support and life satisfaction in spouses of patients with stroke in the chronic phase. *Patient Education and Counseling*. 85(2), e48–e52.

Audulv, A., Asplund, K., & Norbergh, K. G. (2010). Who's in charge? The role of responsibility attribution in self-management among people with chronic illness. *Patient Education and Counseling*, *81*(1), 94–100.

Bandura, A. (1989). Human agency in social cognition theory. *American Psychologist*, 44(9), 1175–1184.

Bandura, A. (1994). Self-efficacy. In V. S. Ramachaudran (Ed.), *Encyclopedia of human behavior* (Vol. 4, pp. 71–81). New York, NY: Academic Press.

Bandura, A. (1995). Exercise of personal and collective efficacy in changing societies. In A. Bandura (Ed.), *Self-efficacy in changing societies* (pp. 1–45). Cambridge, U.K.: Cambridge University Press.

Bandura, A. (1997). The nature and structure of self-efficacy. In A. Bandura (Ed.), *Self-efficacy: The exercise of control*. New York, NY: W.H. Freeman.

Barlow, J. H., Sturt, J., & Hearnshaw, H. (2002). Self-management interventions for people with chronic conditions in primary care: Examples from arthritis, asthma and diabetes. *Health Education Journal, 61*(4), 365–378.

Boden-Albala, B., Litwak, E., Elkind, M. S. V., Rundek, T., & Sacco, R. L. (2005). Social isolation and outcomes post stroke. *Neurology, 64,* 1888–1892.

Bury, M. (2005). The body, health and society. In M. Bury (Ed.), *Health and illness* (pp. 61–79). Cambridge, U.K.: Polity Press.

Bury, M., Newbold, J., & Taylor, D. (2005). *A rapid review of the current state of knowledge regarding lay-led self-management of chronic illness: Evidence review.* London, U.K.: National Institute for Health and Clinical Excellence.

Cadilhac, D. A., Hoffmann, S., Kilkenny, M., Lindley, R., Lalor, E., Osborne, R. H., & Batterbsy, M. (2011). A phase II multicentered, single-blind, randomized, controlled trial of the stroke self-management program. *Stroke, 42*(6), 1673–1679.

Challis, D., Hughes, J., Berzins, K., Reilly, S., Abell, J., & Stewart, K. (2010). *Self-care and case management in long-term conditions: The effective management of critical interfaces.* London, U.K.: HMSO.

Ch'Ng, A. M., French, D., & Mclean, N. (2008). Coping with the challenges of recovery from stroke: Long term perspectives of stroke support group members. *Journal of Health Psychology, 13,* 1136–1146.

Corben, S., & Rosen, R. (2005). *Self-management for long-term conditions: Patients' perspectives on the way ahead.* London, U.K.: King's Fund.

Cott, C. A., Wiles, R., & Devitt, R. (2008). Continuity, transition and participation: Preparing clients for life in the community post-stroke. *Disability and Rehabilitation, 29*(20), 1566–1574.

Coulter, A., & Ellins, J. (2006). *Quality enhancing interventions: Patient-focused interventions: A review of the evidence.* London, U.K.: The Health Foundation and Picker Institute Europe.

Creer, T. L., & Holroyd, K. A. (1997). Self management. In A. Baum, S. Newman, J. Weinman, & C. McManus (Eds.), *Cambridge handbook of psychology, health and medicine* (Vol. 1). Cambridge, U.K.: Cambridge University Press.

Davidson, B., How, T., Worral, L., Hickson, L., & Togher, L. (2008). Social participation for older people with aphasia: The impact of communication disability on friendships. *Topics in Stroke Rehabilitation, 15*(4), 325–340.

de Silva, D. (2011). *Helping people help themselves: A review of the evidence considering whether it is worthwhile to support self-management.* London, U.K.: The Health Foundation.

Department of Health. (2001). *The expert patient: A new approach to chronic disease for the 21st century.* London, U.K.: Department of Health.

Department of Health. (2006). *Supporting people with long term conditions to self care: A guide to developing local strategies and good practice.* London, U.K.: DH Publications Orderline.

Dixon, G., Thornton, E. W., & Young, C. A. (2007). Perceptions of self-efficacy and rehabilitation among neurologically disabled adults. *Clinical Rehabilitation, 21*(3), 230–240.

Ellis-Hill, C., Payne, S., & Ward, C. (2008). Using stroke to explore the Life Thread Model: An alternative approach to understanding rehabilitation following an acquired disability. *Disability and Rehabilitation, 30*(2), 150–159.

Evans, R. L., Hendricks, R. D., Haselkorn, J. K., Bishop, D. S., & Baldwin, D. (1992). The family's role in stroke rehabilitation: A review of the literature. *American Journal of Physical Medicine and Rehabilitation, 71*(3), 135–139.

Ewart, C. K. (1992). The role of physical self efficacy in the recovery from a heart attack. In R. Schwarzer (Ed.), *Self-efficacy: Thought control of action* (Vol. 1, pp. 287–305). Philadelphia, PA: Taylor & Francis.

Gibson, P. G., Powell, H., Wilson, A., Abramson, M. J., Haywood, P., Bauman, A., … Roberts, J. J. L. (2002). Self-management education and regular practitioner review for adults with asthma. Cochrane *Database of Systematic Reviews* (3). doi: 10.1002/14651858.CD001117.

Glass, T. A., Berkman, L. F., Hiltunen, E. F., Furie, K., Glymour, M. M., Fay, M. E., & Ware, J. (2004). The families in recovery from stroke trial (FIRST): Preliminary study results. *Psychosomatic Medicine, 66,* 889–897.

Greenhalgh, T., Campbell-Richards, D., Vijayaraghaven, S., Collard, A., Malik, F., Griffin, M., … Macfarlane, F. (2011). New models of self-management education for minority ethnic groups: Pilot randomised trial of a story-sharing intervention. *Journal of Health Service Research & Policy*, 16(1), 28–36.

Hardeman, W., & Mitchie, S. (2009). Training and quality assurance of self-management interventions. In S. Newman, L. Steed, & K. Mulligan (Eds.), *Chronic physical illness: Self-management and behavioural interventions* (pp. 98–120). Berkshire, U.K.: Open University Press.

Hardeman, W., Sutton, S., Griffin, S., Johnston, M., White, A., Wareham, N. J., & Kinmonth, A. L. (2005). A causal modelling approach to the development of theory-based behaviour change programmes for trial evaluation. *Health Education Research Theory and Practice*, 20(6), 676–687.

Hirsche, R., Williams, B., Jones, A., & Manns, P. (2011). Chronic disease self-management for individuals with stroke, multiple sclerosis and spinal cord injury. *Disability and Rehabilitation*, 33(13–14), 1136–1146.

Holman, H., & Lorig, K. (1992). Perceived self-efficacy in the self-management of chronic disease. In C. Schwarzer (Ed.), *Self-efficacy: Thought control of action* (Vol. 1, pp. 305–324). Washington, DC: Hemisphere Publishing Corporation.

Huijbregts, M. P. J., Myers, A. M., Streiner, D., & Teasell, R. (2008). Implementation, process, and preliminary outcome evaluation of two community programs for persons with stroke and their care partners. *Topics in Stroke Rehabilitation*, 15(5), 503–520. doi:10.1310/tsr1505–503

Imison, C., Naylor, C., Goodwin, N., Buck, D., Curry, N., Addicott, R., & Zollinger-Read, P. (2011). *Transforming our health care system: Ten priorities for commissioners*. London, U.K.: The Kings Fund.

Johnston, M., Bonetti, D., Joice, S., Pollard, B., Morrison, V., Francis, J. J., & Macwalter, R. (2007). Recovery from disability after stroke as a target for a behavioural intervention: Results of a randomized controlled trial. *Disability and Rehabilitation*, 29(14), 1117–1127. doi:779965732 [pii] 10.1080/03323310600950411

Johnston, S. E., Liddy, C. E., & Ives, S. M. (2011). Self-management support: A new approach still anchored in an old model of care. *Canadian Journal of Public Health*, 102(1), 68–72.

Jones, F., & Lennon, S. (2009). A new stroke self-management programme: Preliminary analysis of training for practitioners. *International Journal of Stroke*, 4(s2), 23.

Jones, F., Mandy, A., & Partridge, C. (2008). Reasons for recovery after stroke: A perspective based on personal experiences. *Disability and Rehabilitation*, 30(7), 507–516.

Jones, F., Mandy, A., & Partridge, C. (2009). Changing self-efficacy in individuals following a first time stroke: Preliminary study of a novel self-management intervention. *Clinical Rehabilitation*, 23(6), 522–533. doi:10.1177/0269215508101749

Jones, F., & Riazi, A. (2011). Self-efficacy and self-management after stroke: A systematic review. *Disability and Rehabilitation*, 33(10), 797–810.

Jovicic, A., Holroyd-Leduc, J., & Straus, S. (2006). Effects of self-management interventions on health outcomes of patients with heart failure: A systematic review of randomised controlled trials. *BMC Cardiovascular Disorders*, 6(1), 43.

Kendall, E., Catalano, T., Kuipers, P., Posner, N., Buys, N., & Charker, J. (2007). Recovery following stroke: The role of self-management education. *Social Science and Medicine*, 64, 735–746.

Kendall, E., Ehrlich, C., Sunderland, N., Muenchberger, H., & Rushton, C. (2011). Self-managing versus self-management: Reinvigorating the socio-political dimensions of self-management. *Chronic Illness*, 7, 87–98.

Kendall, E., & Rogers, A. (2007). Extinguishing the social? State sponsored self-care policy and the Chronic Disease Self-Management Programme. *Disability and Society*, 22(2), 129–143.

Kennedy, A., Reeves, D., Bower, P., Lee, V., Middleton, E., Richardson, … Rogers, A. (2007). The effectiveness and cost effectiveness of a national lay-led self care support programme for patients with long-term conditions: A pragmatic randomised controlled trial. *Journal of Epidemiology and Community Health*, 61, 254–261.

Kennedy, A., Rogers, A., & Gately, C. (2005). From patients to providers: Prospects for self-care skills trainers in the National Health Service. *Health & Social Care in the Community*, 13, 431–440.

Kielman, T., Huby, G., Powell, A., Sheikh, A., Price, D., Williams, S., & Pinnock, H. (2010). From support to boundary: A qualitative study of the border between self-care and professional care. *Patient Education and Counseling, 79,* 55–61.

Lake, A. J., & Staiger, P. K. (2010). Seeking the views of health professionals on translating chronic disease self-management models into practice. *Patient Education and Counseling, 79*(1), 62–68.

Langford, A., Sawyer, D., Gioimo, S., Brownson, C., & O'Toole, M. (2007). Patient-centered goal setting as a tool to improve diabetes self-management. *The Diabetes Educator, 33,* 139s–144s.

Lawn, S., McMillan, J., & Pulvirenti, M. (2011). Chronic condition self-management: Expectations of responsibility. *Patient Education and Counseling, 84,* e5–e8.

Lawn, S., & Schoo, A. (2010). Supporting self-management of chronic health conditions: Common approaches. *Patient Education and Counseling, 80,* 205–211.

Lazurus, R. S. (1990). Stress, coping and illness. In H. Friedman (Ed.), *Personality and disease* (pp. 97–120). Oxford, U.K.: John Wiley & Sons.

Levack, W., Dean, S. G., Siegert, R. J., & McPherson, K. (2011). Navigating patient-centred goal setting in inpatient stroke rehabilitation: How clinicians control the process to meet perceived professional responsibilities. *Patient Education and Counseling, 85*(2), 206–213.

Levanthal, H., Benyamini, Y., Brownlee, S., Diefenbach, M., Leventhal, E., Patrick-Miller, L., & Robitaille. (1997). Illness representations: Theory and measurement. In K. J. Petrie & J. A. Weinman (Eds.), *Perceptions of health and illness* (pp. 19–47). Amsterdam, the Netherlands: Harwood Academic Publishers.

Lorig, K. (1986). Development and dissemination of an arthritis patient education course. *Family and Community Health, 9,* 23–32.

Lorig, K., & Holman, H. R. (2003). Self-management education: History, definition, outcomes and mechanisms. *Annals of Behavioral Medicine, 26*(1), 1–7.

Lorig, K., Sobel, D. S., Ritter, P., Laurent, D. D., & Hobbs, M. (2001). Effect of a self-management program on patients with chronic disease. *Effective Clinical Practice, 4*(6), 256–262.

Lorig, K., Sobel, D. S., Stewart, A. L., Byron, W., Bandura, A., Ritter, P., … Holman, H. R. (1999). Evidence suggesting that a chronic disease self-management program can improve health status while reducing hospitalisation: A randomized trial. *Medical Care, 37*(1), 5–14.

Luger, T., Cotter, K. A., & Sherman, A. M. (2009). It's all in how you view it: Pessimism, social relations and life satisfaction in older adults with arthritis. *Aging and Mental Health, 13*(5), 635–647.

Mackenzie, A., Perry, L., Lockhart, E., Cottee, M., Cloud, G., & Mann, H. (2007). Family carers of stroke survivors: Needs, knowledge, satisfaction and competence in caring. *Disability and Rehabilitation, 33*(29), 111–121.

Maclean, N., Pound, P., Wolfe, C., & Rudd, A. (2002). The concept of patient motivation. A qualitative analysis of stroke professionals' attitudes. *Stroke, 33,* 444–448.

McKenna, S., Jones, F., Glenfield, P., & Lennon, S. (2011). "Bridges" – Promoting self-management for stroke survivors in the community: A feasibility randomised controlled trial. *International Journal of Stroke, 6*(s2), 50.

McKevitt, C., Fudge, N., Redfern, J., Sheldenkar, A., Crichton, S., Rudd, A., … Wolfe, C. (2011). Self-reported long-term needs after stroke. *Stroke, 42,* 1398–1403.

Medical Research Council Health Services and Public Health Research Board. (2000). A framework for the development and evaluation of RCTs for complex interventions to improve health.

Mulligan, K., & Newman, S. (2007). Self-management interventions. In S. Ayers, C. Baum, C. McManus, S. Newman, K. Wallston, K. Weinman, & R. West (Eds.), *Cambridge handbook of psychology, health and medicine* (2nd ed., pp. 393–397). Cambridge, U.K.: Cambridge University Press.

Newbold, J., Taylor, D., & Bury, M. (2006). Lay-led self-management in chronic illness: A review of the evidence. *Chronic Illness, 2,* 249–261.

Newman, S., Steed, L., & Mulligan, K. (2004). Self-management interventions for chronic illness. *Lancet, 364*(9444), 1523–1537.

Newman, S., Steed, L., & Mulligan, K. (2009). *Chronic physical illness: Self-management and behavioural interventions.* Berkshire, U.K.: Open University Press.

Phillips, J. (2010). *Self care reduces costs and improves health – The evidence*. London, U.K.: Expert Patients Programme – Community Interest Company.

Rittman, M., Boylstein, C., Hinojosa, R., Hinojosa, M. S., & Haun, J. (2007). Transition experiences of stroke survivors following discharge home. *Topics in Stroke Rehabilitation, 14*(2), 21–31. doi:HX878403X27TP262 [pii] 10.1310/tsr1402-21

Robinson-Smith, G., & Pizzi, E. R. (2003). Maximizing stroke recovery using patient self-care self-efficacy. *Rehabilitation Nursing, 28*(2), 48–51.

Rosewilliam, S., Roskell, C., & Pandyn, A. (2011). A systematic review and synthesis of the quantitative and qualitative evidence behind patient centred goal setting. *Clinical Rehabilitation, 25*, 501–514.

Sabari, J. S., Meisler, J., & Silver, E. (2000). Reflections upon rehabilitation by members of a community based stroke club. *Disability and Rehabilitation, 22*(7), 330–336.

Salter, K., Hellings, C., Foley, N., & Teasell, R. (2008). The experience of living with stroke: A qualitative meta-synthesis. *Journal of Rehabilitation Medicine, 40*, 595–602.

Schreurs, K. M. G., Colland, V. T., Kuijer, R. G., de Ridder, D. T. D., & van Elderen, T. (2003). Development, content, and process evaluation of a short self-management intervention in patients with chronic diseases requiring self-care behaviours. *Patient Education and Counseling, 51*, 133–141.

Smith, J., Forster, A., House, A., Knapp, P., Wright, J. J., & Young, J. (2008). Information provision for stroke patients and their caregivers. *Cochrane Database of Systematic Reviews, 16*(2), CD001919. doi:10.1002/14651858.CD001919.pub2

Taylor, D., & Bury, M. (2007). Chronic illness, expert patients and care transition. *Sociology of Health and Illness, 29*(2), 27–45.

Taylor, G. H., Todman, J., & Broomfield, N. M. (2011). Post-stroke emotional adjustment: A modified social cognitive transition model. *Neuropsychological Rehabilitation, 21*(6), 808–824. doi:10.1080/09602011.2011.598403

Treasure, J., & Maissi, E. (2007). Motivational Interviewing. In S. Ayers, C. Baum, C. McManus, S. Newman, K. Wallston, K. Weinman, & R. West (Eds.), *Cambridge handbook of psychology, health and medicine* (2nd ed., pp. 363–366). Cambridge, U.K.: Cambridge University Press.

Vassilev, I., Rogers, A., Sanders, C., Kennedy, A., Blickem, C., Protheroe, J., ... Morris, R. (2011). Social networks, social capital and chronic illness self-management: A realist review. *Chronic Illness, 7*(1), 60–86.

Watkins, C., Auton, M. F., Deans, C. F., Dickinson, H. A., Jack, C. I., Lightbody, C. E., ... Leathley, M. J. (2007). Motivational interviewing early after acute stroke: A randomized, controlled trial. *Stroke, 38*(3), 1004–1009.

Wilson, P., Kendall, S., & Brooks, F. (2007). The Expert Patients Programme: A paradox of patient empowerment and medical dominance. *Health & Social Care in the Community, 15*(5), 426–438.

Zoffman, V., Harder, I., & Kirkevold, M. (2008). A person-centred communication and reflection model: Sharing decision-making in chronic care. *Qualitative Health Research, 18*(5), 670–685.

15

Goal Setting in Paediatric Rehabilitation

Lesley Wiart

CONTENTS

15.1 Introduction

In Chapter 3, Siegert and colleagues described how patients in a rehabilitation environment evaluate their current situation and determine the discrepancy between their current and previous state. Patients seek information to determine what is possible and what activities and attributes would help them regain the state of their idealized self. Parents of children with disabilities face unique challenges as they often lack a reference point for their child's potential; it can be difficult for them to know what is possible for their children. While the adult with a sustained injury works to regain their previous level of functioning, parents of children with developmental disabilities create their vision of the future based on what they imagine is possible for their child.

This chapter is an overview of issues specific to goal setting in rehabilitation for children with disabilities and their families in the context of family-centred service delivery. Goal setting with families with children with disabilities can be complex due to the multitude of services that families access in different environments, changing priorities as children age and the shifting of responsibility for goal setting to the child as they become able to identify their own rehabilitation priorities. The case scenario of Maria demonstrates some of the challenges as well as some strategies for goal setting that can result in a more coordinated approach to rehabilitation service delivery (see Box 15.1). Topics explored in this chapter include goal setting and family-centred care, goals that are important to children with disabilities and their families, family participation in

BOX 15.1   CASE STUDY

Maria is 5 years old and has a diagnosis of spastic diplegic cerebral palsy. She is transitioning from a preschool programme for children with disabilities where she received occupational therapy, physical therapy and speech language pathology services on a weekly basis. The school has requested occupational therapy and physical therapy consultation at school. Maria's mother has requested occupational and physical therapy services from home care to address concerns at home which include difficulty ascending and descending stairs of their two-level home. At school, Maria walks with a walker in the classroom and uses a wheelchair for travelling longer distances and outdoors (Gross Motor Function Classification System [Palisano et al., 1997] Level III). Maria uses her wheelchair to keep up with the other students in the hallway and uses her walker in the classroom. She does require some assistance with the majority of fine motor tasks. For example, she is able to colour with large crayons once she is assisted with the preparation of the crayon and paper (Manual Ability Classification System [Eliasson et al., 2006] Level III). The school-based occupational therapist and physical therapist observed Maria at school. At the end of the visit, the therapists met with the teacher to make some recommendations to support Maria's participation in her educational programme. The teacher asked the therapist to participate in the goal setting process for the individual programme plan (IPP) which would involve all members of the team, including Maria's parents and the home care therapists. As a standard requirement for the home care programme, the therapists used the COPM (Law, Baptiste, et al., 2005) to identify goals for Maria. Maria and her parents completed the COPM interview together, and Maria was able to articulate some challenges she experienced at home and at school, particularly in regard to developing friendships. Her parents also raised some additional problems that were focused on managing the stairs at home and decreased independence with self-care tasks. The five problems that were identified as priorities with the COPM were the following:

1. Decreased independence with self-care skills (brushing teeth and hair and washing face in the morning)
2. Difficulty with ascending and descending stairs at home
3. Challenges with making friends
4. Difficulty with getting in and out of the car independently
5. Challenges with managing food utensils independently

The IPP meeting began with a review of the priority problem areas identified by the COPM process. Once Maria's parents had the opportunity to explain why the problem areas identified were important to them, the discussion focused on how the family goals could be incorporated into her educational goals. For example, it was agreed that the development of friendships and the use of eating utensils are also very relevant at school, and both areas should be addressed in the IPP. The discussion ensued about implementation of strategies to address the goals at home and at school. Although improving her ability to move up and down the stairs independently was a goal for Maria's family, it was agreed by all that Maria would continue to take the elevator at school and use her wheelchair in the hallways in order to conserve energy for her academic pursuits, to be able to keep up with her classmates in the hallway and to make the transition between classrooms efficient. At home, the home care therapists would work with Maria to address transfers in and out of the family vehicle, stair mobility, self-care skills and feeding. The school and home care therapists discussed how they could collaborate to ensure they are working together and communicating effectively.

This scenario highlights several issues that need to be considered when setting therapeutic goals in paediatric rehabilitation. In this example, the home care therapists used a formalized process for goal setting and demonstrated a family-centred approach to goal setting by using the COPM and ensuring that the discussion about educational goals considered the issues that were important to Maria and her family. The team worked collaboratively to identify the goals and established one set of goals that could be addressed, as appropriate, in different environments. Although the education system and the health-care programme had separate requirements for goal setting processes and documentation, the family, therapists and teacher collaborated to ensure the goals were meaningful to Maria and her family, integrating the goal-setting processes as much as possible and collaborating to implement strategies to address the goals. The goal-setting process provided the foundation for collaboration between therapists working in different service sectors so that therapeutic efforts towards achieving Maria's goals were coordinated.

goal setting, the use of individualized goal-setting tools in paediatrics, current evidence for the effects of goal setting on child outcomes, using the International Classification of Functioning, Disability and Health (ICF) (World Health Organization, 2001) in goal setting with families and collaborative goal setting as a strategy for increasing continuity of care for families.

15.2 Goal Setting and Family-Centred Care

Family-centred care has become a prominent and widely accepted approach to service delivery in paediatrics. Collaborative decision making between families and service providers lays the foundation for family-centred practice, and families are acknowledged as the experts on their children's needs. The uniqueness of families is respected (King, Teplicky, King, & Rosenbaum, 2004; Shelton & Stepanek, 1994), and families have different resources and opportunities to participate in decision making in regard to their child's rehabilitation (Dodd, Saggers, & Wildy, 2009). In paediatric rehabilitation, therapists often maintain long-term relationships with families. Therefore, therapists must be flexible with goal setting as family values, beliefs and priorities can change (Wiart, Ray, Darrah, & Magill-Evans, 2010) and responsibility for goal setting shifts from parents to the child over time. Ultimately, a family-centred approach to rehabilitation involves identification of therapy goals based on the goals that are important to families.

15.3 What Rehabilitation Goals Are Important to Children and Families?

Surprisingly, there is very little research describing the goals that parents of children with disabilities have for their children. Hayashi and Frost (2006) reported on the administration of an individualized goal-setting tool, the Canadian Occupational Performance Measure (COPM) (Law, Baptiste, et al., 2005), with 1559 parents of children who access paediatric rehabilitation services. Eighty percent of parents identified issues related to leisure activities, and 65.4% identified issues related to socialization (i.e. visiting, phone calls and parties). Hayashi and Frost also conducted qualitative, focus group interviews with 10 guardians and four children with disabilities. The focus group with the guardians indicated that enhancing socialization and acceptance by others were the most important goals they had regarding their children. Other qualitative studies indicate that parents consider belonging to a community, choice, independence, personal control, participation in age-appropriate activities and interpersonal relationships to be important outcomes for their children (Giangreco, Cloninger, & Iverson, 1998; Goddard, Lehr, & Lapadat, 2000; Wiart et al., 2010).

Siebes et al. (2007) reported on the goals of five parents of children with cerebral palsy which focused on functional abilities of their children including self-care skills, mobility and communication skills. In a retrospective chart review of 121 medical records of children with cerebral palsy, Knox (2008) identified 12 areas of concern identified by parents and therapists: activities of daily living, hand function, eating/drinking, floor mobility, sitting, standing/walking, transfers, stiffness, communication, therapy, visual perception and behaviour. Overall, existing research with children and youth and their families suggests that families are focused on functional therapy goals that lead to increased participation in activities that are meaningful to them. While the nature of the child's disability may influence the path families take to achieve these goals, the overarching goals of parents of children with disabilities are not different from those of parents of children without disabilities; they want their children to develop their functional skills, lead fulfilling lives and be accepted and valued by others. The need to ensure that tasks and activities are meaningful for children and the influence of individual family values, beliefs and contexts highlight the importance of individualized goal setting and meaningful family engagement in the goal-setting process.

Most of the research evaluating paediatric rehabilitation goals focuses on parent goals; research on the goals of children and youth themselves is sparse. Shikako-Thomas et al. (2009) conducted a study on factors that contribute to quality of life of adolescents with cerebral palsy (aged 12–16 years). The predominant theme was the importance of the relationship between personal interests and preferences (intrinsic factors) and opportunities to participate in those activities (extrinsic factors) (Shikako-Thomas et al., 2009). One of the main findings of this research was the key role of differential valorization, or the value that individuals attribute to any particular task or activity. This concept is important because the value attributed to a task or activity influences the activities individuals choose to pursue, their motivation to engage in those activities as well as how successfully they engage in those tasks or activities. This research highlights the importance of individualized goal setting since the value that individuals place on various activities is subjective and variable.

The concept of differential valorization suggests that perhaps the importance of self-selection of meaningful activities has not been emphasized enough in conceptual frameworks used in rehabilitation. For example, the ICF (World Health Organization, 2001), the most prominent conceptual framework used in paediatric rehabilitation, attributes discrepancies between what the child can do (capacity) and what they actually do (performance) to the presence of contextual barriers. As Morris (2009) points out, the ICF model does not emphasize the importance of choice and intrinsic motivation for participation in selected activities or roles.

Morris (2009) also suggests that capability theory could be used to a greater extent in paediatric rehabilitation. Capability theory was originally developed by Sen (1992), an economist dedicated to studying the facilitation of economic growth in developing nations (Siegert & Ward, 2010). Capability theory was further developed by Nussbaum (2000), a professor of law and ethics who emphasized the importance of personal choice and core human entitlements out of respect for human dignity. Capability, according to Sen (1999), describes *achieved functioning* that is moderated by individual capability, opportunity and choice. There is recognition that individuals have different aims (inter-end variation) that lead individuals to do things they value (Sen, 1999). While capability theory was developed in fields external to rehabilitation, it is embedded in social justice and basic human rights and therefore has direct implications for rehabilitation. For example, as Siegert and Ward pointed out, capability theory would encourage a focus on things important for leading a happy or fulfilling life since it emphasizes the rights of individuals to choose to participate in activities that are meaningful and important to them. Clearly, the need for more emphasis on personal choice and motivation in paediatric rehabilitation becomes obvious when we consider that all individuals have activities in which they could participate but they choose not to. This would shift the emphasis from the traditional therapeutic focus on task performance towards considering performance in the context of what the child is motivated to do. Exploring the theoretical relationships between individual capacity, opportunity and personal choice highlights the need to work with the individual for whom goals are being established to ensure that therapeutic activities align with the activities that are desired by the child and their family.

15.4 Family Participation in the Goal-Setting Process

Research suggests that engaging in formalized goal-setting processes with families may result in increased engagement in the rehabilitation programme (Øien, Fallang, & Østensjø, 2010) since the child and their family are more motivated to participate in therapy (Ekstrom-Ahl, Johansson, Granat, & Carlberg, 2005). Family involvement may also increase parental perceptions of self-efficacy because parents can focus on discrete, targeted goals rather than general developmental goals that may lead to feelings of guilt because they feel they are not doing enough for their child (Øien et al., 2010). For example, in a study comparing goal-directed functional therapy and activity-focused therapy (Löwing, Bexelius, & Brogren Carlberg, 2009), family and preschool staff reported feeling relieved that they could focus on targeted goals instead of feeling responsible for all aspects of the child's development. A focus on specific goals also enables families to celebrate their child's achievements (Wiart et al., 2010). Celebrating goal achievement can be particularly important when children with disabilities make important and meaningful gains in abilities that may not represent a significant milestone from the perspective of parents of children without disabilities.

Individualized goal-setting tools can provide systematic processes for identifying goals that are meaningful to families. Meaningful family engagement in goal setting can encourage a functional approach to intervention as parents and children are likely to identify functional and meaningful therapy goals (Østensjø, Øien, & Fallang, 2008). Despite the emphasis on goal-directed approaches to paediatric rehabilitation, research suggests that formalized approaches to goal setting are not yet common practice among rehabilitation service providers (Darrah, Wiart, Magill-Evans, Ray, & Andersen, 2012) as challenges with the widespread use of formalized goal setting in rehabilitation practice have been reported in the literature. Reported challenges include inadequate documentation of goals (Nijhuis, Reinders-Messelink, de Blécourt, Boonstra, et al., 2008), lack of programme expectations for the use of standardized goal-setting processes (Darrah et al., 2012) and lack of parental involvement in the goal-setting process (Nijhuis et al., 2007; Wiart et al., 2010). In a Canadian study that involved interviews with programme managers about their practices related to goal setting (Darrah et al., 2012), only 11 of 47 (23.4%) of the programmes had implemented formalized goal-setting processes. In a retrospective chart review conducted in the Netherlands where a national framework for team collaboration and goal documentation, the rehabilitation activities profile (Roelofsen, Lankhorst, & Bouter, 2001), has been implemented, the charts of 24% of children did not include documented goals (Nijhuis, Reinders-Messelink, de Blécourt, Ties, et al., 2008).

The research that does include the use of individualized goal-setting tools suggests that goals are primarily identified by parents and that children have limited involvement in setting their own goals for rehabilitation. Limited involvement of children may be due to the assumption that identification of goals would be too challenging for a child. However, some literature suggests that children as young as 5 years can be active participants in setting their own goals (Missiuna & Pollock, 2000), and limitations with children's involvement in setting their own goals may be attributed more to the methods that have been used to obtain their input rather than the child's ability to participate in goal setting (Missiuna, Pollock, Law, Walter, & Cavey, 2006). Engaging children in setting their own goals can result in goals that are more meaningful to the child and result in greater feelings of autonomy and control over their own successes (Sands & Doll, 1996). Children and their parents may not always have the same goal priorities, and therefore collaborative goal setting with families involves consideration of multiple perspectives with increasing responsibility for the child to set their own goals over time. For example, children between 5 and 8 years of age may focus more on self-care and leisure activities, while parents are more focused on academic tasks such as printing and drawing (Missiuna & Pollock, 2000). Other research has demonstrated that the goals of adolescents and older school-aged children may differ from those of their parents (McGavin, 1998). McGavin reported that parents were more concerned about issues related to self-care skills and low physical activity levels, while adolescents were more concerned about lack of independence with mobility skills and lack of close relationships with peers. While some children may be able to articulate what their goals are, children with more significant cognitive impairments may not be able to clearly articulate their goals. However, parents and therapists can still involve these children in goal identification by observing the child to determine which activities they enjoy and appear to be motivating to them.

The following section is an overview of three tools for collaborative goal setting with parents and children: the COPM (Law, Baptiste, et al., 2005), goal attainment scaling (GAS) (Kiresuk & Sherman, 1968) and the perceived efficacy and goal-setting system (PEGS) (Missiuna, Pollock, & Law, 2004). Individualized goal-setting tools have potential for more widespread use in paediatrics due to the family-centred approach to goal setting and the ability of the tools to address heterogeneous goals that are often identified by multi-disciplinary teams across a variety of settings (Steenbeek, Ketelaar, Galama, & Gorter, 2007).

15.4.1 Canadian Occupational Performance Measure

The COPM is based on the Canadian model of occupational performance (Townsend, 1997), a theoretical framework for occupational therapy that outlines functioning within the domains of self-care, productivity and leisure. It is a client-centred, goal-setting tool and an individualized outcome measure originally developed for use with adults receiving occupational therapy services. However, its use has expanded across a broad range of clinical areas and disciplines (Esnouf, Taylor, Mann, & Barrett, 2010; Harvey et al., 2011; Padankatti et al., 2011). The COPM is increasingly being used in research to evaluate the achievement of outcomes that are important from the perspectives of parents of children with disabilities and has become the most common goal-setting tool discussed in the paediatrics literature (Tam, Teachman, & Wright, 2008). Administration of the COPM involves a systematic process for client goal identification and prioritization via a semi-structured interview process used to identify problems and rate their importance. The child and/or parent rates their performance in the prioritized problem areas and satisfaction with performance on a 10-point scale pre- and post-rehabilitation intervention. A change score of two points or greater is considered to be clinically significant (Law, Baptiste, et al., 2005).

Several research studies have used the COPM with children with disabilities (Law, Majnemer, et al., 2005; Stewart & Neyerlin-Beale, 2000; Tam, Archer, Mays, & Skidmore, 2005), and clinicians maintain that children as young as five or six can identify and prioritize goals (Law, Baptiste, et al., 2005). There is some evidence that the COPM is valid and reliable when conducted with parents of children with disabilities (Cusick & Lannin, 2007; Verkerk, Wolf, Louwers, Meester-Delver, & Nollet, 2006). Although the COPM provides important information about the child's or parents' perspectives on goal attainment, combining the COPM with GAS or other individualized goal-setting tools and outcome measures may provide a more thorough assessment of child progress because both subjective ratings of performance and more objective measurement of functional status are considered (Doig, Fleming, Kuipers, & Cornwell, 2010; Tam et al., 2008; Wallen, O'Flaherty, & Waugh, 2004).

15.4.2 Goal Attainment Scaling

GAS is increasingly being used in paediatric rehabilitation research to measure achievement of individualized goals (Steenbeek et al., 2007; Tam et al., 2008) and has been used in several studies to evaluate treatment effectiveness (Desloovere et al., 2012; O'Connor & Stagnitti, 2011; Pfeiffer, Koenig, Kinnealey, Sheppard, & Henderson, 2011; Wallen et al., 2011). Once the goals are established, gradations of goal achievement are developed on a five-point scale from negative two to positive two with the baseline scored as negative two and the expected outcome at zero. There is evidence to support the reliability and validity of GAS with paediatric populations (Law, Dai, & Siu, 2004; Palisano & Gowland, 1993; Palisano, Haley, & Brown, 1992; Stephens & Haley, 1991). In a study conducted to evaluate utility of the GAS for use with children with cerebral palsy, GAS demonstrated adequate responsiveness to change following a conductive education intervention (Law et al., 2004). While GAS can be used in a family-centred manner by ensuring the goals are identified by families, in practice, the literature suggests that goals are primarily identified by clinicians or researchers (Tam et al., 2008). Children with disabilities as young as 8 years of age are able to participate in the identification of goals for GAS (Mitchell & Cusick, 1998). Identified limitations of GAS include challenges with identifying discrete levels, scales that address multiple dimensions, establishing goals that are too *easy* (Schlosser, 2004) and the potential for a floor effect if the child regresses since the lowest rating represents performance at baseline (Law et al., 2004). See Chapter 8 for further details.

15.4.3 Perceived Efficacy and Goal-Setting System

The PEGS (Missiuna et al., 2004) was developed by occupational therapists to engage children with disabilities in the process of setting their own goals. The PEGS is a client-centred individualized goal-setting tool and an outcome measure developed specifically for use in paediatrics for children aged 5–8 years (Missiuna et al., 2004). The authors of the PEGS highlight the importance of self-identification of goals, particularly since perceived self-efficacy (i.e. one's judgement of one's own capabilities to plan and act towards competent task performance) affects the choice of activities and the effort one puts towards task achievement and persistence (Missiuna et al., 2004).

The PEGS includes 24 items (12 gross motor and 12 fine motor) that children would commonly engage in on a daily basis divided into three subscales: self-care, school/productivity and leisure. The items are presented to the child with two pictorial representations of a child performing the task competently and one picture of the child performing the task less competently. The child is asked how much he or she is like the child on the card, and then the child sorts the cards in order of activities for which they feel they are most to least competent. Following this rating process for the 24 items, the child is asked if there are any other things that were not discussed that he or she would like to improve on during therapy; identified tasks are added to the items that the child rated that they were not competent. The therapist then conducts an interview with the child whereby the child's goal priorities are established.

A pilot study conducted with 37 children and their parents to evaluate feasibility of the PEGS and compare goals and perceived child competence in performance of daily tasks from the perspective of the child and their parents suggested that children were able to successfully establish goals for therapy and prioritize the goals. Therapists reported that children were engaged and understood the instructions. Administration of the PEGS takes between 10 and 20 min. Although parents generally perceived the child to be less competent than the children themselves, parents and the child agreed on competence for 10 of the 12 gross motor items and 7 of the 12 fine motor items (Missiuna & Pollock, 2000).

15.5 Effects of Goal Setting on Child Outcomes

While research linking family-identified goals to improved child outcomes is promising, results remain inconclusive due to the lack of research in this area and combined interventions that make it impossible to determine the unique contributions that goal setting makes towards the studied outcomes. However, parents have reported that setting functional therapy goals encourages translation of therapy activities into the home (McGibbon Lammi & Law, 2003) and increases engagement and motivation to participation in rehabilitation (Ekstrom-Ahl et al., 2005; Øien et al., 2010). In a randomized controlled trial to compare the effectiveness of traditional physical therapy for children with cerebral palsy and therapy focused on parent-identified goals and functional skills attainment (Ketelaar, Vermeer, Hart, Petegem-van Beek, & Helders, 2001), the functional skills group had more improvement in self-care and motor skills. In a prospective cohort study comparing activity-focused and goal-directed approaches to therapy, the goal-directed therapy group demonstrated greater improvements on the functional and caregiver assistance scales of the mobility and self-care domains of the Pediatric Evaluation of Disability Inventory (PEDI) (Haley, Coster, Ludlow, Haltiwanger, & Andrellos, 1992) over the course of a 12-week intervention period (Löwing et al., 2009). The goal-directed therapy group also improved more than the activity therapy group on the caregiver assistance scale of the social function domain. While the results suggest positive effects of goal setting, there were two other key differences between the two groups. The goal-directed group also attended regular group meetings for therapy and received parent education at the beginning of the intervention, while the activity-focused group did not. In a randomized controlled trial to compare child- versus context-focused intervention (which included the use of the COPM) for children with cerebral palsy (Law et al., 2011), the two approaches were determined to be equally as effective. Both groups improved on the functional skills and caregiver assistance scales of the PEDI and the gross motor function measure (Russel, Rosenbaum, Avery, & Lane, 2002) after 6 months of intervention, and there were no differences between groups on lower extremity range of motion, the assessment of preschool children's participation (King et al., 2004) or the psychological empowerment scale (Akey, Marquis, & Ross, 2000). A repeated measures design study conducted with 22 children with cerebral palsy to determine the effects of goal-directed, intensive, activity-focused physiotherapy, resulted in improvements in gross motor function, self-care and functional skills.

In summary, while the research on the effects of goal-directed therapy is promising, it is impossible to disentangle the contribution of goal setting from other aspects of the interventions evaluated. Additional research is required to explore the unique contribution that goal setting makes to engagement in therapy, child and family motivation, self-efficacy and improved child and family outcomes.

15.6 Using the International Classification of Functioning, Disability and Health in Setting Goals with Families

The ICF (World Health Organization, 2001) has received a great deal of attention as a guiding conceptual framework and common language to describe the functioning of individuals with health conditions and disabilities. The focus on functional abilities instead of deficits and the representation of the complex interactions between the individual and the environment that affect functioning have led to its uptake, at least at a conceptual level, in rehabilitation. Subsequent to the publication of the original version, the World Health Organization published a child and youth version of the ICF, the ICF-CY (Lollar & Simeonsson, 2005). While the conceptual framework of the ICF-CY is the same as the original version, the child and youth version contains additional codes that are specific to children that address developmental skills and school-related activities. The purpose of this section is to explore how the ICF-CY can be used to assist in goal setting in paediatric rehabilitation.

Clinicians can introduce the conceptual framework of the ICF when setting goals with families so that they consider the broad range of goals that may be relevant to them. In addition, using the ICF can stimulate therapists' reflection on the assumed relationships between intervention strategies and outcomes (Darrah, Wiart, & Magill-Evans, 2008). For example, parents may want their child to move around more efficiently at school so that he or she can participate in social activities with peers. This goal may be achieved through interventions aimed at reducing environmental barriers to mobility, social interventions aimed at fostering understanding and positive interactions with peers (both reducing environmental barriers) and direct physical therapy aimed at improving walking speed and endurance (components of activity). Clinically, making explicit some of the assumed relationships between interventions and goals may be useful in order to facilitate reflection about the multiple influences on functioning and the evidence base to support the theoretical links between components of the ICF (Darrah, 2008). The ICF can also be used to track types of goals. In a recent study (Darrah et al., 2008), physical and occupational therapists were asked to develop therapy goals based on clinical case scenarios. While the exercise is somewhat artificial due to the absence of family input, the results indicated that most therapists focused on activity level goals, while more therapists working with younger children identified goals at the component of body function/structure. At a programme level, aggregate data on how goals are categorized into ICF components may be useful. For example, if a particular service mandate is to enhance participation at home and community, understanding the nature of goals according to the ICF components would provide information as to the extent to which rehabilitation goals and interventions are focused on achieving participation.

15.7 Conclusions

While it may be ideal for the same therapists to work with a child across multiple environments, rehabilitation service delivery systems are often still divided into traditional silos of health, education and social services. Families of children with disabilities often experience fragmentation of service delivery because they receive services from multiple professionals across settings and service sectors such as education and health (Giangreco, 1995). Parents of children with disabilities often spend a considerable amount of time and effort finding, learning about, and coordinating services for their children (Ray, 2002). Collaborative goal setting with the entire service delivery team can be used as a strategy to decrease service fragmentation and ensure a common set of goals (Ahl, Johansson, Granat, & Carlberg, 2005). Programmes that frequently work together can integrate goal setting processes to facilitate cohesive service delivery for families. In addition to the potential for enhancing collaboration among all members of the team, collaborative goal-setting processes ensure that families do not need to participate in multiple goal setting processes for the different services they access. For example, one family may participate in setting rehabilitation goals with therapists at school and with the therapists at a local rehabilitation centre. While integrated goal-setting processes across agencies or programmes require inter-agency collaboration and agency-level integration of goal-setting processes (King & Meyer, 2006), therapists may be able to coordinate processes even when agencies require separate goal-setting processes and documentation. Successful integration of goal-setting processes can decrease stress for families and ensure that the team is working towards achieving the same outcomes and can facilitate collaboration with other paediatric service providers (Øien et al., 2010).

In summary, collaborative goal setting with families is an exciting opportunity to engage children and families in working towards rehabilitation outcomes that are meaningful to them. The goal-setting tools reviewed in this chapter can provide systematic processes for doing so. While formalized goal-setting processes may not yet be implemented in practice, there is great potential for operationalizing the principles of family-centred care by ensuring that rehabilitation goals are important and meaningful for children with disabilities and their families.

References

Ahl, L. E., Johansson, E., Granat, T., & Carlberg, E. B. (2005). Functional therapy for children with cerebral palsy: An ecological approach. *Developmental Medicine & Child Neurology*, *47*(9), 613–619.

Akey, T. M., Marquis, J. G., & Ross, M. E. (2000). Validation of scores on the Psychological Empowerment Scale: A measure of empowerment for parents of children with a disability. *Educational & Psychological Measurement*, *60*(3), 419–438.

Cusick, A., & Lannin, N. (2007). Adapting the Canadian Occupational Performance Measure for use in a paediatric clinical trial. *Disability & Rehabilitation*, *29*(10), 761–766.

Darrah, J. (2008). Using the ICF as a framework for clinical decision making in pediatric physical therapy. *Advances in Physiotherapy*, *10*(3), 146–151.

Darrah, J., Wiart, L., & Magill-Evans, J. (2008). Do therapists' goals and interventions for children with cerebral palsy reflect principles in contemporary literature? *Pediatric Physical Therapy*, *20*(4), 334–339.

Darrah, J., Wiart, L., Magill-Evans, J., Ray, L., & Andersen, J. (2012). Are family-centred principles, functional goal setting and transition planning evident in therapy services for children with cerebral palsy? *Child: Care, Health & Development*, *38*(1), 41–47.

Desloovere, K., Schörkhuber, V., Fagard, K., Van Campenhout, A., De Cat, J., Pauwels, P., ... Molenaers, G. (2012). Botulinum toxin type A treatment in children with cerebral palsy: Evaluation of treatment success or failure by means of goal attainment scaling. *European Journal of Paediatric Neurology*, *16*(3), 229–236.

Dodd, J., Saggers, S., & Wildy, H. (2009). Constructing the 'ideal' family for family-centred practice: Challenges for delivery. *Disability & Society*, *24*(2), 173–186.

Doig, E., Fleming, J., Kuipers, P., & Cornwell, P. L. (2010). Clinical utility of the combined use of the Canadian occupational performance measure and goal attainment scaling. *American Journal of Occupational Therapy*, *64*(6), 904–914.

Ekstrom-Ahl, L. E., Johansson, E., Granat, T., & Carlberg, E. B. (2005). Functional therapy for children with cerebral palsy: An ecological approach. *Developmental Medicine & Child Neurology*, *47*(9), 613–619.

Eliasson, A. C., Krumlinde-Sundholm, L., Rösblad, B., Beckung, E., Arner, M., ... Rosenbaum, P. (2006). The Manual Ability Classification System (MACS) for children with cerebral palsy: Scale development and evidence of validity and reliability. *Developmental Medicine & Child Neurology*, *48*(7), 549–554.

Esnouf, J. J. E., Taylor, P. N., Mann, G. E., & Barrett, C. L. (2010). Impact on activities of daily living using a functional electrical stimulation device to improve dropped foot in people with multiple sclerosis, measured by the Canadian occupational performance measure. *Multiple Sclerosis*, *16*(9), 1141–1147.

Giangreco, M., Cloninger, C., & Iverson, V. (1998). *Choosing outcomes and accommodations for children*. Baltimore, MD: Paul H. Brookes.

Giangreco, M. F. (1995). Related services decision-making: A foundational component of effective education for students with disabilities. *Physical & Occupational Therapy in Pediatrics*, *15*(2), 47–67.

Goddard, J. A., Lehr, R., & Lapadat, J. C. (2000). Parents of children with disabilities: Telling a different story. *Canadian Journal of Counselling*, *34*(4), 273–289.

Haley, S., Coster, W., Ludlow, L. H., Haltiwanger, J. T., & Andrellos, P. J. (1992). *Pediatric evaluation of disability inventory: Development, standardization, and administration manual*. Boston, MA: Trustees of Boston University, Center for Rehabilitation Effectiveness.

Harvey, L. A., Ristev, D., Hossain, M. S., Hossain, M. A., Bowden, J. L., Boswell-Ruys, C. L., ... Ben, M. (2011). Training unsupported sitting does not improve ability to sit in people with recently acquired paraplegia: A randomised trial. *Journal of Physiotherapy, 57*(2), 83–90.

Hayashi, R., & Frost, C. J. (2006). Being, belonging, and becoming: Examining rehabilitation service delivery to children with disabilities and their families. *Journal of Social Work in Disability & Rehabilitation, 4*(4), 39–56.

Ketelaar, M., Vermeer, A., Hart, H. T., Petegem-van Beek, E., & Helders, P. J. M. (2001). Effects of a functional therapy program on motor abilities of children with cerebral palsy. *Physical Therapy, 81*(9), 1534–1545.

King, G., Law, M., King, S., Hurley, P., Hanna, S., Kertoy, M., ... Young, N. (2004). *Children's assessment of participation and enjoyment (CAPE) and preferences for activities of children (PAC)*. San Antonio, TX: Harcourt Assessment.

King, G., & Meyer, K. (2006). Service integration and co-ordination: A framework of approaches for the delivery of co-ordinated care to children with disabilities and their families. *Child: Care, Health & Development, 32*(4), 477–492.

King, S., Teplicky, R., King, G., & Rosenbaum, P. (2004). Family-centered service for children with cerebral palsy and their families: A review of the literature. *Seminars in Pediatric Neurology, 11*(1), 78–86.

Kiresuk, T. J., & Sherman, R. E. (1968). Goal attainment scaling: A general method for evaluating comprehensive community mental health programs. *Community Mental Health Journal, 4*(6), 443–453.

Knox, V. (2008). Do parents of children with cerebral palsy express different concerns in relation to their child's type of cerebral palsy, age and level of disability? *Physiotherapy, 94*(1), 56–62.

Law, L. S. H., Dai, M. O. S., & Siu, A. (2004). Applicability of goal attainment scaling in the evaluation of gross motor changes in children with cerebral palsy. *Hong Kong Physiotherapy Journal, 22*, 22–28.

Law, M., Baptiste, S., Carswell, A., McColl, M., Polatajko, H., & Pollock, N. (2005). *Canadian occupational performance measure* (4th ed.). Ottawa, Ontario, Canada: CAOT Publications ACE.

Law, M., Majnemer, A., McColl, M. A., Bosch, J., Hanna, S., Wilkins, S., ... Stewart, D. (2005). Home and community occupational therapy for children and youth: A before and after study. *Canadian Journal of Occupational Therapy, 72*(5), 289–297.

Law, M. C., Darrah, J., Pollock, N., Wilson, B., Russell, D. J., Walter, S. D., ... Galuppi, B. (2011). Focus on function: A cluster, randomized controlled trial comparing child- versus context-focused intervention for young children with cerebral palsy. *Developmental Medicine & Child Neurology, 53*(7), 621–629.

Lollar, D. J., & Simeonsson, R. J. (2005). Diagnosis to function: Classification for children and youths. *Journal of Developmental & Behavioral Pediatrics, 26*, 323–330.

Löwing, K., Bexelius, A., & Brogren Carlberg, E. (2009). Activity focused and goal directed therapy for children with cerebral palsy – Do goals make a difference? *Disability & Rehabilitation, 31*(22), 1808–1816.

McGavin, H. (1998). Planning Rehabilitation: A comparison of issues for parents and adolescents. *Physical & Occupational Therapy in Pediatrics, 18*(1), 69–82.

McGibbon Lammi, B., & Law, M. (2003). The effects of Family-Centred Functional Therapy on the occupational performance of children with cerebral palsy. *Canadian Journal of Occupational Therapy, 70*(5), 285–297.

Missiuna, C., & Pollock, N. (2000). Perceived efficacy and goal setting in young children. *Canadian Journal of Occupational Therapy, 67*(2), 101–109.

Missiuna, C., Pollock, N., & Law, M. (2004). *Perceived efficacy and goal setting system (PEGS)*. San Antonio, TX: Psychological Corporation.

Missiuna, C., Pollock, N., Law, M., Walter, S., & Cavey, N. (2006). Examination of the Perceived Efficacy and Goal Setting System (PEGS) with children with disabilities, their parents, and teachers. *American Journal of Occupational Therapy, 60*(2), 204–214.

Mitchell, T., & Cusick, A. (1998). Evaluation of a client-centred paediatric rehabilitation programme using goal attainment scaling. *Australian Occupational Therapy Journal, 45*(1), 7–17.

Morris, C. (2009). Measuring participation in childhood disability: How does the capability approach improve our understanding? *Developmental Medicine & Child Neurology, 51*(2), 92–94.

Nijhuis, B. J. G., Reinders-Messelink, H. A., de Blécourt, A. C. E., Boonstra, A. M., Calamé, E. H. M., Groothoff, J. W., ... Postema, K. (2008). Goal setting in Dutch paediatric rehabilitation. Are the needs and principal problems of children with cerebral palsy integrated into their rehabilitation goals? *Clinical Rehabilitation, 22*(4), 348–363.

Nijhuis, B. J. G., Reinders-Messelink, H. A., de Blécourt, A. C. E., Olijve, W. G., Haga, N., Groothoff, J. W., ... Postema, K. (2007). Towards integrated paediatric services in the Netherlands: A survey of views and policies on collaboration in the care for children with cerebral palsy. *Child: Care, Health & Development, 33*(5), 593–603.

Nijhuis, B. J. G., Reinders-Messelink, H. A., de Blécourt, A. C. E., Ties, J. G., Boonstra, A. M., Groothoff, J. W., ... Postema, K. (2008). Needs, problems and rehabilitation goals of young children with cerebral palsy as formulated in the rehabilitation activities profile for children. *Journal of Rehabilitation Medicine, 40*(5), 347–354.

Nussbaum, M. (2000). *Women and human development: The capabilities approach.* Cambridge, U.K.: Cambridge University Press.

O'Connor, C., & Stagnitti, K. (2011). Play, behaviour, language and social skills: The comparison of a play and a non-play intervention within a specialist school setting. *Research in Developmental Disabilities, 32*(3), 1205–1211.

Øien, I., Fallang, B., & Østensjø, S. (2010). Goal-setting in paediatric rehabilitation: Perceptions of parents and professional. *Child: Care, Health & Development, 36*(4), 558–565.

Østensjø, S., Øien, I., & Fallang, B. (2008). Goal-oriented rehabilitation of preschoolers with cerebral palsy – A multi-case study of combined use of the Canadian Occupational Performance Measure (COPM) and the Goal Attainment Scaling (GAS). *Developmental Neurorehabilitation, 11*(4), 252–259.

Padankatti, S. M., Macaden, A. S., Cherian, S. M., Thirumugam, M., Pazani, D., Kalaiselvan, M., ... Srivastava, A. (2011). A patient-prioritized ability assessment in haemophilia: The Canadian Occupational Performance Measure. *Haemophilia, 17*(4), 605–611.

Palisano, R. J., & Gowland, C. (1993). Validity of goal attainment scaling in infants with motor delays. *Physical Therapy, 73*(10), 651–660.

Palisano, R. J., Haley, S. M., & Brown, D. A. (1992). Goal attainment scaling as a measure of change in infants with motor delays. *Physical Therapy, 72*(6), 432–437.

Palisano, R. J., Rosenbaum, P., Walter, S. D., Russell, D., Wood, E., & Galuppi, B. (1997). Development and reliability of a system to classify gross motor function in children with cerebral palsy. *Developmental Medicine & Child Neurology, 39*, 214–223.

Pfeiffer, B. A., Koenig, K., Kinnealey, M., Sheppard, M., & Henderson, L. (2011). Effectiveness of sensory integration interventions in children with autism spectrum disorders: A pilot study. *American Journal of Occupational Therapy, 65*(1), 76–85.

Ray, L. D. (2002). Parenting and childhood chronicity: Making visible the invisible work. *Journal of Pediatric Nursing, 17*(6), 424–438.

Roelofsen, E. E., Lankhorst, G. J., & Bouter, L. M. (2001). Simultaneous development and implementation of the Children's Rehabilitation Activities Profile: A communication instrument for pediatric rehabilitation. *Disability & Rehabilitation, 23*(14), 614–622.

Russel, D. J., Rosenbaum, P. L., Avery, L. M., & Lane, M. (2002). *Gross motor function measure user's manual* (Vol. 159). London, U.K.: Mac Keith Press.

Sands, D. J., & Doll, B. (1996). Fostering self-determination is a developmental task. *Journal of Special Education, 30*(1), 58–76.

Schlosser, R. W. (2004). Goal attainment scaling as a clinical measurement technique in communication disorders: A critical review. *Journal of Communication Disorders, 37,* 217–239.

Sen, A. (1992). *Inequality re-examined.* Oxford, U.K.: Oxford University Press.

Sen, A. (1999). *Development as freedom.* Westminster, MD: Alfred A Knopf Incorporated.

Shelton, T., & Stepanek, J. (1994). *Family-centered care for children needing specialized health and developmental services* (3rd ed.). Bethesda, MD: Association for the Care of Children's Health.

Shikako-Thomas, K., Lach, L., Majnemer, A., Nimigon, J., Cameron, K., & Shevell, M. (2009). Quality of life from the perspective of adolescents with cerebral palsy: "I just think I'm a normal kid, I just happen to have a disability". *Quality of Life Research, 18*(7), 825–832.

Siebes, R. C., Ketelaar, M., Gorter, J. W., Wijnroks, L., De Blécourt, A. C. E., Reinders-Messelink, H. A., & Vermeer, A. (2007). Transparency and tuning of rehabilitation care for children with cerebral palsy: A multiple case study in five children with complex needs. *Developmental Neurorehabilitation, 10*(3), 193–204.

Siegert, R. J., & Ward, T. (2010). Dignity, rights and capabilities in rehabilitation. *Disability & Rehabilitation, 32*(25), 2138–2146.

Steenbeek, D., Ketelaar, M., Galama, K., & Gorter, J. W. (2007). Goal attainment scaling in paediatric rehabilitation: A critical review of the literature. *Developmental Medicine & Child Neurology, 49*(7), 550–556.

Stephens, T. E., & Haley, S. M. (1991). Comparison of two methods for determining change in motorically handicapped children. *Physical & Occupational Therapy in Pediatrics, 11*(1), 1–17.

Stewart, S., & Neyerlin-Beale, J. (2000). The impact of community paediatric occupational therapy on children with disabilities and their carers. *British Journal of Occupational Therapy, 63*(8), 373–379.

Tam, C., Archer, J., Mays, J., & Skidmore, G. (2005). Measuring the outcomes of word cueing technology. *Canadian Journal of Occupational Therapy, 72*(5), 301–308.

Tam, C., Teachman, G., & Wright, V. (2008). Paediatric application of individualised client-centred outcome measures: A literature review. *British Journal of Occupational Therapy, 71*(7), 286–296.

Townsend, E. A. (1997). *Enabling occupation: An occupational therapy perspective.* Ottawa, Ontario, Canada: CAOT Publications.

Verkerk, G., Wolf, M., Louwers, A., Meester-Delver, A., & Nollet, F. (2006). The reproducibility and validity of the Canadian Occupational Performance Measure in parents of children with disabilities. *Clinical Rehabilitation, 20*(11), 980–989.

Wallen, M., Ziviani, J., Naylor, O., Evans, R., Novak, I., & Herbert, R. D. (2011). Modified constraint-induced therapy for children with hemiplegic cerebral palsy: A randomized trial. *Developmental Medicine & Child Neurology, 53*(12), 1091–1099.

Wallen, M. A., O'Flaherty, S. J., & Waugh, M. C. A. (2004). Functional outcomes of intramuscular botulinum toxin type a in the upper limbs of children with cerebral palsy: A phase II trial. *Archives of Physical Medicine & Rehabilitation, 85*(2), 192–200.

Wiart, L., Ray, L., Darrah, J., & Magill-Evans, J. (2010). Parents' perspectives on occupational therapy and physical therapy goals for children with cerebral palsy. *Disability & Rehabilitation, 32*(3), 248–258.

World Health Organization. (2001). *International classification of functioning, disability and health.* Geneva, Switzerland: World Health Organization.

16

Use of Goals as a Focus for Services for Community-Dwelling Older People

John G.M. Parsons, Stephen Jacobs and Matthew J.G. Parsons

CONTENTS

16.1 Introduction

This chapter will explore the use of goal setting as a tool to focus the delivery of rehabilitation for older people in home-care settings within New Zealand. The chapter begins with a description of the changing demographics across Organization for Economic Co-operation and Development (OECD) countries over the next 20 years. Following this, the concept of successful ageing and related concepts will briefly be presented. Together with principles already discussed elsewhere in this book, these key concepts form the basis for the use of goal setting among the current cohort of older people accessing health services.

Over the last 10–15 years, there has been considerable emphasis on a model of quality improvement in home-care service delivery within New Zealand. The model, called *restorative home care*, focuses on restoration and maintenance of older people's physical function, aiding compensation for impairments, so that the highest level of function is achieved. The model integrates principles from medicine, nursing, goal facilitation and rehabilitation to improve functional outcomes for older people. It is anticipated that through the use of progressive restorative programmes, the achievement of relevant goals are facilitated by exposure to appropriate services and engagement of support workers for older people. In order to develop goals that are person-centred, there needs to be some mutuality between the health professional and the client when identifying goals. The participation of the older person in the goal-setting process is to enhance adherence to and achievement of the goal. This chapter will conclude with a description of the experience of the use of goal setting within the context of restorative home care.

16.2 Demographic Changes in OECD Countries

Improving the ability of health and welfare systems to respond to the needs of older people (age 65+) is among the greatest challenges of our time. Among developed countries, the next 20 years will see growth in those over 65 years of age and a more rapid increase in the proportions of people over 75 years. Maximizing the health and well-being of older people is a major public issue. Consequently, the growth in this age group is anticipated to have a considerable impact on health and disability resources. Physical inactivity and disuse plays a major role in a number of age-related conditions such as diabetes, sarcopaenia (muscle loss) and heart disease. Many researchers and clinicians describe the harm associated with *wrapping older people in cotton wool* and much of this deterioration is linked to deconditioning and disuse (McMurdo, 1999). Preclinical disability is recognizable (Fried, Ferrucci, Darer, Williamson, & Anderson, 2004; Guralnik, Ferrucci, Simonsick, Salive, & Wallace, 1995; Idler & Kasl, 1995; Jagger, Arthur, Spiers, & Clarke, 2001; Langlois et al., 1996; Reuben, Rubenstein, Hirsch, & Hays, 1992; Reuben et al., 2004; Vita, Terry, Hubert, & Fries, 1998), and there is significant potential to forestall the development of disability both with health-promoting interventions such as physical activity (Gill et al., 2002; Kerse, Elley, Robinson, & Arroll, 2005) and appropriate nutrition. Improvement in abilities in those already with functional decline is also possible (Nelson et al., 2004). Thus, there is strong evidence that older people have considerable potential to recover functional capacity.

16.3 Successful Ageing

The concept of successful, healthy, optimal, active, productive ageing (or positive ageing) is supported by longitudinal, cross-sectional and quasi-experimental studies. An empirical definition of and a set of strategies for successful ageing was provided by Rowe and Kahn (1999) based on the data from the MacArthur Foundation Study of Successful Aging. The concept of successful ageing refers to the resilience of people who succeed in achieving a positive balance between gains and losses during ageing. This view is supported by studies that show that despite the difficult and often inevitable losses that result from ageing, most older people maintain a subjective feeling of well-being (Diener, Suh, Lucas, & Smith, 1999; Kunzmann, Little, & Smith, 2000; Smith, Fleeson, Geiselmann, Settersten, & Kunzmann, 1999). Prior to Rowe and Kahn, Baltes and Baltes (1990) published *Successful Aging*, which took a bio-psychosocial perspective and described a process of selective optimization and compensation (SOC) for ageing with success. Consideration of the SOC model allows for the conceptualization that ageing is a dynamic balance between gains and losses, so the model is highly congruent with contemporary evidence concerning goal facilitation.

16.4 Selective Optimization with Compensation Model

The SOC model of ageing (Baltes & Baltes, 1990) proposes a system of three adaptive processes: selection, optimization and compensation. *Selection* denotes a restriction of involvement in activities in response to lost capacity. *Optimization* refers to efforts to augment or enrich one's reserves in order to continue functioning (e.g. physical activity). *Compensation* involves efforts to meet goals by new means (e.g. modifying behaviours, using assistive devices). When considering the strategies employed by an older person who has an increasing degree of disability, it is important to consider these three processes. Fiksenbaum, Greenglass, and Eaton (2006) agreed that as people age, they have to cope with regular and frequent failure in attaining the action goals they set for themselves.

In addition, the SOC model suggests that as people age, they experience an increase in stressful life changes such as loss of a spouse, retirement or forced relocation (Bisconti, 1999). Additional stressors common among older people include reduced income, illness, loss of a driver's licence and/or becoming a carer for a family member who is ill (Schulz & Heckhausen, 1996). For many older people, these stressors steadily accumulate, resulting in significant frustration in their aspirations to maintain a normal adult lifestyle and increasing their dependence on others. They may also mean older people are unable to engage in desired activities to obtain gratification in social relationships which results in life dissatisfaction.

While the SOC model acknowledges losses as an inevitable part of the ageing process, it also suggests that the older individual is able to continue to generate positive outcomes. One of the key elements of the model is that people create environments which make success possible while effectively dealing with losses due to ageing.

To achieve congruence between their actual and desired life course, individuals must either try to modify the course of personal development to align with personal goals and aspirations (assimilative mode) or adjust personal goals to the constraints they are facing (accommodative model). Brandtstadter and colleagues (Brandtstädter & Renner, 1990; Brandtstädter, Wentura, & Rothermund, 1999) argued that individuals will engage in assimilative activities as long as they see a reasonable chance that such behaviours will help them achieve their goals.

16.5 Goal Setting and Older People

In health contexts, goal-setting opportunities are often not exploited to the degree that they could be (Baker, Marshak, Rice, & Zimmerman, 2001). Even when goal setting is used, health professionals sometimes view this as a foreign process for clients. This often results in goals being set by the health professional for the client (Bradley, Bogardus, Tinetti, & Inouye, 1999; Harwood, 2010; Holliday, Antoun, & Playford, 2005; Playford, Dawson, Limbert, Smith, & Ward, 2000), contrary to the principles of person-centred care. It is also clear that effective goal setting with older people requires skill (Bogardus et al., 2001; Davies, Laker, & Ellis, 2008; Lee, Arthur, & Avis, 2008; Stolee, Zaza, Pedlar, & Myers, 1999). The increased prevalence of cognitive impairment, communication difficulties and multiple co-morbidities provide added complexity to the process.

In addition, clinical experience often highlights the tension between the wishes of the older person's family or carers and the ability of a service provider to work towards an older person's goals. Bogardus et al. (2001) found that agreement between an older person, their carer and their physician regarding their goals for intervention was low (kappa 0.19–0.28). Given the multiple problems frequently encountered in working with older people, a focus on their aspirations and goals can assist all parties to attend to the active role older people can take in shaping their own futures (Rapkin & Fischer, 1992a, 1992b). Attention has also been drawn to the benefits of goal setting as a means of allowing judgements to be made about the effectiveness of particular services for the older person (Rockwood, Stolee, Howard, & Mallery, 1996).

Despite evidence of positive outcomes from goal setting, some studies report that older people are less likely to prefer an active role in clinical decision making than younger age groups (Arora & McHorney, 2000; Ekdahl, Andersson, & Friedrichsen, 2009). However, the evidence shows that using client-driven goals to direct rehabilitation for older people is strongly recommended (Bradley et al., 2000; Holahan & Chapman, 2002; Inglis, 2007; Schulman-Green, Naik, Bradley, McCorkle, & Bogardus, 2006). The remainder of the chapter will explore the use of goal setting as a focus for rehabilitation services provided to older people receiving a new model of home care.

16.6 Home Care and Functional Outcomes for Older People

Home care has traditionally involved home help to meet domestic needs. However, due to the increasingly complex needs of community-dwelling older people, services have shifted to providing domestic, personal and health-care services (Fleming & Taylor, 2007). The overarching goal of home care is to 'provide high quality, appropriate and cost-effective care to individuals that will enable them to maintain their independence and the highest quality of life' (Havens, 1999, p. 1). Fundamentally, home care is viewed as having three key objectives:

1. To substitute for acute care hospitalization
2. To substitute for long-term care institutionalization
3. To prevent the need for institutionalization and maintain individuals in their own home and community (Havens, 1999)

A report prepared for the World Health Organization (WHO) defined home care as

> ...the provision of health services by formal and informal caregivers in the home in order to promote, restore and maintain a person's maximal level of comfort, function and health including care toward a dignified death. Homecare services can be classified into preventive-promotive, therapeutic, rehabilitative/restorative, long-term maintenance and palliative care categories. (Havens, 1999, p. 1)

In New Zealand, home-care services provide personal care and household management to promote and maintain the independence of older people living at home (Ministry of Health, 2003). A systematic review, identifying 26 studies, examined the typical characteristics of home care (Thome et al., 2003). The reviewers found home care aimed to improve quality of life, increase functional ability and maintain independence allowing the person to remain at home. Through assessment, support is determined by the older person's needs and hospital care is minimized by assisting the individual at their home. However, there is extensive support for the view that health services delivered in an older person's home are often delivered at a critical juncture in an individual's functional status. Between 25% and 50% of older people who are hospitalized lose some of their functional abilities during their hospital stay (Gillick, Serrell, & Gillick, 1982; Inouye et al., 1993). Three months after a hospitalization, 66% of those who lose function while in hospital will have still not regained their previous level of functioning (Boyd et al., 2009; Sager & Rudberg, 1998; Sager et al., 1996). Traditional models of home care often do not operate on the premise that they can assist older people to regain or maintain functional capacity.

A recent cross-sectional observational study of over 4000 older people explored quality indicators for home care across 11 European countries (Bos et al., 2007). Across Europe, the most common quality problems identified were *failure to action rehabilitation potential in ADLs, no therapies [occupational therapy and physiotherapy] involved in service delivery* and *inadequate pain control* (Bos et al., 2007, p. 325). The authors commented on the issue of *rehabilitation potential*, observing that many European home-care agencies do not provide exercise or physical therapies to their clients.

Patmore and McNulty (2005a, 2005b) completed a study in England exploring person-centred flexible home care, finding that older people differ considerably in their preferences and values. Therefore, home care needs to be flexible in order to identify and meet older people's preferences. There is also a growing awareness that what matters most to older people is not just health in its narrowest interpretation but including a concern for choice, autonomy, independence and community integration among many others. Given that traditional home-care service models are invariably delivered with a traditional biomedical focus, it is not surprising that these areas which are of high importance to the older person are so often omitted. The use of goal setting as an approach to identify an older person's beliefs and preferences and to structure services to meet these goals is one strategy to address these shortcomings in service delivery.

Although home care has the potential to have a major influence on improving this situation, it often focuses more on treating disease and *taking care* of the client than on helping clients to regain functioning and independence. In Australia, a more independence- and recovery-focused model of home care is often called the *active service model* (Lewin & Vandermeulen, 2010; Lewin, Vandermeulen, & Coster, 2006; Ryburn, Wells, & Foreman, 2009); in the United Kingdom, it is called *re-ablement* (Glendinning & Newbronner, 2008; Patmore & McNulty, 2005; Pilkington, 2008; Rabiee & Glendinning, 2011); while *restorative home support* is the preferred term within New Zealand (King, Parsons, & Robinson, 2012; King, Parsons, Robinson, & Jörgensen, 2011; Parsons, Rouse, Robinson, Sheridan, & Connolly, 2012, 2013; Parsons & Parsons, 2012b) and the United States (Baker, Gottschalk, Eng, Weber, & Tinetti, 2001; Baker, Marshak, et al., 2001; Nadash & Feldman, 2003; Parsons, Senior, et al., 2012; Tinetti et al., 2002; Tinetti, Charpentier, Gottschalk, & Baker, 2012).

16.7 Use of Goal Setting as a Focus for the Implementation of Restorative Home Care

Within New Zealand, restorative home support has been developing over the past 10 years, during which time several key components of a restorative model have been identified and developed. First, there needs to be involvement of the older person, their family and home-care staff in setting goals and reaching agreement on the process for reaching the goals. This needs to encompass the use of a self-care progress report to document agreed goals, establish the client's baseline function, standardize the assessment of clients, clarify care responsibility across the multiple providers and track clients' progress towards their goals. Second, training needs to be provided for home-care nurses, therapists and support workers in rehabilitation and in geriatric medicine, with attainment of the client's own goals highlighted. In addition, there needs to be a reorientation of the focus of the home-care team from primarily treating disease and *taking care* of clients to maximizing function and comfort and working as an integrated inter-professional team with shared goals. Finally, there needs to be comprehensive assessment and diagnosis leading to the development of a multifaceted treatment plan that includes various combinations of exercise, behavioural changes, environmental adjustments and adaptive equipment, counselling and support and training and education of the older person, family and friends (Baker, Gottschalk, et al., 2001; Francis & Netten, 2003; Harris-Kojetin, Lipson, Fielding, Kiefer, & Stone, 2004; Nadash & Feldman, 2003; Stone, 2001; Stone & Wiener, 2001; Tinetti et al., 2002).

A standardized goal-setting process has been recognized as integral to this. The process (see Figure 16.1) needs to be integrated with a comprehensive assessment tool and also has to be structured to allow for the generation of support plans based on the goals identified by the older person.

Goal setting fits within an overall model of restorative home care that can assist governments to achieve effective and sustainable health and support services for their ageing populations. Internationally, the concept of ageing in place has been the objective in a number of policies and has undergone shifts in its interpretation during this period. The first major advance occurred in 1994 when OECD ministers reached a consensus that people should be able to continue living in their own place of residence in their later years. In the event that this is no longer possible, the alternative would be for older people to live in a 'sheltered and supportive environment which is as close to their community as possible, in both the social and geographical sense' (OECD, 1994, p. 18). Within New Zealand, ageing in place is defined as the ability of people to 'make choices in later life about where to live, and receive the support to do so' (Dalziel, 2001, p. 10). Despite this broad categorization, ageing in place often refers to the ability of older people to remain dwelling in the community, and residential care in the form of either rest homes or hospitals is specifically excluded.

Jacobs (2010) and Jacobs, Rouse, and Parsons (in press) identified factors key to the successful implementation of the New Zealand government's vision for ageing in place, as presented in the New Zealand Health of Older People Strategy (Ministry of Health, 2002). These factors are presented in Figure 16.2 as a conceptual framework for optimizing the quality of services provided to older people.

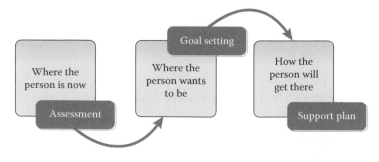

FIGURE 16.1
The assessment–goal setting–support plan development continuum.

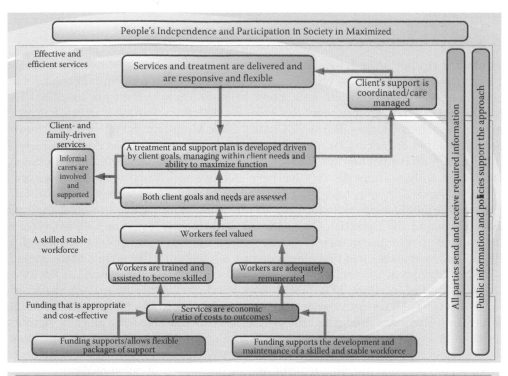

Effective and efficient services
- Clients are targeted to appropriate services (domestic support – short and long term, low needs, significant needs, critical needs and supported discharge)
- Reviews undertaken every three months
- Positive trusting relationship between assessing agency and home care provider
- Coordinated care (appropriate liaison and integration of services with primary care and allied health)
- Geographical alignment of assessing and coordinating agencies with primary care
- Appropriate ratio of clients to coordinators

Client- and family-driven services
- Social and community reintegration (social role valorization)
- Supporting self-management principles through empowerment techniques such as goal facilitation
- Comprehensive geriatric assessment (*INTER*RAI)
- Appropriate carer assessment
- Ensuring services are matched to client aspirations

A skilled stable workforce
- Reduced staff turnover
- Guaranteed hours for support workers
- Appropriate salary levels, linked to competency with career progression opportunities
- Enhanced supervision and delegation of support workers
- Appropriate competency levels (HBSS: Low needs – coaching/motivational level and significant/critical needs – health professional; assessing agency: health professional)
- Education: Support workers (National Standardized Training using experiential learning techniques); assessors and coordinators (post graduate, case reviews, in service education)

Funding that is appropriate and cost-effective
- Existing community resources are utilized
- Communities are supported to develop local solutions
- Funding models support flexibility and responsiveness
- Client recovery is maximized and services reduced to reflect reduced need
- Service provision reflects client needs

FIGURE 16.2
Theoretical model for the delivery of services for older people. (Reproduced from Jacobs, S.P., Implementation as a systematic manageable process rather than a Pandora's box of confusion: Reshaping community home care services for older people, Doctoral dissertation, The University of Auckland, Auckland, New Zealand, 2010. With permission.)

16.8 TARGET Approach

A number of studies have shown that there is a propensity to invest heavily in services that focus on assessment of the health of older people, without concomitant consideration of how to deliver effective health-care intervention to improve their life situation. There is an inherent but indefensible belief that comprehensive assessment is in itself a panacea (Clarkson, Venables, Hughes, Burns, & Challis, 2006; Mountain & Pighills, 2003; Stewart, Challis, Carpenter, & Dickinson, 1999). The potential for a standardized goal-setting tool to be integrated with comprehensive assessment tools to ensure that assessment findings are implemented within service delivery has been recognized within the model of restorative home care. Various attempts have been made to standardize goal setting in rehabilitation. The most commonly used tools for goal setting with older people are goal attainment scaling (GAS) and the Canadian Occupational Performance Measure (COPM). GAS was initially developed for use in mental health settings but has been applied in many different health-care contexts, including older person's rehabilitation (Boersma, Maes, Joekes, & Dusseldorp, 2006; Bravo, Dubois, & Roy, 2005; Forbes, 1998; Gordon, Powell, & Rockwood, 1999; Rockwood et al., 1996, 2003; Stolee, Rockwood, Fox, & Streiner, 1992; Stolee et al., 1999). Use of the GAS involves open-ended exploration of self-identified goals in an interview process. The main strength of the GAS is its responsiveness to clinically significant changes in goal attainment (Forbes, 1998). The main limitation of GAS is the difficulty of its implementation – intensive training is required to enable clinicians to select precise treatment goals and to define realistic and distinct levels of outcome (Smith, Cardillo, Smith, & Amezaga, 1998). (See Chapter 7 for more details on GAS.)

The COPM (Law et al., 1990) uses an interview process to elicit open-ended patient-identified goals. The COPM focuses on occupational performance problems in self-care, productivity and leisure. However, it does not examine which occupations are rewarding to the client or what support systems are needed for the client to carry out these occupations (Spencer & Davidson, 1998).

Given these important issues, there was significant potential to develop a new structured goal facilitation tool. To this end, the Towards Achieving Realistic Goal for Elders Tool (TARGET) (Parsons, 2010; Parsons & Parsons, 2012a; Parsons, Senior, et al., 2012) was developed by clinicians with an in-depth knowledge of the tools previously mentioned. It has been used clinically in a number of organizations within New Zealand to allow services in the community to be structured around the goals identified by older people. It provides a way to ensure that the principles of person-centred care are integrated within the delivery of services. The TARGET process involves five stages. An overview of these stages are presented in Figure 16.3 and described in the following texts in detail.

16.8.1 Stage 1: Assessment: Where the Person Is Now

The first stage of the TARGET process involves assessment of the older person's situation at the time of referral. To illustrate the TARGET process within the context of restorative home care in New Zealand, the case of Agnes Foster is now presented. The local area health board received a referral from Agnes' general practitioner following a visit from Agnes' daughter, who complained of increased stress levels associated with a decline in Agnes' functional ability. An overview of Agnes' initial presentation is provided in Box 16.1.

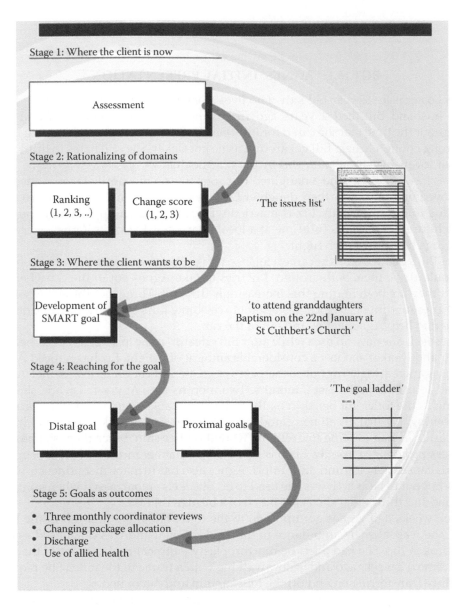

Stage 1: Where the client is now

Assessment

Stage 2: Rationalizing of domains

Ranking (1, 2, 3, ..)

Change score (1, 2, 3)

'The issues list'

Stage 3: Where the client wants to be

Development of SMART goal

'to attend granddaughters Baptism on the 22nd January at St Cuthbert's Church'

Stage 4: Reaching for the goal

'The goal ladder'

Distal goal

Proximal goals

Stage 5: Goals as outcomes

- Three monthly coordinator reviews
- Changing package allocation
- Discharge
- Use of allied health

FIGURE 16.3

The TARGET process. (From Parsons, J.G.M. and Parsons, M.J.G.: The effect of a designated tool on person-centred goal identification and service planning among older people receiving homecare in New Zealand. *Health Social Care Commun.* 2012. 20(6). 653–662. Copyright Wiley-VCH Verlag GmbH & Co. KGaA. Reproduced with permission.)

16.8.2 Stage 2: Rationalization of Domains

Following assessment, *areas of difficulty* are identified in an *issues list*. These areas are functions that the older person is concerned about or finds hard to complete. While it is appreciated that this potentially reinforces a deficit model of ageing, a strengths-based focus can be seen to work using the same model.

BOX 16.1 AGNES' INITIAL PRESENTATION

Agnes Foster is an 87-year-old lady who lives alone in her three-bedroom house.

Her husband Bill died 4 years ago from cancer. Agnes remained fit and well throughout the time that she cared for Bill. She thinks that her years of farming made her strong enough to help Bill get around as he got sicker. She still hates to think how thin her lovely big strong man was by the time he died.

Agnes has three sons and a daughter. Her sons live on the family farm. Agnes and Bill moved up to live near their daughter Liz 6 years ago when they retired from the farm due to Bill's ill health. Liz is married with three grown-up children and four grandchildren. She works full-time at a local pharmacy. Liz visits Agnes every day and brings her dinner each night.

After Bill's death, Agnes became a lot less active. She never had a driver's licence as Bill would drive them both around. Liz tries to take Agnes out in the car when she can but they are both finding this increasingly difficult. Three months ago when Liz took Agnes for dinner at a local restaurant to celebrate Liz's 60th birthday, one of Liz's sons had to help Agnes get in and out of the car.

Agnes feels she gave up for a while after Bill's death, so she lost her appetite, became weaker and weaker and lost a considerable amount of weight. Liz has noticed Agnes becoming increasingly frail over the past year. One indication of this is that Agnes has had four falls in the last 6 months. Two months ago, Agnes fell while she was walking to the toilet, cut her shin badly and was not able to get up until Liz arrived that evening. Liz had to call her grandson to help get Agnes back into her chair. The district nurses had to come to dress the wound on her shin. Since then, she has had the dressing changed weekly. Liz has also noticed that her mum is often constipated and this causes her pain and discomfort. Agnes also has urinary incontinence, which causes her not to be as active as she used to be. She feels embarrassed when going out in public and thinks that she is too much of a burden on Liz.

Three weeks ago, Agnes got up to go to the toilet one night and fell in the bathroom. She was taken by ambulance to the local hospital and was diagnosed as having a broken hip. She had a left hemiarthroplasty (surgical replacement of the head of her femur) 2 weeks ago and is now walking with a frame to the toilet. She requires assistance transferring on and off the toilet and in and out of bed.

After her operation, Agnes has developed a delirium from which she has not fully recovered, so at times she is confused. On her discharge from hospital, Liz wants Agnes to come and live with her. Prior to this hospital admission, Liz has been cooking her mum a meal each day and bringing it round. However, with Agnes' appetite so poor nowadays, she never finished the meals.

Liz thinks that the time has come where her mum needs to come to live with her. Liz has also been finding that while Agnes has always been extremely house-proud, Liz now has to do all the housework. This is becoming more and more difficult for Liz as she has a bad back. She is scared she will hurt herself and then her mother would be in a worse situation. Agnes refuses to go anywhere but back to her own home.

TABLE 16.1

Summary and Prioritization of Agnes' Areas of Concern

All Areas of *Difficulty or Concern* Identified by Agnes	Areas Ranked as of *High Importance* by Agnes	Areas *Most Needing Change* according to Agnes
Walking outside		Walking outside
Climbing stairs	Climbing stairs	
Getting in and out of the car	Getting in and out of the car	Getting in and out of the car
Walking on uneven ground	Walking on uneven ground	
Travelling on public transport		
Washing small items of clothing		
Housework		
Shopping		
Showering/bathing		Showering/bathing
Washing clothes		
Taking drinks from one room to the next	Taking drinks from one room to the next	
Going out socially	Going out socially	Going out socially
Driving		
Pain		

After identifying areas of difficulty, these areas are then *ranked* first in terms of how *important* it is for the older person to be able to undertake the task and second in terms of how much they would like to *change* their ability to undertake the task. This process involves reflective listening, with the assessor stating the issues arising from the assessment to the older person and providing them with an opportunity to identify which issues are most important to them and which ones they wish to work on changing. A simple three-point scale (1, no change/not important; 2, a little change/important; and 3, a lot of change/very important) is used to assist with identification of the most pressing issues.

Returning again to the example of Agnes, Table 16.1 presents a summary of all areas of difficulty or concerns from Agnes' point of view, along with identification of those areas considered (1) of high importance and (2) most needing of change. This forms the basis of the conversation between the assessor and Agnes to assist Agnes to identify a goal around which her service provision can be structured. The scoring for importance and areas needing change are useful for identifying areas that Agnes may wish to focus on as part of her service provision.

16.8.3 Stage 3: Goal Setting: Where the Person Wants to Be

Following the ranking of issues, goals are then selected. This includes the documentation of a distal goal (i.e. long-term or primary goal) that is specific, measurable, attainable, realistic and time oriented. In Figure 16.3, Agnes' distal goal is stated as being 'to attend granddaughter's baptism at St Cuthbert's church on 22nd January'. This distal goal is then broken into proximal goals (i.e. short-term goals) through a process of activity breakdown, which may include addressing areas of deficit that would prevent the older person from attaining their goal (e.g. falls risk, decreased muscle strength, difficulty with showering and other personal cares). It is appreciated that a large number of older people do not recognize the word *goal* as being appropriate to them – a recognition of where they are now, where they want to get to and how they are going to get there without focusing on specific

BOX 16.2   DISCUSSION OF POSSIBLE GOALS WITH AGNES

Interviewer: OK Agnes, I can now see the areas that you see as being important to you. They were getting in and out of the car, showering yourself and going out socially. Is there anything that you would like to work towards that relates to those areas?

Agnes: No, I don't think so dear.

Interviewer: Well we spoke about how you like to go out in the car with your family. Is that something we could work towards?

Agnes: Well I did want to get to my granddaughters baptism but I really don't see how I could get there. I am just not up to it anymore.

Interviewer: Well I am not so sure Agnes. If that is something you would like to work towards, then we can work out how you would get there. Shall we do that?

Agnes: If that would be possible, then that would be marvellous.…

terms has been found in clinical practice to have more meaning for the current cohort of older people. This concept allows for consideration of both proximal and distal goals within the context of the older person's current abilities.

TARGET was developed to be used in conjunction with other tools and scales utilized by health professionals in their clinical practice. TARGET is solely a conduit for presenting the findings of these other scales and tools to the client in such a way that areas of deficit can be discussed. If the older person wishes to address these issues, solutions can then be developed.

In the case of Agnes, climbing stairs, walking on uneven ground, getting in and out of the car, taking drinks from one room to the next, showering independently and going out socially were all identified as being important areas that Agnes wished to focus on. Part of the conversation leading to Agnes verbalizing her goal is illustrated in Box 16.2.

Often, in practice, the process of talking about the needs and wishes of the older person leads to them formulating their goal very early on in the TARGET process. In other cases, they require prompting and guidance to discuss the areas that they have highlighted as being important to them.

16.8.4 Stage 4: Reaching for the Goal: How the Person Will Get There

This step moving on from formulation of the goal to working out how to achieve it is often the most difficult of all, as it involves the identification of the steps necessary for the older person to get from their present state of functioning to the state in which their goal is reached. This is done in the form of a ladder. As can be seen from the case of Agnes, there were several areas to work on to allow her to reach her goal (see Figure 16.4).

Extensive work in New Zealand and Australia has shown that identification of the goal and the required steps to attain that goal is not enough to change the tasks and activities prescribed in the support plan. Traditionally, this document has described the precise activities to be completed by the support worker, which often involve assisting with activities of daily living and housework tasks. Changing the emphasis to reflect the required flexibility and rehabilitative focus inherent in the goal ladder is vital. This also has to occur in an efficient manner that does not significantly impact on the time required to formulate the support plan.

To sit at front row of granddaughters baptism on 21st March next year
To be able to walk 15 m with her stick and one person helping by 28th February
To be able to manage continence for 4 h by 31st January
To be able to walk to car and get in with a little help by Christmas this year
To make lunch independently in 3 months' time
To be independent with showering in 3 months' time
To be able to defrost and heat meals on wheels with help of support worker in 2 weeks
To have pain less than 3/10 when she first gets up in the morning by next week

FIGURE 16.4
Goal ladder for Agnes Foster.

Since 2010, the University of Auckland, in collaboration with Canterbury District Health Board in New Zealand, has been working on a system to allow for the development of support plans that allow for the required evolution of the identified goals into flexible and individualized activities. The system (called SORT – Strategies to Optimize Recovery) uses the WHO's International Classification of Functioning, Disability and Health (ICF) (World Health Organization, 2001) as a framework for a database of graded functional and support tasks to be undertaken by the support worker (and includes over 1000 tasks). For each step on the goal ladder, a corresponding domain of the ICF is determined. Following this, the ICF domains are used to produce individually tailored support plans. For each domain, there is a drop-down list of activities. Activities appropriate for the client are chosen and automatically inserted into the support plan. Prompts relating to the activities will also appear to ensure that the safety of the client and support worker is maximized. The support plan produced will be in a Microsoft Word© document and therefore will be able to be modified by the clinician to ensure that individual tailoring of service provision is maintained. The process is summarized in Figure 16.5.

16.8.5 Stage 5: Goals as Outcomes

The use of goals as outcomes has been the focus of considerable interest within the field of rehabilitation research. As highlighted by a number of studies, the ability to use goals in this way relies on the skill of the person working with the client to identify meaningful and measurable goals (Bovend'Eerdt, Botell, & Wade, 2009; Siegert, 2010; Teal, Haidet, Balasubramanyam, Rodriguez, & Naik, 2012). There is significant potential for the use of TARGET in this way, and a study exploring the use of a three-point measure of success in goal attainment at regular client review (1, not achieved; 2, partly achieved; and 3, fully achieved) has been published (Parsons & Parsons, 2012b). However, it is also important to consider the ability of the use of a standardized approach to goal identification to influence other activities that can be used as outcomes for the quality of service delivery and provision. A number of studies and evaluations have identified that the use of TARGET enhanced the development of these activities relating to quality enhancement within home care. These include the development of individually tailored rehabilitation plans that are categorized using the WHO ICF model (World Health Organization, 2001) as a measure of the integration of assessment and the identification of client goals into service planning and delivery (Parsons, Rouse, et al., 2012), the measurement of the use of allied health in

Suggested structure of SORT (Strategies to Optimize Resources Toolkit)

Goal ladder entered in free text (informed by completed assessment)	To sit at front row of grandson's wedding on 21st March 2011	Drop down menu of selected ICF domains (e.g. pain, walking, caring for others)
	To be able to walk 15 m with her stick and one person's helping by February 2011	
	To be able to manage continence for 4 h by January 2011	
	To be able to walk to car and get in with a little help by Christmas 2010	
Compulsory completion of demographic information and casemix level	To be able to carry drinks and meal on trolley from kitchen to armchair in 3 months time	
	To be independent with showering in 3 months	
	To be able to defrost and heat meals on wheels with the help of support worker in 2 weeks	

Process	Example
1. ICF domains for each step on the goal ladder listed	1. To be independent with showering in 3 months will generate the ICF domain 'washing'
2. Choose from list of activities for each ICF domain	2. Under the domain washing are around 10 activities relating to the person's functional ability to undertake washing and showering; this would include: shower top half independently with support worker washing bottom half; shower with support worker providing supervision; shower independently with support worker in the house
3. Generation of a list of issues to attend to in relation to each activity	3. In the case of showering the list would include: consider referral to OT; is there a step into the shower; is there a need for adaptive equipment
4. User modified careplan produced which has options for printing, emailing or faxing	4. The careplan generated is in Microsoft Word and so some modification to ensure that it is individually tailored to the client is possible

FIGURE 16.5
SORT process. (From Parsons, J. and Parsons, M., *Strategies for Optimising Recovery Tool*, The University of Auckland, Auckland, New Zealand, 2012.)

response to the alignment of services to the goals identified by the client (Parsons, Rouse, et al., 2012, 2013) and service costs and staff turnover (King et al., 2011, 2012).

16.8.6 Other Considerations

As described in Figure 16.2, the implementation of a restorative model of home care that has goal setting as a focus also requires close attention to other factors. The first of these is funding. Operating a model that uses the assessment–goal setting–support plan development model described here has required the development of innovative funding models that allow for the delivery of services that are flexible to meet individual client's goals and needs. The workforce also needs to be trained to become skilled through nationally recognized standardized training programmes and to feel valued so that staff retention is high. There is ongoing development and evolution of the model, as the goals identified and the resulting support plan need to form the basis for ongoing dialogue between the members of the core team (home-care coordinator, client, family and support worker) as well as with other members of the health-care team delivering services to the client (e.g. general practitioner, allied health staff and district nursing).

16.9 Conclusion

Government policies and strategies across developed countries aspire to effectively support older people to remain in their home. Furthermore, not only is there evidence demonstrating numerous clinical benefits, but remaining at home is clearly the preferred choice of older people. However, the resultant effect has been substantial increase in demand and expenditure for home-care services. Despite the fact that home care provides indispensable assistance to community-dwelling older people, there is a plethora of evidence revealing that the current provision is fraught with issues. The forecast increasing ageing of our population, including the rapid increase of the oldest old, will result in a higher prevalence of chronic illness and disability with community-dwelling older people exhibiting increasingly complex needs. Consequently, improving the quality of provision and creating sustainable home-care services to meet the needs of these older people is imperative.

The role of a standardized goal-setting tool integrated within a continuum of comprehensive assessment leading to individualized support plans that allow for the necessary flexibility in service provision has been demonstrated in this chapter. However, the need to embed such service development within a coherent and comprehensive health services model has also been highlighted.

References

Arora, N. K., & McHorney, C. A. (2000). Patient preferences for medical decision making: Who really wants to participate? *Medical Care, 38*(3), 335–341.

Baker, D. I., Gottschalk, M., Eng, C., Weber, S., & Tinetti, M. E. (2001). The design and implementation of a restorative care model for home care. *Journal of American Geriatric Society, 41*, 257–263.

Baker, S., Marshak, H. H., Rice, G. T., & Zimmerman, G. J. (2001). Patient participation in physical therapy goal setting. *Physical Therapy, 81*(5), 1118–1126.

Baltes, P. B., & Baltes, M. M. (1990). *Successful aging: Perspectives from the behavioral sciences.* Cambridge, U.K.: Cambridge University Press.

Bisconti, T. L. (1999). Perceived social control as a mediator of the relationships among social support, psychological well-being, and perceived health. *The Gerontologist, 39*(1), 94–103.

Boersma, S. N., Maes, S., Joekes, K., & Dusseldorp, E. (2006). Goal processes in relation to goal attainment: Predicting health-related quality of life in myocardial infarction patients. *Journal of Health Psychology, 11*(6), 927.

Bogardus, S., Bradley, E. H., Williams, C. S., Maciejewski, P. K., van Doorn, C., & Inouye, S. K. (2001). Goals for the care of frail older adults: Do caregivers and clinicians agree? *American Journal of Medicine, 110*(2), 97–102.

Bos, J. T., Frijters, D. H. M., Wagner, C., Carpenter, G. I., Finne-Soveri, H., Topinkova, E., ... Bernabei, R. (2007). Variations in quality of Home Care between sites across Europe, as measured by Home Care Quality Indicators. *Aging-Clinical & Experimental Research*, 19(4), 323–329.

Bovend'Eerdt, T. J., Botell, R. E., & Wade, D. T. (2009). Writing SMART rehabilitation goals and achieving goal attainment scaling: A practical guide. *Clinical Rehabilitation*, 23(4), 352–361.

Boyd, C. M., Ricks, M., Fried, L. P., Guralnik, J. M., Xue, Q. L., Xia, J., & Bandeen-Roche, K. (2009). Functional decline and recovery of activities of daily living in hospitalized, disabled older women: The women's health and aging study I. *Journal of the American Geriatrics Society*, 57(10), 1757–1766.

Bradley, E. H., Bogardus, S. T., Tinetti, M. E., & Inouye, S. K. (1999). Goal-setting in clinical medicine. *Social Science & Medicine*, 49(2), 267–278.

Bradley, E. H., Bogardus, S. T., van Doorn, C., Williams, C. S., Cherlin, E., & Inouye, S. K. (2000). Goals in geriatric assessment are we measuring the right outcomes? *The Gerontologist*, 40(2), 191–196.

Brandtstädter, J., & Renner, G. (1990). Tenacious goal pursuit and flexible goal adjustment: Explication and age-related analysis of assimilative and accommodative strategies of coping. *Psychology and Aging*, 5(1), 58–67.

Brandtstädter, J., Wentura, D., & Rothermund, K. (1999). Intentional self-development through adulthood and later life: Tenacious pursuit and flexible adjustment of goals. In J. Brandtstädter & R. M. Lerner (Eds.), *Action and self-development: Theory and research through the life-span* (pp. 373–400). Thousand Oaks, CA: SAGE Publications, Inc.

Bravo, G., Dubois, M. F., & Roy, P. M. (2005). Using goal attainment scaling to improve the quality of long-term care: A group-randomized trial. *International Journal for Quality in Health Care*, 17(6), 511–519.

Clarkson, P., Venables, D., Hughes, J., Burns, A., & Challis, D. (2006). Integrated specialist assessment of older people and predictors of care-home admission. *Psychological Medicine*, 36(7), 1011–1021.

Dalziel, L. (2001). *The New Zealand positive ageing strategy*. Wellington, New Zealand: Ministry of Social Policy.

Davies, S., Laker, S., & Ellis, L. (2008). Promoting autonomy and independence for older people within nursing practice: A literature review. *Journal of Advanced Nursing*, 26(2), 408–417.

Diener, E., Suh, E. M., Lucas, R. E., & Smith, H. L. (1999). Subjective well-being: Three decades of progress. *Psychological Bulletin*, 125(2), 276–302.

Ekdahl, A. W., Andersson, L., & Friedrichsen, M. (2009). "They do what they think is the best for me." Frail elderly patients' preferences for participation in their care during hospitalization. *Patient Education and Counseling*. 80(2): 232–240.

Fiksenbaum, L. M., Greenglass, E. R., & Eaton, J. (2006). Perceived social support, hassles, and coping among the elderly. *Journal of Applied Gerontology*, 25(1), 17.

Fleming, G. and B. J. Taylor (2007). Battle on the home care front: Perceptions of home care workers of factors influencing staff retention in Northern Ireland. *Health & Social Care in the Community*, 15(1), 67–76.

Forbes, D. (1998). Goal attainment scaling. A responsive measure of client outcomes. *Journal Gerontological Nursing*, 24(12), 34–40.

Francis, J., & Netten, A. (2003). *Home care workers: Careers, commitments and motivations*. Kent, U.K.: University of Kent at Canterbury, Personal Social Services Research Unit.

Fried, L., Ferrucci, L., Darer, J., Williamson, J. D., & Anderson, G. (2004). Untangling the concepts of disability, frailty, and comorbidity: Implications for improved targeting and care. *Journals of Gerontology Series A: Biological Sciences & Medical Sciences*, 59(3), 255–263.

Gill, T., Baker, D., Gottschalk, M., Peduzzi, P., Allore, H., & Byers, A. (2002). A program to prevent functional decline in physically frail, elderly persons who live at home. *New England Journal of Medicine*, 347, 1068–1074.

Gillick, M. R., Serrell, N. A., & Gillick, L. S. (1982). Adverse consequences of hospitalization in the elderly. *Social Science and Medicine*, 16(10), 1033–1038.

Glendinning, C., & Newbronner, E. (2008). The effectiveness of home care reablement: Developing the evidence base. *Journal of Integrated Care, 16*(4), 32–39.

Gordon, J., Powell, C, & Rockwood, K. (1999). Goal attainment scaling as a measure of clinically important change in nursing home patients. *Age & Ageing, 28*(3), 275–281.

Guralnik, J., Ferrucci, L., Simonsick, E., Salive, M., & Wallace, R. (1995). Lower-extremity function in persons over the age of 70 years as a predictor of subsequent disability. *New England Journal of Medicine, 332*, 566–561.

Harris-Kojetin, L., Lipson, D., Fielding, J., Kiefer, K., & Stone, R. I. (2004). *Recent findings on front-line long-term care workers: A research synthesis 1999–2003*. Washington, DC, U.S. Department of Health and Human Services, Assistant Secretary for Planning and Evaluation, Office of Disability, Aging and Long-Term Care Policy.

Harwood, M. (2010). Rehabilitation and indigenous peoples: The Maori experience. *Disability & Rehabilitation, 32*(12), 972–977.

Havens, B. (1999). *Home-based and long-term care: Home care issues at the approach of the 21st century from a world health organization perspective.* Manitoba, Canada, World Health Organization.

Holahan, C., & Chapman, J. R. (2002). Longitudinal predictors of proactive goals and activity participation at age 80. *Journals of Gerontology Series B: Psychological Sciences & Social Sciences, 57*(5), P418–P425.

Holliday, R. C., Antoun, M., & Playford, E. D. (2005). A survey of goal-setting methods used in rehabilitation. *Neurorehabilitation and Neural Repair, 19*(3), 227.

Idler, E. L., & Kasl, S. V. (1995). Self-ratings of health: Do they also predict change in functional ability? *Journals of Gerontology Series B: Psychological Sciences & Social Sciences, 50*(6), S344–S353.

Inglis, A. (2007). *Client-centered goal setting for older people in rest homes: Prospective descriptive study.* Auckland, New Zealand: The University of Auckland.

Inouye, S. K., Wagner, D. R., Acampora, D., Horwitz, R. I., Cooney, L. M., & Tinetii, M. E. (1993). A controlled trial of a nursing-centered intervention in hospitalized elderly medical patients: The Yale Geriatric Care Program. *Journal of the American Geriatrics Society, 41*(12), 1353–1360.

Jacobs, S. P. (2010). *Implementation as a systematic manageable process rather than a Pandora's Box of confusion: Reshaping community home care services for older people* (Doctoral dissertation). The University of Auckland, Auckland, New Zealand.

Jacobs, S. P., Rouse, P., & Parsons, M. (in press). Leading change within health services: The theory behind a systematic process for leading the implementation of new services within a network structure. *Leadership in Health Services.*

Jagger, C., Arthur, A., Spiers, N., & Clarke, M. (2001). Patterns of onset of disability in activities of daily living with age. *Journal of the American Geriatric Society, 49*, 404–409.

Kerse, N., Elley, C. R., Robinson, E., & Arroll, B. (2005). Is physical activity counseling effective for older people? A cluster randomized, controlled trial in primary care. *Journal of the American Geriatrics Society, 31*, 817–820.

King, A. I. I., Parsons, M., & Robinson, E. (2012). A restorative home care intervention in New Zealand: Perceptions of paid caregivers. *Health & Social Care in the Community, 20*(1): 70–79.

King, A. I. I., Parsons, M., Robinson, E., & Jörgensen, D. (2011). Assessing the impact of a restorative home care service in New Zealand: A cluster randomised controlled trial. *Health & Social Care in the Community, 20*(4), 365–374.

Kunzmann, U., Little, T. D., & Smith, J. (2000). Is age-related stability of subjective well-being a paradox? Cross-sectional and longitudinal evidence from the Berlin Aging Study. *Psychology and Aging, 15*(3), 511–526.

Langlois, J., Maggi, S., Harris, T., Simonsick, E., Ferruci, L., Pavan, M., ... Enzi, G. (1996). Self-report of difficulty in performing functional activities identifies a broad range of disability in old age. *Journal of the American Geriatrics Society, 44*, 1421–1428.

Law, M., Baptiste, S., McColl, M., Opzoomer, A., Polatajko, H., & Pollock, N. (1990). The Canadian occupational performance measure: An outcome measure for occupational therapy. *Canadian Journal of Occupational Therapy, 57*(2), 82–87.

Lee, L.-L., Arthur, A., & Avis, M. (2008). Using self-efficacy theory to develop interventions that help older people overcome psychological barriers to physical activity: A discussion paper. *International Journal of Nursing Studies, 45*(11), 1690–1699.

Lewin, G., & Vandermeulen, S. (2010). A non-randomised controlled trial of the Home Independence Program (HIP): An Australian restorative programme for older home-care clients. *Health & Social Care in the Community, 18*(1), 91–99.

Lewin, G., Vandermeulen, S., & Coster, C. (2006). Programs to promote independence at home: How effective are they? *Journal of the British Society of Gerontology, 16*(3), 24–26.

McMurdo, M. (1999). Exercise in old age: Time to unwrap the cotton wool. *British Journal of Sports Medicine, 33*, 295–296.

Ministry of Health. (2002). *Health of older people strategy.* Wellington, New Zealand: Ministry of Health.

Mountain, G., & Pighills, A. (2003). Pre-discharge home visits with older people: Time to review practice. *Health & Social Care in the Community, 11*(2), 146–154.

Nadash, P. B. P., & Feldman, P. (2003). The effectiveness of a "Restorative" model of care for home care patients. *Home Healthcare Nurse, 21*(6), 421–423.

Nelson, M. E., Layne, J. E., Bernstein, M. J., Nuernberger, A., Castaneda, C., Kaliton, D., … Fiatarone Singh, M. A. (2004). The effects of multidimensional home-based exercise on functional performance in elderly people. *Journals of Gerontology Series A: Biological Sciences & Medical Sciences, 59*(2), 154–160.

OECD. (1994). *Caring for frail elderly people: New directions in care.* Paris, France: Organisation for Economic Co-operation and Development.

Parsons, J. (2010). *Do older people set goals? A study to determine the impact of a goal facilitation tool on home based support services* (Doctoral dissertation). The University of Auckland, Auckland, New Zealand.

Parsons, J., & Parsons, M. (2012a). *Strategies for optimising recovery tool.* Auckland, New Zealand: The University of Auckland.

Parsons, J., Rouse, P., Robinson, E. M., Sheridan, N., & Connolly, M. J. (2012). Goal setting as a feature of homecare services for older people: Does it make a difference? *Age and Ageing, 41*(1), 24–29.

Parsons, J., Rouse, P., Robinson, E. M., Sheridan, N., & Connolly, M. J. (2013). Restorative home care, physical function and social support. *Archives of Physical Medicine & Rehabilitation, 94*(6), 1015–1022.

Parsons, J. G. M., & Parsons, M. J. G. (2012b). The effect of a designated tool on person-centred goal identification and service planning among older people receiving homecare in New Zealand. *Health & Social Care in the Community, 20*(6), 653–662.

Parsons, M., Senior, H. E., Kerse, N., Chen, M., Jacobs, S., Vanderhoorn, S., … Anderson, C. (2012). The Assessment of Services Promoting Independence and Recovery in Elders Trial (ASPIRE): A pre-planned meta-analysis of three independent randomised controlled trial evaluations of ageing in place initiatives in New Zealand. *Age and Ageing, 41*(6), 722–728.

Patmore, C., and McNulty, A. (2005a). *Caring for the whole person: Home care for older people which promotes well-being and choice.* York, U.K.: University of York.

Patmore, C., & McNulty, A. (2005b). *Making home care for older people more flexible and person-centred: Factors which promote this.* York, U.K.: Social Policy Research Unit.

Pilkington, G. (2008). Homecare re-ablement: Why and how providers and commissioners can implement a service. *Journal of Care Services Management, 2*(4), 354–367.

Playford, E., Dawson, L., Limbert, V., Smith, M., & Ward, C. D. (2000). Goal setting in rehabilitation: Report of a workshop to explore professionals perceptions of goal-setting. *Clinical Rehabilitation, 14*(5), 491–496.

Rabiee, P., & Glendinning, C. (2011). Organisation and delivery of home care re-ablement: What makes a difference? *Health & Social Care in the Community, 19*(5), 495–503.

Rapkin, B. D., & Fischer, K. (1992a). Framing the construct of life satisfaction in terms of older adults' personal goals. *Psychology and Aging, 7*(1), 138–149.

Rapkin, B. D., & Fischer, K. (1992b). Personal goals of older adults: Issues in assessment and prediction. *Psychology and Aging, 7*(1), 127–137.

Reuben, D. B., Rubenstein, L. V., Hirsch, S. H., & Hays, R. D. (1992). Value of functional status as a predictor of mortality: Results of a prospective study. *American Journal of Medicine, 93*(6), 663–669.

Reuben, D. B., Seeman, T. E., Keeler, E., Hayes, R. P., Bowman, L., Sewall, A., ... Guralnik, J. M. (2004). The effect of self-reported and performance-based functional impairment on future hospital costs of community-dwelling older persons. *Gerontologist, 44*(3), 401–407.

Rockwood, K., Howlett, S., Stadnyk, K., Carver, D., Powell, C., & Stolee, P. (2003). Responsiveness of goal attainment scaling in a randomized controlled trial of comprehensive geriatric assessment. *Journal of Clinical Epidemiology, 56*(8), 736–743.

Rockwood, K., Stolee, P., Howard, K., & Mallery, L. (1996). Use of goal attainment scaling to measure treatment effects in an anti-dementia drug trial. *Neuroepidemiology, 15*(6), 330–338.

Rowe, J. W., & Kahn, R. L. (1999). Successful aging. In K. Dychtwald (Ed.), *Healthy aging: Challenges and solutions* (pp. 27–44). Gaithersburg, MD: Aspen Publishers.

Ryburn, B. D. P., Wells, Y., & Foreman, P. (2009). Enabling independence: Restorative approaches to home care provision for frail older adults. *Health & Social Care in the Community, 17*(3), 225.

Sager, M. A., Franke, T., Inouye, S. K., Landefeld, C. S., Morgan, T. M., Rudberg, M. A., ... Winograd, C. H. (1996). Functional outcomes of acute medical illness and hospitalization in older persons. *Archives of Internal Medicine, 156*(6), 645–652.

Sager, M. A., & Rudberg, M. A. (1998). Functional decline associated with hospitalization for acute illness. *Clinics in Geriatric Medicine, 14*(4), 669–679.

Schulman-Green, D. J., Naik, A. D., Bradley, E. H., McCorkle, R., & Bogardus, S. T. (2006). Goal setting as a shared decision making strategy among clinicians and their older patients. *Patient Education and Counselling, 63*(1–2), 145–151.

Schulz, R., & Heckhausen, J. (1996). A life span model of successful aging. *American Psychologist, 51*(7), 702–714.

Siegert, R. (2010). Goal-setting in rehabilitation: Perhaps it is rocket science. *Journal of the Australian Rehabilitation Nurse Association, 13*(1), 4–8.

Smith, A., Cardillo, J. E., Smith, S. C., & Amezaga, A. M. (1998). Improvement scaling (rehabilitation version): A new approach to measuring progress of patients in achieving their individual rehabilitation goals. *Medical Care, 36*(3), 333–347.

Smith, J., Fleeson, W., Geiselmann, B., Settersten, R. A., Jr., & Kunzmann, U. (1999). Sources of well-being in very old age. In P. B. Baltes & K. U. Mayer (Eds.), *The Berlin Aging Study: Aging from 70 to 100* (pp. 450–471). Cambridge, U.K.: Cambridge University Press.

Spencer, J. C., & Davidson, H. A. (1998). The Community Adaptive Planning Assessment: A clinical tool for documenting future planning with clients. *American Journal of Occupational Therapy, 52*(1), 19–30.

Stewart, K., Challis, D., Carpenter, I., & Dickinson, E. (1999). Assessment approaches for older people receiving social care: Content and coverage. *International Journal of Geriatric Psychiatry, 14*(2), 147–156.

Stolee, P., Rockwood, K., Fox, R. A., & Streiner, D. L. (1992). The use of goal attainment scaling in a geriatric care setting. *Journal of the American Geriatrics Society, 40*(6), 574–578.

Stolee, P., Zaza, C., Pedlar, A., & Myers, A. M. (1999). Clinical experience with goal attainment scaling in geriatric care. *Journal of Aging and Health, 11*(1), 96.

Stone, R. I. (2001). Research on frontline workers in long-term care. *Generations, 25*(1), 49–57.

Stone, R. I., & Wiener, J. (2001). *Who will care for us? Addressing the long-term care workforce crisis.* Washington, DC: The Urban Institute and the American Association of Homes and Services for the Aging.

Teal, C. R., Haidet, P., Balasubramanyam, A. S., Rodriguez, E., & Naik, A. D. (2012). Measuring the quality of patients' goals and action plans: Development and validation of a novel tool. *BMC Medical Informatics and Decision Making, 12*(1), 152.

Thome, B., et al. (2003). Home care with regard to definition, care recipients, content and outcome: systematic literature *review. Journal of Clinical Nursing, 12*(6), 860–872.

Tinetti, M. E., Baker, D., Gallo, W. T., Nanda, A., Charpentier, P., & O'Leary, J. (2002). Evaluation of restorative care vs usual care for older adults receiving an acute episode of home care. *Journal of the American Medical Association, 287*(16), 2098–2105.

Tinetti, M. E., Charpentier, P., Gottschalk, M., & Baker, D. I. (2012). Effect of a restorative model of posthospital home care on hospital readmissions. *Journal of the American Geriatrics Society, 60*(8), 1521–1526.

Vita, A. J., Terry, R. B., Hubert, H. B., & Fries, J. F. (1998). Aging, health risks, and cumulative disability. *New England Journal of Medicine, 338*, 1035–1041.

World Health Organisation. (2001). *International classification of functioning, disability and health.* Geneva, Switzerland: World Health Organisation.

17

Goals and Goal Setting for People with Aphasia, Their Family Members and Clinicians

Sue Sherratt, Linda Worrall, Deborah Hersh, Tami Howe and Bronwyn Davidson

CONTENTS

17.1 Introduction

According to Playford, Siegert, Levack, and Freeman (2009), professionals understand goal setting to be a 'process of discussion and negotiation in which the individual and staff determine the key priorities for rehabilitation for that individual' (p. 335). Most terms used to describe goal setting and patient-centredness (e.g. participation, involvement, agreement, interaction, collaboration, partnership, negotiation, sharing) incorporate the concept of at least two parties participating in a discussion about goals. However, for people with aphasia, participation may, at best, be challenging and, at worst, be virtually impossible. In many cases, there are likely to be three parties involved rather than two, because families may need to take a more prominent role in the process.

People with aphasia are a unique health population; aphasia (also known as dysphasia) is a language disorder usually occurring after a stroke which affects comprehension, expression, reading, writing and numeracy. These are people whose thought processes are not usually affected; they have the same thoughts, feelings and opinions as they did prior to their stroke but experience the frustration of not being able to easily or completely translate these into language and thereby communicate with others. Clients with aphasia have expressed this by saying 'Mind – fine, mouth – sometimes' (Newcastle Aphasia Group, 2009) or 'Upstairs very smart. Downstairs crap' (pointing to his head and then his mouth) (Worrall et al., 2011, p. 315).

Despite public knowledge of aphasia being limited (Code et al., 2001; Flynn, Cumberland, & Marshall, 2009; McCann, Tunnicliffe, & Anderson, 2012; Sherratt, 2011), this disorder affects approximately 25%–35% of individuals who have a stroke (Dickey et al., 2010; Engelter et al., 2006). Therefore, approximately one million people in the United States (the same incidence as Parkinson's disease) (National Institute of Neurological Disorders and Stroke, 2010) and around 80,000 people in Australia are living with aphasia (Australian Institute of Health and Welfare, 2010). Aphasia is also associated with more severe strokes, more severe disabilities and a higher mortality rate (Dickey et al., 2010). These individuals are often older and also more likely to be discharged to long-term care or rehabilitation (Dickey et al., 2010).

It is of significance regarding goal setting to take into account the additional effects that aphasia has on the individual concerned, the effect on his or her quality of life as well as the effect on his or her family and friends. Aphasia is known to have devastating effects on all domains of quality of life (Barry & Douglas, 2000; Cruice, Worrall, Hickson, & Murison, 2003; Parr, 2007). People's sense of identity may be crushed (Brumfitt, 1993; Shadden, 2005; Shadden, Haggstrom, & Koski, 2008), and they may feel that their personal strengths and abilities have been diminished. Their competence may be questioned due to their difficulties in normal communication (Shadden et al., 2008). Their relationships with others, particularly family and friends, may deteriorate or disappear (Dalemans, De Witte, Wade, & Van den Heuvel, 2008; Hilari & Northcott, 2006). The lack of closer, more intimate relationships may contribute to decreased life satisfaction and well-being (Lyon, 2004; Parr, 1994). Participation in employment, hobbies and activities they previously enjoyed may no longer be possible and usually decrease post-stroke (Hilari et al., 2010; Natterlund, 2010). New activities may be limited or hindered by the very nature of the disorder. People with aphasia are also at a greater risk of depression (up to 70%) than those without it (Kauhanen et al., 2000). These factors will all impinge on the ability of the person with aphasia to reflect on and express his or her priorities for rehabilitation. Aphasia also is a predictor of longer hospital stays and greater use of rehabilitation services (Dickey et al., 2010). It could be argued that these people have a greater need for relevant goal setting as they have an increased potential impact on the health and care system.

In the relatively few general rehabilitation goal-setting studies that have included people with aphasia (e.g. Armstrong, 2008; Leach, Cornwell, Fleming, & Haines, 2010), difficulties in participating in, or contributing to, the goal-setting process have been considered a major barrier. A key factor is the additional time required to discuss and explore goal options and for clients needs and priorities to be expressed and understood (Armstrong, 2008).

17.2 Goals and Rehabilitation: Finding Out What People with Aphasia, Their Family Members and Their Treating Clinicians Want

In view of the particular needs of this group, and the fact that no previous studies of rehabilitation goal setting had focused specifically on them, we investigated what people with aphasia and their families wanted from aphasia rehabilitation. We conducted in-depth interviews with 50 people with aphasia and 48 family members across three cities in Australia (for more details, see Howe et al., 2012; Worrall et al., 2011). We asked participants about their experiences of having aphasia, or having a family member with aphasia, their goals at different points post-onset, their rehabilitation experiences and what services they would have wanted. We also interviewed 36 treating speech–language pathologists regarding 84* separate goal-setting experiences specifically with the participants with aphasia in this study to explore their experiences of providing therapy, their goals for the person with aphasia and their family members, their perceptions of the goals of their clients and their experiences of goal setting (for additional details, see Sherratt et al., 2011). Qualitative content analysis (Graneheim & Lundman, 2004) was conducted on all interview data using NVivo qualitative data analysis software (QSR International Pty Ltd, 2011) and MS Word software programs.

17.2.1 People with Aphasia

Due to their communication impairment, goal setting with people with aphasia can be a long and convoluted process for everyone involved. In addition, these clients may have coexisting issues related to their cognitive capacity. The complex and abstract nature of aphasia and its effects may be demanding for these clients and their families. Clients may also feel disempowered when dealing with this unfamiliar disorder. Knowledge of the collated goals of a range of people with aphasia can guide aphasia rehabilitation services at various stages of recovery.

The 50 participants with aphasia interviewed in this study comprised 24 males and 26 females with a mean age of 63.9 ± 10.8 years. They had had aphasia for a mean duration of 54.9 ± 43.6 months and scored a mean Western Aphasia Battery Aphasia Quotient (Kertesz, 1982) of 69.6 (±24.2). Nine broad categories of goals were derived from the data (Worrall et al., 2011). First, most participants expressed the desire to be *normal* and to return to the security of their pre-stroke life. Second, all participants with aphasia spoke of the importance of regaining their communication. They described the feelings of frustration, hopelessness, isolation and depression at not being able to talk. Many highlighted aphasia as being of higher priority to them than physical impairments, in contrast to the health-care system's focus on physical impairments. They also expressed a wide range of communication needs which extended far beyond immediate practicalities. People with aphasia spoke about the need for communication to be relevant to real life. Third, one of the most commonly reported goals was that of acquiring information about aphasia and stroke for themselves and their family. Other information needs related to their prognosis, expectations about the stages of rehabilitation, services available to them and the nature of therapy itself.

Fourth, participants wanted speech–language therapy that met their needs at different stages of rehabilitation; the need for more frequent treatment that continued longer was also expressed. Fifth, they highlighted their need for control and independence by wanting to do things for themselves, be part of the decision making of their care, and to obtain information from other sources.

Sixth, many people reported feeling disempowered by their aphasia and wanted to regain dignity and respect, with acknowledgement of their competency. Some sought

---

* Some SLPs were interviewed concerning more than one of the participants with aphasia who were being treated at different stages of rehabilitation.

respect by highlighting their premorbid skills and accomplishments. Seventh, these participants had social, leisure and work goals, which ranged from conversing with their family, chatting with friends and extended to strong desires to return to employment or to volunteer work.

Eighth, a number of people spoke of wanting to contribute to society, particularly to improving the lives of people with aphasia, helping students and increasing public awareness of aphasia. Finally, entwined with communication-related goals, were the prioritisation of goals related to physical function and health. These goals included keeping fit, going for walks and managing other health conditions.

These nine broad categories of goals included goals in areas of social life, work and leisure as well as altruism which are not so well recognized in rehabilitation. While some spoke positively about the services that they received, others spoke negatively about their experiences of the health services, including speech–language pathology. The subtle differences in the accounts of these people with aphasia reflect the widespread impact of a communication impairment on all relationships and its spillover effect on social, leisure and work goals.

The relationship of these clients to speech–language pathologists and other health service providers may have been negatively affected by their impaired communication. This may have disadvantaged them in obtaining or accessing appropriate information and services. This finding encourages services to place the relationships between service provider and user at the centre of treatment (Worrall et al., 2010).

The goals of people with aphasia identified in this study could all be relate to components of the World Health Organization's International Classification of Functioning, Disability and Health (ICF), particularly to the activities and participation dimensions (for further discussion, see Worrall et al., 2011). This indicates that goals across the ICF spectrum are important to people with aphasia and that rehabilitation services need to address these priorities. Environmental factors such as friendship were mentioned by some participants as being important in recovery. Effective services to maintain friendships and reinforce positive relationships with health professionals would address the social isolation, anxiety and depression that are major sequelae of aphasia (Cruice et al., 2003).

17.2.1.1 Case Example

Eleanor was only 39 years old when she had her stroke. She had been working as a nurse. She was interviewed for our study 4 years later, and by this time, her communication was still moderately impaired. Eleanor recalled that the most important thing for her in the early stages, both in hospital and during her 3 months of rehabilitation, was to get home. Despite all the services on offer during that time, she described that period as *bad* and lonely. She refused visits from friends because she did not want them to see her there or like that. In addition to the goal of getting home, she wanted to speak and to get back to her work in nursing. Eleanor described her therapy as *hard* work, and when she showed the interviewer her workbooks, it was evident that her therapist had clearly set out her goals there: speaking, understanding more, writing and compensatory use of gesture to convey her message. While these were well-justified impairment-level goals, they only partially captured the broader goals that Eleanor had regarding returning to work and living independently. Since that time, Eleanor has taken on volunteer work. She felt that her experiences were deeply influenced by her health training and by being a younger person with aphasia, and she remained steadfast in her desire to continue with speech–language therapy and to go back to nursing itself.

We interviewed two of Eleanor's speech–language pathologists for this study. Sarah described spending a lot of time talking to Eleanor about her goals. She talked about 'coming up with a wish list but then also coming up with a list of things that were do-able so that you're not setting someone up to fail…'. Sarah offered therapy thrice a week for a while but was aware of the limits of her hospital outpatient service to address Eleanor's longer-term vocational needs. So Eleanor was transferred to another community-based service. There she had therapy with Martha who recalled that Eleanor arrived with very clear ideas of what she wanted, rejecting impairment-level tasks in favour of functional goals and conversational skills. Martha worked with Eleanor to negotiate her volunteering opportunities and a range of functional language-based tasks to help her to continue to live independently. Eleanor still remains frustrated by her inability to return to nursing but her volunteering keeps her busy and in contact with people.

17.2.2 Family Members

Aphasia affects not only the individual but also his or her family. In fact, family members of people with aphasia are affected more negatively following a stroke than the relatives of those without aphasia (Bakas, Kroenke, Plue, Perkins, & Williams, 2006). However, studies exploring the rehabilitation goals of the family members for their family member with aphasia, as well as goals for themselves, have involved small samples or focused solely on spouses or on family members' needs rather than their goals. In a summary of previous research, Levack, Siegert, Dean, and McPherson (2009) concluded that, generally in adult rehabilitation, family members have been sidelined in collaborative goal setting. The focus for clinicians has been predominantly on the needs of the client and not those of their family members.

In our large multi-centre investigation described earlier, 48 family members were interviewed after being nominated by their relatives with aphasia. The family members comprised 36 female and 12 male family members, aged from 24 to 83 years. Twenty-eight family members were spouses or de facto partners, five were siblings, four were daughters, three were sons, two were parents and six were other relatives (e.g. sister-in-law).

Analysis revealed that these relatives had seven categories of goals for themselves: to be included in rehabilitation, to be provided with hope and positivity, to be able to communicate and maintain a relationship with the person with aphasia, to be given information, to be given support, to take care of their own well-being and to cope with new responsibilities (for a more in-depth discussion of family members' goals, see Howe et al., 2012).

Most family members wanted to be included in rehabilitation, particularly during the early stages, not simply given updates on progress. They felt that being included would give them a better understanding of therapy, how to help, meet other people with aphasia and feel *useful*. Some relatives wanted to be involved so that they could reinforce the speech–language pathologist's goals and provide background information. A few were reportedly not permitted to observe therapy and those whose family member with aphasia lived alone were not always included in the rehabilitation process.

Some family members spoke about the importance of being provided with a sense of hope and positivity, especially in the immediate period post-stroke. They did 'not want false hopes of course, but [they] didn't want no hope'. Hope was considered to be an important motivating factor but participants indicated that many health professionals had been negative. Most family members talked of wanting to be able to communicate with their relative, and some stated they wished they had received some specific training. More specifically, some relatives wanted to maintain their relationship with the person with aphasia in a positive and satisfying way.

The majority of participants expressed the need for information about aphasia, stroke and rehabilitation services. Some were not aware of a disorder called *aphasia* and were confused about the terms *dysphasia* and *aphasia*. Family members wanted verbal information but others wanted written information to refer to later. The information should preferably be in *layman's terms* and provided pre-emptively and perhaps repeated over time. Family members also expressed concern about the level of information that was provided to them.

Most participants identified general, psychosocial and financial support as a goal for themselves in both the short and long term. Some wanted support in a group setting, whereas others preferred one-to-one support. Some participants indicated the need to have their own space and time apart from their relative with aphasia. A few requested long-term respite care so that they could have longer breaks. Many participants had concerns about the negative emotional impact on them in the initial stages. A few participants reported goals relating to their own physical well-being.

Being able to cope with the new responsibilities that had arisen was expressed as a goal by many participants. These responsibilities included financial concerns and new roles (interpreting communication to others, keeping their relative stimulated, incorporating their relative in financial decisions, etc.). Some family members were trying to cope with other caring responsibilities as well as their relative with aphasia. Balancing responsibilities when the person with aphasia lived alone was considered more difficult.

Some aspects of these seven categories of goals have been reported previously (Avent et al., 2005; Denman, 1998; Le Dorze & Signori, 2010; Michallet, Le Dorze, & Tetreault, 2001), but this more comprehensive study includes the perspectives of a number of different types of relatives, not just spouses. Being involved in the rehabilitation of a relative with aphasia may be particularly problematic due to the latter's inability to easily communicate the content and process of rehabilitation. The current study suggests that some family members perceive that inclusion of family members is not happening to the extent that is required. The goals of family members noted here represent what they wanted for themselves. The issue of whether speech–language pathologists are able or wish to set goals for family members to achieve for themselves is debatable. Although it has been specifically recommended that clinicians do not set goals for family members to achieve alone (McMillan & Sparkes, 1999; Randall & McEwen, 2000), this decision may depend on the treatment context, service provisions and/or clinicians' choice.

In addition to goals for themselves, family members also expressed goals they had for their family member with aphasia. A number of the categories overlapped with those identified by the family members as goals for themselves (e.g. improving communication, information). Analysis of data from interviews with family members revealed nine broad categories of goals for the person with aphasia. They were recovery and understanding the future, communication, social contact, stimulation, independence, information, services, hope and positivity and health concerns, both physical and emotional. Family members expressed their concerns regarding recovery and what to expect in the future. While the individuals were in the hospital early on, family members talked about the importance of the person with aphasia getting back home. Others talked about them returning to normal, while some family members highlighted the importance of improving their quality of life and making sure they were happy.

Most family members stressed the importance of improved communication for the person with aphasia. Some relatives wanted an improvement in communication so that the person with aphasia could express their basic needs. Others wished that the person with aphasia's communication could sufficiently recover so that the latter could use the telephone or join in group conversations. Some family members hoped for improved communication so that the person with aphasia could discuss complex issues or manage their own finances.

The significance of social contact for the person with aphasia was emphasized by many relatives. The nature of the social contact ranged from the person with aphasia having the chance to be connected to others in a similar situation to developing and maintaining friendships with people outside of the family. Family members of younger individuals with aphasia wanted their relative to have the opportunity to socialize with people of a similar age.

Relatives of people with aphasia highlighted the importance of stimulation *to alleviate the boredom*. As well as leisure activities, relatives wanted activities available for the individuals with aphasia to keep their *mind[s] challenged*. Family members also wanted their relative with aphasia to gain as much independence as possible. Independence ranged across a continuum, from the relative being able to be left on their own at home during the day to being able to go to the shops or use public transportation on their own. Goals for independence sometimes clashed with safety concerns (e.g. 'I would rather see him get out, be independent... and maybe something terrible happens down the track but at least he's had a shot').

Many family members identified concerns with the services that were available. Difficulties with health systems extended across the continuum of care and included all aspects of health care. Family members spoke about understaffing, and limited, or a lack of, facilities and services in general. Regarding speech–language pathology, family members wanted this to be more intensive (e.g. 'have intensive things right from the word go'), more frequent (e.g. 'to go one day a week is just not good enough'), more relevant (e.g. 'we couldn't find a group... for some kind of bonding with her age group') and ongoing/limitless (e.g. 'it's got to be ongoing, on the communication side of it'). Some family members reported that they had to become advocates for their relative with aphasia in order to ensure that they received the appropriate services. For people who lived alone pre-stroke, family members were often concerned about the lack of appropriate accommodation options available. In addition to their own information needs, family members also wanted the individuals with aphasia to receive information, particularly about aphasia, what they should expect in their recovery and what services were available to them.

As noted earlier, family members considered hope and positivity to be a crucial aspect of stroke and aphasia care for themselves but also particularly to keep their relative with aphasia motivated (*to give them the hope to try for themselves*).

Finally, both the physical and emotional health of the person with aphasia was of concern to their family members. Some stated that their initial concern was that the relative with aphasia would survive. Other concerns include physical issues (e.g. mobility, seizures, swallowing) and mental and emotional health problems (e.g. depression). By becoming aware of the similarities and differences between the goals of individuals with aphasia and their family members, clinicians can provide better services for this population.

17.2.2.1 Case Example

Darren was the main carer for his wife, Margaret, who was nearly 73 years old when she had her stroke. At over 3 years post-onset, Margaret had persistent moderate–severe expressive and receptive language difficulties. Darren was protective of her and had firm ideas about what she needed to help her recovery. He had removed her, against advice, 3 weeks post-stroke from her inpatient rehabilitation facility where she had received at least daily speech–language therapy, saying that the therapists there were too young and were not helping her. Because she had recovered a reasonable level of physical function, Darren brought Margaret home and quickly tried to organize outpatient therapy at their local community health service. Darren's goals for himself were for information and support. For Margaret, he wanted conversation and social opportunities, for her to return to her old domestic duties, especially the cooking, and help to manage her depression. Over a 3-year period, the couple saw three speech–language pathologists, who set the following goals:

- SP1: Harriet's goals: clear yes/no, basic receptive skills, increased basic vocabulary, word repetition, to give information and encourage attendance at a group
- SP2: Claire's goals: talking with family/friends, reading the bible, listening skills, household tasks, group, education, and respite for Darren
- SP3: Vicky's goals: comprehension and expression ability, educating their friends as conversation partners, strategies for conversation repair, attendance at a group

Although there is some overlap between Darren's goals and those of the therapists, a key difference was that Darren did not believe that his wife had any comprehension issues. He maintained that Margaret understood everything and that it was only her expression which was affected. Darren withdrew her early from treatment with Harriet, a move which did not surprise this therapist at all. Claire, the second therapist, saw the couple for about 2 years and they were only transferred on to Vicky, the third therapist, because Claire changed jobs and Vicky also ran an aphasia group which they attended. Darren was complimentary about the latter two therapists, despite the fact that there were overlaps with what they did and what Harriet had tried to do, in particular in relation to Margaret's work on comprehension. In our interviews with the therapists, Claire reported that her goal for Darren was that he would become more realistic in his expectations for speech–language therapy. Vicky said she now offered short bursts of therapy in order to give the couple a sense of hope because Margaret had *plateaued*. All three therapists encouraged attendance at an aphasia group and all commented on Margaret's passivity in goal setting and their recognition of Darren as the goal-setting partner. This case demonstrates that not only are goals important in therapy but so are *how* they are negotiated and the relationships between the parties. All three therapists recognized the need to work on comprehension: Claire couched reading comprehension within work on bible reading, something Margaret was keen to do, and worked carefully on Darren's ability to accept Margaret's deficits. Vicky varied the emphasis on comprehension and expression, to maintain hope and limit a sense of failure. They also stressed the need for the couple to remain socially connected.

17.2.3 Speech–Language Pathologists

Although the term *goal* is frequently used both within and outside of rehabilitation, the concept of goal itself may be problematic to clients and their family members. Even among clinicians, there is confusion and a lack of consensus as to its definition (Levack, Dean, McPherson, & Siegert, 2006), as well as how the goal-setting process should take place (Playford et al., 2000). In our study, we asked speech–language pathologists specifically what their definition of a goal was (Hersh, Sherratt, et al., 2012). Clinicians often commented that in fact a goal was difficult to explain. An analysis of their comments fell broadly into six overlapping general categories. Firstly, goals were described as something that clients wished to achieve so that their wishes acted as the foundation for choices made about therapy. Secondly, comments included in the definition incorporated the aspects of the acronym SMART, that is, specific, measurable, achievable, realistic and time-bound (McLellan, 1997; Schut & Stam, 1994). This reflected a professional perspective of needing to achieve short-term, measurable outcomes which suited the often restricted timeframes for which services were available. Similarly, Levack, Dean, Siegert, and McPherson (2011) found that certain goals in stroke rehabilitation (short time frames and physical functioning) were *privileged* by clinicians; these goals followed the recommendations to be SMART. Goals relating to psychological and social issues or to broader aspects of life after stroke were not set. The similar results from these two separate studies of stroke rehabilitation (for people with and without aphasia in two different countries) suggest that these findings may be widespread in adult rehabilitation. Thirdly, goals were conceptualized as a series of steps or subgoals en route towards an overarching goal; these steps could more easily be translated into discrete therapy tasks. The fourth category reflected speech–language pathologists' tendencies to define goals according to whether they were impairment goals or functional goals and to assume that goals were more likely to be impairment-focused in the acute stage of rehabilitation when the medical model was prominent and functional later down the recovery track. In the fifth category, clinicians expressed the idea of goals as a contract that provided a means to judge how efficient therapy was. These goals were therefore explicit, specific and often aligned to professional rather than client priorities. Finally, clinicians reported that they had implicit goals which were not expressed or written down. Sometimes, these goals were a *silent agenda* that may have involved such things as changing the perceptions or attitudes of the client and/or family member or helping to improve people's confidence, or ability to adjust, what one therapist described as *feeling goals*.

Despite the challenges involved in goal setting, clinicians may have no clear framework to guide them and little specific training in the process (Van De Weyer, Ballinger, & Playford, 2010). Although goal setting has advantages to the clinician (enhanced teamwork, greater workplace efficiency, more structured treatment and increased client motivation) (Doig, Fleming, Cornwell, & Kuipers, 2009; Levack, Taylor, et al., 2006), client-centred goal setting is time-consuming and establishing a meaningful relationship is demanding (Levack, Dean, et al., 2006; Scobbie, Dixon, & Wyke, 2011).

Speech–language pathologists have expressed concern about the appropriateness of the aphasia therapy they are providing (Morris, Howard, & Kennedy, 2004). The research literature has failed to describe what exactly speech–language pathologists are striving for with people with aphasia and their families. The family can be considered as much a client as the person with aphasia (Cruice, Worrall, & Hickson, 2006), and yet people with aphasia and their family members report only rarely participating in goal setting (Byng, Cairns, & Duchan, 2002). Furthermore, only one-fifth of aphasia treatment time was estimated to be aimed at the family and other significant people (Johansson, Carlsson, & Sonnander, 2011).

The 36 speech–language pathologists interviewed were predominantly female (2 males, 34 females), reflecting the 97% female domination of the speech–language pathology workforce in Australia (Speech Pathology Australia, 2002). They worked in six clinical settings, namely, acute and post-acute inpatient and outpatient rehabilitation, private practice, domiciliary (individual therapy in client's own home) and community groups. Almost 80% of the clinicians interviewed worked in either in- or outpatient rehabilitation.

These speech–language pathologists described their goals both generally and with specific reference to those particular people with aphasia that they had treated. As would be expected, speech–language pathologists reported that they formulated goals according to their clients' communication needs (for additional details, see Sherratt et al., 2011). Verbal/ expressive communication was usually the focus and the goals often related to speaking or to comprehension. Some clinicians reported having goals that targeted communication in specific modalities like writing and reading. Other aspects of communication were rarely mentioned. For some speech–language pathologists, the method or activities were reported, rather than the actual goal.

The speech–language pathologists identified and described a number of goals relating to coping and participation. Some clinicians emphasized the importance of establishing a trusting relationship because goals could not otherwise be met. Facilitating participating in social activities for the person with aphasia was naturally an important overarching goal, with family or friends. Support for the person with aphasia, support from these clients and facilitating support networks and a supportive environment were emphasized. In a few cases, clinicians reported that their support goals included acting as an advocate for the person with aphasia in family meetings, guardianship decisions and other legal discussions or *interpreting* medical information. Speech–language pathologists also included facilitation of client-to-client contact, particularly within a group setting.

Goals relating to educating the client were frequently expressed. This was usually in the form of discussion, supplemented by written material. Many clinicians considered this to be a priority goal in treatment. Education incorporated information on aphasia, stroke, rehabilitation and prognosis and sometimes included educating their clients about broader aspects of life (e.g. healthy eating, exercise, depression). The educational goals varied depending on the rehabilitation setting and the needs of the client. The provision of information also served to empower the client and maximize their independence.

Evaluation of the client was also reported as a goal for clinicians. This included formal and informal assessment, monitoring progress, feedback from the client and the relevance of therapy. Formal assessments were used to monitor and evaluate progress. A few speech–language pathologists reported having no goals for their clients, usually in the early stages of treatment or if the clinician was a locum.

A substantial number of speech–language pathologists acknowledged having no goals for family members. For some clinicians, there was no opportunity to include family members due to distance or transport issues or the family member's lack of time/exhaustion. A number of clinicians were restricted in their contact with family members due to the therapeutic setting, therapist's personal preferences or the wishes of the person with aphasia. A few speech–language pathologists emphasized the importance of having family members involved in the rehabilitation process.

The most frequently reported goal of clinicians for family members was education related to aphasia, stroke and the rehabilitation process. A wide variety of verbal and written information was provided to the family in either generic or personally tailored forms. In community settings, information was often sent directly to family members, particularly for those relatives of people with aphasia living alone.

Communication training for family members was noted by clinicians. This included strategies for facilitating communication and strategies for overcoming communication breakdown. Another area of focus were goals relating to coping, support and participation factors for the family members; thus, clinicians supported family members by means of counselling as well as self-care strategies. At times, this involved facilitating contact with external counselling networks or support groups. In some cases, family members provided support to the clinicians by facilitating therapy attendance of the person with aphasia.

17.2.3.1 Case Example

Edwina, an 82-year-old woman with mild–moderate aphasia following a stroke, was an inpatient in rehabilitation when her husband died relatively suddenly. She did not return to the rehabilitation unit after her husband's funeral. She subsequently attended speech–language therapy at an outpatient rehabilitation unit.

Amidst this grief, her only child, Jane, wanted individualized treatment for her mother that was tailored to her mother's health difficulties and also to her mother's 'funny attitude to life'. Jane strongly advocated for her family's right to make health-care decisions and also felt that it was critical for the family to participate in treatment ('I wanted people… to stop treating us as one of a hundred and treat us as *the* one in the hundred, so that – so that we were all involved'). She wanted to participate in her mother's speech–language therapy sessions but was not included. She also wanted support for herself. She felt that she was perceived as being difficult and that it would have been easier if she had been more compliant and did not 'upset their [the clinicians'] routine'. She wanted to be given hope regarding her mother's prognosis but was only told what her mother could not and would not ever be able to do (e.g. walk or talk).

Edwina did not remember goals being discussed but she wanted to read and also have conversations about current events. She was adamant that she did not want to name flash cards or do writing. Edwina did not feel she could refuse to do the therapy tasks given to her. However, she threw her therapy sheets away 'because it was so silly'. Edwina was upset because other health professionals only worried about her arm and her leg, whereas she wanted help with her communication.

Gwen, the clinician, felt that Edwina, due to her grief, was not ready for therapy or goal setting. Nevertheless, Gwen reported that Edwina's goal was to improve her verbal output. Gwen tried to make therapy functional and flexible and 'sometimes I'd just let her have a bit of a chat… and a bit of a cry'. However, Gwen's therapy notes record that 'patient's writing improving to be able to write four to five letter words… then copy and then write with the non-dominant hand'. Gwen stated that she encouraged Jane to attend her mother's therapy sessions but Jane would usually sit outside. Gwen also tried to involve Jane in communication partner training 'not on an official level but a little bit of that sort of thing'.

Gwen stated that she was *devastated* when Edwina discharged herself from therapy because she *had enough*. Gwen felt that it was a challenge for Edwina to attend therapy and that the timing of the therapy was not ideal. Gwen wanted Edwina to continue having therapy because she saw *glimmers of some motivation and some improvement*.

This example indicates how real-life events (in this case, the death of the client's husband) can have a significant effect on the treatment experiences of a person with aphasia, their family and their treating clinician. Although the client had goals, she did not feel it was appropriate to refuse to participate in the (*silly*) therapy tasks she was given. Her daughter, Jane, wanted to be involved in her mother's treatment but felt excluded, unsupported and without hope. The clinician tried to provide functional therapy tasks as well as support Edwina in her grief. The lack of transparency in the needs and goals of the three stakeholders in this example resulted in a frustrating, dissatisfying and unproductive rehabilitation experience for those involved. Gwen, the clinician, summed this up by stating 'we didn't achieve a lot really'.

17.3 Tensions in the Goal-Setting Process

Triangulating the perspectives of the three stakeholders in aphasia goal setting (people with aphasia, their family members and their treating speech–language pathologists) enabled us to gain a unique view of both the matches and mismatches manifested in this process. A comparison of the categories of goals for the person with aphasia (by the participants with aphasia themselves, their family members and their speech–language pathologists) is shown in Table 17.1 and of the categories of goals for the family members (for the family members themselves and by the speech–language pathologists) in Table 17.2.

A comparison between the goals of the clients (person with aphasia and their family member) and those of the speech–language pathologists revealed an overlap in the goals identified by all three parties (e.g. the need for information). However, it is apparent that there were also a significant number of goals identified by the clients which were not expressed by the clinicians. In a few cases, clinicians had goals that were not expressed by either of the client groups. A closer examination of the mismatched goals between the

TABLE 17.1

Categories of Goals for Participants with Aphasia

People with Aphasia for Themselves	Family Member for the Person with Aphasia	Speech–Language Pathologists for the Person with Aphasia
Communication	Communication	Communication
Information	Information	Education
Control and independence	Independence	
Dignity and respect		Coping and participation
Return to pre-stroke life	Recovery and understanding the future	Evaluation
Social, leisure and work	Social contact	Participation
Altruism and contribution to society	Stimulation	
Physical function and health	Health concerns (physical and emotional) Services Hope and positivity	Coping and participation

TABLE 17.2

Categories of Goals for Family Members

Family Member for Themselves	Speech–Language Pathologists for the Family Member
Communicate with the individual and maintenance of their relationship	Communication training
Information	Education
Support	Coping, support and participation
Coping with new responsibilities	Coping
Own well-being	
Hope	
	Participation
Be included in rehabilitation	

two client groups and the clinicians yielded six sources of tension: relationships, hope, communication and translation of identity, unmet needs, influence of context and the translation of goals.

Firstly, the significance of a good relationship with their health professionals, particularly their speech–language pathologist, was stressed by the people with aphasia and their family members, thereby highlighting the centrality of the relationships in contemporary health care (Hughes, Bamford, & May, 2008). For both groups of clients, a constructive and respectful relationship with their clinician was considered to be a critical a *priori* aspect of their rehabilitation; they wanted a relationship that was of value in itself, not merely to act as the necessary foundation for treatment. Older clients have reported that they are not able to discuss personal goals until rapport with their clinicians had been developed (Schulman-Green, Naik, Bradley, McCorkle, & Bogardus, 2006). Speech–language pathologists envisaged the relationship in a different light; they wanted to develop sufficient rapport with clients to ensure the effectiveness of treatment. Therefore, clients considered the relationship as a separate indispensable entity, while clinicians felt this connection to be a necessary underpinning of therapeutic tasks and activities. Some clinicians mentioned particular instances in which rapport had not been adequately established, resulting in limited progress for the client with aphasia. Worrall et al. (2010) have argued that the 'relationship between speech-language pathologists and clients is paramount to successful aphasia rehabilitation, and that managing relationship tensions well is an essential part of the process of therapy' (p. 295). Studies have shown that relationship-centred care results in clients displaying higher satisfaction, better adherence to prescriptions and better physical and psychological health (Frankel & Quill, 2005; Williams, Frankel, Campbell, & Deci, 2000). Family members also spoke of their relationship with the person with aphasia; if these relationships are positive and supportive, clients reportedly have better physical and psychological health and use health care more sparingly (Williams et al., 2000).

Being given hope was the second area of mismatch or tension identified in this study. Hope was considered to be important by the participants with aphasia and their family members. Hope was significant in the way that prognoses were conveyed to them (e.g. 'I think we kept our hope up but we weren't being given any encouragement by anybody' – family member). Clients and family members spoke of the devastating effect when hope was taken away (e.g. 'how dare they take that hope away by saying… I mean that's just kills everything' – family member). Hope also gave the family members motivation to continue focusing on their relative's rehabilitation.

In contrast, while some speech–language pathologists talked about the importance of hope, others discussed the need for acceptance of the disability by the client and their family (e.g. his wife 'wanted him back to normal… and I was wanting her to understand the depth and breadth of aphasia and dyspraxia'). We found that the professionals expressed a desire for acceptance or adjustment, thereby sending a message to clients and families that the aphasia was not going to resolve entirely; this was a difficult message for them to cope with in the light of their hopes for the future and full recovery.

The third tension was communication and the translation of identity. As would be expected, increasing communicative competence was a goal of all participants. Participants with aphasia wanted to reclaim a range of communication competencies, from expressing basic needs to reading books to taking part in conversations on simple and complex topics with their family and friends. Family members also talked about the desire to improve their communication with the person with aphasia, as well as wanting the individual to have a meaningful life. Although speech–language pathologists spoke about communication goals, they often used different language to describe their goals (e.g. 'So it would have been things like practising yes/no questions, working on semantic processing, eliciting automatic speech, and those kinds of, sub goals as well'). In other words, speech–language pathologists were focused on language tasks and transactional language for message sending and receiving. Clients appeared to want both message sending transactional and social interactional language which would allow them to assert their identities, establish and maintain satisfying relationships and function socially.

The fourth tension, unmet needs, included the focus of the people with aphasia on their requirement for information and services. Family members also reported unmet needs, particularly a lack of timely presented information and support. Speech–language pathologists had expert knowledge about aphasia and its effects but were not always providing the personalized and relevant information which people with aphasia and families wanted. People with aphasia and their family members considered aphasia as a family problem and highlighted the need for greater recognition of the impact of aphasia on family members. Family members wanted the opportunity to be involved in rehabilitation; however, speech–language pathologists were at times unable or unwilling to include family members in rehabilitation.

The influence of context was the fifth tension. People with aphasia and family members expressed concerns or goals depending on the stage of their rehabilitation or degree of acceptance of their disability, rather than the context of treatment. For example, in hospital, some clients with aphasia expressed the generalized goal of wanting to go home or return to *normal*. Speech–language pathologists often talked about the influence of context in goal setting, particularly the setting and constraints of their workplace. Hence, speech–language pathologists viewed the home environment as the best place for goal setting but were required to do goal setting in the hospital environment. People with aphasia who were in hospital merely wanted to go home, thereby creating a tension between the goals of the speech–language pathologists and the person with aphasia in hospital. Financial and time constraints can create an environment in which goal setting is restricted (Schulman-Green et al., 2006). Clinicians were often bound by their working context (hospital, clinic, community) in terms of the nature and frequency of treatment, whereas the clients with aphasia were focusing on adjustment, no matter what the context was. Once the client was at home or in the community, speech language pathologists found it easier to set real-life goals.

The sixth tension arose around the involvement of family members in treatment. Family members wanted to participate in the therapy sessions with the clients with aphasia. Many family members felt strongly that they should be part of this process to enable them to understand aphasia and learn relevant communication strategies. Some clinicians wanted family members to be involved so that they could contribute to the therapeutic process. However, misunderstandings arose, with clinicians inviting family to attend sessions but the latter not feeling included (e.g. 'no, they took mum away and did it with mum and then they'd come and tell me afterwards what was wrong with her'). Some family members and speech–language pathologists were ambivalent about family involvement in therapy; some family members did not feel welcome or else considered a therapy session to be an opportunity for respite, while clinicians at times found treatment sessions difficult when family members attended.

The final tension which arose is the translation of goals. Speech–language pathologists discussed the difficulties in translating goals and the tensions that arose during this process. The clients with aphasia and their family members tended to identify broad goals like 'I want to get back to how I was before'. Clinicians frequently reported prescriptive subgoals (e.g. 'it is actually pretty hard to set goals with people with aphasia particularly if [it] …is severe, because the kind of processes that we need to go through are very… a very linguistic based discussion') which some clients found hard to understand (e.g. 'I couldn't quite see where my girl was going with me'). A more transparent process of translating broad client goals into specific goals would provide the clients with a clearer understanding and acceptance of more specific goals.

Tensions arise when the perspectives of people with aphasia and their families are not known to speech–language pathologists and vice versa. Our research has identified areas of tension between therapists and clients in goal setting. To address these tensions and to achieve collaborative and appropriate goal setting in rehabilitation, the process of goal setting and ways of achieving mutual understanding between clinicians, people with aphasia and their families need attention and clarification. Current goal-setting frameworks may not be sufficiently relevant or applicable to these specific clients and therapists. An innovative, evidence-based and *SMARTER* goal-setting process (discussed in the following section) may offer a modus operandi that can be applied across the continuum of care.

17.4 Enhancing the Rehabilitation Goal-Setting Experience in the Context of Aphasia

The acronym of SMART has dominated goals and goal setting in rehabilitation (Wade, 2009b); however, SMART goals may not always meet the needs of clients in rehabilitation (Playford et al., 2009) and tend to be too rigid (Wade, 2009a). Also, there is no single agreed SMART approach to goal setting (Levack et al., 2012) and the SMART paradigm encourages clinicians to emphasize impairment goals that are easier to measure and report (Leach et al., 2010).

Based on the three-way findings of our project on goal setting and aphasia, the SMARTER goal-setting framework was developed, that is, the goal-setting *process* should be shared, monitored, accessible, relevant, transparent, evolving and relationship-centred (Hersh, Worrall, Howe, Sherratt, & Davidson, 2012). This framework does not seek to replace SMART on the grounds that the two acronyms address different things. The acronym SMART is really about the *nature* of the goals themselves, for example, that they should be specific and measurable. The acronym SMARTER instead provides a structure for a more collaborative goal-setting *process*. It emphasizes that the way in which goals are negotiated is important and warrants more attention. Each aspect of SMARTER helps to create an overall framework which captures what the participants in our study described as necessary to support the setting of rehabilitation goals.

The principle of *shared* decision making is inextricably entwined with all aspects of the goal-setting process. All stakeholders in the process indicated their desire to be involved in decisions about therapy. Shared goal setting is founded on accessible information, preparation and discussion. The term *shared* also incorporates effective collaboration with other professionals in order to address people's goals more holistically.

The term *monitored* highlights two key issues. Firstly, it denotes continuous evaluation so that the goal-setting process becomes an iterative process, guiding therapy based on appraisal and feedback. Secondly, monitoring shifts the emphasis from assessment requiring a numeric form to valuing change through a range of creative measures including both quantitative and qualitative assessments, for example, client self-evaluation or family evaluation. The issue of communication access is reflected in the term *accessible*. Information needs to be in an aphasia-friendly format which incorporates additional time, total communication, supported conversation or adaptations of documents. The *relevance* of therapy to people's lives was agreed upon by clinicians and clients. For therapy to be relevant, the goal setting needs to be shared and worked through together. Relevance can be established through ensuring that therapy addresses language use and social communication that holds meaning for the person with aphasia and their communication partners. The connection between goals and therapy needs to be *transparent*. Therefore, there should be clear, accessible records of agreed goals and subgoals and an understanding of the rationale for the therapy approach needed to achieve them. Various creative ways can be used to achieve this transparency, such as goals lists, using metaphor and analogy to explain subgoals and using hierarchies of everyday activities. The goal-setting process emphasizes that goals change with time as recovery occurs and as people encounter different challenges of living with aphasia, that is, goals are *evolving*. People with aphasia reported having different priorities at different stages of their recovery and this highlights the need to revise and revisit goals regularly and providing the opportunity for clients to ask for changes in therapy goals, direction or process. By preparing clients more fully at the beginning of the therapy process, they will be able to be more aware and tuned into their evolving goals over time. The final term, *relationship-centred*, emphasizes the centrality of the relationship to goal setting with people with aphasia. Beach and Inui (2006) asserted that both therapists and clients bring aspects of themselves to the relationship and each party affects the other. Our research findings demonstrate the underlying importance of relationships to all stakeholders in rehabilitation (Worrall et al., 2010).

17.5 Conclusions

In this chapter, we have summarized the findings of the first, large study in Australia which explored goal setting in aphasia rehabilitation from the perspectives of people with aphasia, their family members and their speech–language pathologists. Our interest was what each of these groups wanted from the process, and we had the opportunity to gather their stories, experiences and opinions. Goals for rehabilitation and recovery are individual for the person with aphasia and their family. We suggest that the process for professionals of finding out what these are, and how they change in time, is one that demands time, patience, clear accessible communication and a respectful, supportive and empathetic relationship with both clients and family members. Relevant, timely and quality aphasia therapy rests on a flexible goal-setting process which incorporates SMARTER values, for which all parties are prepared and equally involved.

References

Armstrong, J. (2008). The benefits and challenges of interdisciplinary, client-centred, goal setting in rehabilitation. *New Zealand Journal of Occupational Therapy*, 55(1), 20–25.

Australian Institute of Health and Welfare. (2010). *Chronic Disease Indicators database*. Retrieved 28 December 2010, from http://www.aihw.gov.au/cdi/index.cfm.

Avent, J., Glista, S., Wallace, S., Jackson, J., Nishioka, J., & Yip, W. (2005). Family information needs about aphasia. *Aphasiology*, 19(3/4/5), 365–375.

Bakas, T., Kroenke, K., Plue, L. D., Perkins, S. M., & Williams, L. S. (2006). Outcomes among family caregivers of aphasic versus nonaphasic stroke survivors. *Rehabilitation Nursing*, 31(1), 33–42.

Barry, S. S., & Douglas, J. M. (2000). The social integration of individuals with aphasia. *International Journal of Speech-Language Pathology*, 2(2), 77–91.

Beach, M. C., & Inui, T. (2006). Relationship-centered care: A constructive reframing. *Journal of General Internal Medicine*, 21, S3–S8.

Brumfitt, S. (1993). Losing your sense of self. *Aphasiology*, 7(6), 569–575.

Byng, S., Cairns, D., & Duchan, J. (2002). Values in practice and practising values. *Journal of Communication Disorders*, 35, 89–106.

Code, C., Simmons-Mackie, N., Armstrong, E., Stiegler, L., Armstrong, J., Bushby, E., … Webber, A. (2001). The public awareness of aphasia: An international survey. *International Journal of Language & Communication Disorders*, 36(Suppl.), 1–6.

Cruice, M., Worrall, L., & Hickson, L. (2006). Perspectives of quality of life by people with aphasia and their family: Suggestions for successful living. *Topics in Stroke Rehabilitation*, 13(1), 14–24.

Cruice, M., Worrall, L., Hickson, L., & Murison, R. (2003). Finding a focus for quality of life with aphasia: Social and emotional health, and psychological well-being. *Aphasiology*, 17(4), 333–353.

Dalemans, R. J. P., De Witte, L. P., Wade, D. T., & Van den Heuvel, W. J. A. (2008). A description of social participation in working-age persons with aphasia: A review of the literature. *Aphasiology*, 22(10), 1071–1091.

Denman, A. (1998). Determining the needs of spouses caring for aphasic partners. *Disability and Rehabilitation*, 2(11), 411–423.

Dickey, L., Kagan, A., Lindsay, M. P., Fang, J., Rowland, A., & Black, S. (2010). Incidence and profile of inpatient stroke-induced aphasia in Ontario, Canada. *Archives of Physical Medicine and Rehabilitation*, 91(2), 196–202.

Doig, E., Fleming, J., Cornwell, P., & Kuipers, P. (2009). Qualitative exploration of a client-centered, goal-directed approach to community-based occupational therapy for adults with traumatic brain injury. *American Journal of Occupational Therapy*, 63(5), 559–568.

Engelter, S. T., Gostynski, M., Papa, S., Frei, M., Born, C., Ajdacic-Gross, V., … Lyrer, P. A. (2006). Epidemiology of aphasia attributable to first ischemic stroke: Incidence, severity, fluency, etiology, and thrombolysis. *Stroke*, 37(6), 1379–1384.

Flynn, L., Cumberland, A., & Marshall, J. (2009). Public knowledge about aphasia: A survey with comparative data. *Aphasiology*, 23(3), 393–401.

Frankel, R. M., & Quill, T. (2005). Integrating biopsychosocial and relationship-centered care into mainstream medical practice: A challenge that continues to produce positive results. *Families, Systems & Health*, 23(4), 413–421.

Graneheim, U. H., & Lundman, B. (2004). Qualitative content analysis in nursing research: Concepts, procedures and measures to achieve trustworthiness. *Nurse Education Today*, 24(2), 105–112.

Hersh, D., Sherratt, S., Howe, T., Worrall, L., Davidson, B., & Ferguson, A. (2012). An analysis of the "goal" in aphasia rehabilitation. *Aphasiology*, 26(8), 971–984.

Hersh, D., Worrall, L., Howe, T., Sherratt, S., & Davidson, B. (2012). *SMARTER* goal setting in aphasia rehabilitation. *Aphasiology*, 26(2), 220–233.

Hilari, K., & Northcott, S. (2006). Social support in people with chronic aphasia. *Aphasiology*, 20(1), 17–36.

Hilari, K., Northcott, S., Roy, P., Marshall, J., Wiggins, R. D., Chataway, J., & Ames, D. (2010). Psychological distress after stroke and aphasia: The first six months. *Clinical Rehabilitation*, 24(2), 181–190.

Howe, T., Davidson, B., Worrall, L., Hersh, D., Ferguson, A., Sherratt, S., & Gilbert, J. (2012). 'You needed to rehab…families as well': Family members' own goals for aphasia rehabilitation. *International Journal of Language & Communication Disorders*, 47(5), 511–521.

Hughes, J., Bamford, C., & May, C. (2008). Types of centredness in health care: Themes and concepts. *Medicine, Health Care and Philosophy*, 11(4), 455–463.

Johansson, M. B., Carlsson, M., & Sonnander, K. (2011). Working with families of persons with aphasia: A survey of Swedish speech and language pathologists. *Disability and Rehabilitation*, 33(1), 51–62.

Kauhanen, M.-L., Korpelainen, J. T., Hiltunen, P., Nieminen, P., Sotaniemi, K. A., & Myllyla, V. V. (2000). Domains and determinants of quality of stroke caused by brain infarction. *Archives of Physical Medicine and Rehabilitation, 81,* 1541–1546.

Kertesz, A. (1982). *Western aphasia battery.* New York, NY: Grune & Stratton.

Le Dorze, G., & Signori, F. (2010). Needs, barriers and facilitators experienced by spouses of people with aphasia. *Disability and Rehabilitation, 32*(13), 1073–1087.

Leach, E., Cornwell, P., Fleming, J., & Haines, T. (2010). Patient centered goal-setting in a subacute rehabilitation setting. *Disability and Rehabilitation, 32*(2), 159–172.

Levack, W. M. M., Dean, S. G., McPherson, K. M., & Siegert, R. J. (2006). How clinicians talk about the application of goal planning to rehabilitation for people with brain injury: Variable interpretations of value and purpose. *Brain Injury, 20*(13), 1439–1449.

Levack, W. M. M., Dean, S. G., Siegert, R. J., & McPherson, K. M. (2011). Navigating patient-centered goal setting in inpatient stroke rehabilitation: How clinicians control the process to meet perceived professional responsibilities. *Patient Education and Counseling, 85*(2), 206–213.

Levack, W. M. M., Siegert, R. J., Dean, S. G., McPherson, K., Hay-Smith, E. J. C., & Weatherall, M. (2012). Goal setting and activities to enhance goal pursuit for adults with acquired disabilities participating in rehabilitation [Protocol]. *Cochrane Database of Systematic Reviews,* Issue 4. Art. No.: CD009727.

Levack, W. M. M., Siegert, R. J., Dean, S. G., & McPherson, K. M. (2009). Goal planning for adults with acquired brain injury: How clinicians talk about involving family. *Brain Injury, 23*(3), 192–202.

Levack, W. M. M., Taylor, K., Siegert, R. J., Dean, S. G., McPherson, K. M., & Weatherall, M. (2006). Is goal planning in rehabilitation effective? A systematic review. *Clinical Rehabilitation, 20*(9), 739–755.

Lyon, J. G. (2004). Evolving treatment methods for coping with aphasia approaches that make a difference in everyday life. In J. Duchan & S. Byng (Eds.), *Challenging aphasia therapies.* Hove, U.K.: Psychology Press.

McCann, C., Tunnicliffe, K., & Anderson, R. (2012). Public awareness of aphasia in New Zealand. *Aphasiology, 27*(5), 568–580.

McLellan, D. L. (1997). Introduction to rehabilitation. In B. A. Wilson & D. L. McLellan (Eds.), *Rehabilitation studies handbook.* Cambridge, U.K.: Cambridge University Press.

McMillan, T. M., & Sparkes, C. (1999). Goal planning and neurorehabilitation: The Wolfson Neurorehabilitation Centre approach. *Neuropsychological Rehabilitation, 9*(3–4), 241–251.

Michallet, B., Le Dorze, G., & Tetreault, S. (2001). The needs of spouses caring for severely aphasic persons. *Aphasiology, 15*(8), 731–747.

Morris, J., Howard, D., & Kennedy, S. (2004). The value of therapy: What counts? In J. F. Duchan & S. Byng (Eds.), *Challenging aphasia therapies: Broadening the discourse and extending the boundaries* (pp. 134–157). Hove, U.K.: Psychology Press.

National Institute of Neurological Disorders and Stroke. (2010). *Disorders A-Z.* Retrieved 28 December 2010, from http://www.ninds.nih.gov/disorders/disorder_index.htm.

Natterlund, B. S. (2010). A new life with aphasia: Everyday activities and social support. *Scandinavian Journal of Occupational Therapy, 17*(2), 117–129.

Newcastle Aphasia Group. (2009). *About aphasia.* Newcastle, New South Wales, Australia: HNEH Community Stroke Team.

Parr, S. (1994). Coping with aphasia: Conversations with 20 aphasic people. *Aphasiology, 8*(5), 457–466.

Parr, S. (2007). Living with severe aphasia. *Aphasiology, 21*(1), 98–123.

Playford, E. D., Dawson, L. K., Limbert, V., Smith, M. C., Ward, C. D., & Wells, R. (2000). Goal-setting in rehabilitation: Report of a workshop to explore professionals' perceptions of goal-setting. *Clinical Rehabilitation, 14,* 491–496.

Playford, E. D., Siegert, R., Levack, W. M. M., & Freeman, J. (2009). Areas of consensus and controversy about goal setting in rehabilitation: A conference report. *Clinical Rehabilitation, 23*(4), 334–344.

QSR International Pty Ltd. (2011). *NVivo qualitative data analysis software* (Version 9). Doncaster, Victoria, Australia: QSR International Pty Ltd.

Randall, K. E., & McEwen, I. R. (2000). Writing patient-centered functional goals. *Physical Therapy, 80*, 1197–1203.

Schulman-Green, D. J., Naik, A. D., Bradley, E. H., McCorkle, R., & Bogardus, S. T. J. (2006). Goal setting as a shared decision making strategy among clinicians and their older patients. *Patient Education and Counselling, 63*(1), 145–151.

Schut, H. A., & Stam, H. J. (1994). Goals in rehabilitation teamwork. *Disability and Rehabilitation, 16*(4), 223–226.

Scobbie, L., Dixon, D., & Wyke, S. (2011). Goal-setting and action planning in the rehabilitation setting: Development of a theoretically informed practice framework. *Clinical Rehabilitation, 25*, 468–482.

Shadden, B. B. (2005). Aphasia as identity theft. *Aphasiology, 19*(3), 211–223.

Shadden, B. B., Haggstrom, A., & Koski, P. R. (2008). *Neurogenic communication disorders: Life stories and the narrative self*. San Diego, CA: Plural Publishing.

Sherratt, S. (2011). Written media coverage of aphasia: A review. *Aphasiology, 25*(10), 1132–1152

Sherratt, S., Worrall, L., Pearson, C., Howe, T., Hersh, D., & Davidson, B. (2011). "Well it has to be language-related": Speech-language pathologists' goals for people with aphasia and their families. *International Journal of Speech-Language Pathology, 13*(4), 317–328.

Speech Pathology Australia. (2002). *Labour force survey*. Melbourne, Victoria, Australia: Speech Pathology Australia.

Van De Weyer, R. C., Ballinger, C., & Playford, E. D. (2010). Goal setting in neurological rehabilitation: Staff perspectives. *Disability and Rehabilitation, 32*(17), 1419–1427.

Wade, D. (2009a). Adverse effects of rehabilitation – An opportunity to increase quality and effectiveness of rehabilitation. *Clinical Rehabilitation, 23*(5), 387–393.

Wade, D. (2009b). Goal setting in rehabilitation: An overview of what, why and how. *Clinical Rehabilitation, 23*(4), 291–295.

Williams, G. C., Frankel, R. M., Campbell, T. L., & Deci, E. L. (2000). Research on relationship-centered care and healthcare outcomes from the rochester biopsychosocial program: A self-determination theory integration. *Families, Systems & Health, 18*(1), 79.

Worrall, L., Davidson, B., Hersh, D., Ferguson, A., Howe, T., & Sherratt, S. (2010). The evidence for relationship-centred practice in aphasia. *Journal of Interactional Research in Communication Disorders, 1*(2), 277–300.

Worrall, L., Sherratt, S., Rogers, P., Howe, T., Hersh, D., Ferguson, A., & Davidson, B. (2011). What people with aphasia want: Their goals according to the ICF. *Aphasiology, 25*(3), 309–322.

18

Goal Setting in Stroke Rehabilitation: Theory, Practice and Future Directions

Sheeba Rosewilliam, Anand D. Pandyan and Carolyn A. Roskell

CONTENTS

18.1 Overview of Stroke Rehabilitation

Stroke (cerebrovascular accident) is a major cause of death and disability (Department of Health, 2007; World Health Organization, 2000). It is estimated that 15 million people globally will have a stroke each year, and of these, 5 million will die and another

5 million will be left permanently disabled (World Health Organization, 2000). A stroke results from death of neurones in the brain following a loss of blood supply. Either a block or a bleed in a blood vessel within the brain can lead to a stroke. Following a stroke, a person can present with a variety of sensory–motor and cognitive symptoms such as problems in control of motor function, sensory disturbances, memory, perception, reasoning and concentration. These symptoms reflect the area of brain tissue damaged and also the ability of the brain to compensate for the effects of the damage. Superimposed on these biomedical issues, the consequences of stroke are influenced by the person's psychological and social circumstances such as their confidence, motivation, family support and social support mechanisms. As a result, each person with stroke manifests with a unique presentation of symptoms which require an individualized approach to management.

Natural recovery occurs following stroke, and most of the restitution in function takes place in the first 3 months following stroke (Skilbeck, Wade, Hewer, & Wood, 1983). Recovery tends to slow down or plateau after this period and is typically based more on compensation for impairments than restitution at an anatomical or physiological level. The path of recovery can be influenced by a variety of factors such as early identification of stroke symptoms, access to hyper-acute care (Horn et al., 2005; Indredavik, Bakke, Slørdahl, Rokseth, & Håheim, 1999; Stroke Unit Trialists Collaboration, 1997) with effective interventional procedures (International Stroke Trial-3 Collaborative Group, 2012) and rehabilitation protocols (early mobilization and forced use of limb) (Johansson, 2000).

Many current innovations in acute treatment have reduced mortality rates and improved functional independence following stroke. In the long term, the recovery of function can be influenced by a variety of other factors such as age (with older patients having a poorer prognosis) and other co-morbidities such as post-stroke arthritis, diabetic neuropathy and sarcopaenia (Bagg, Pombo, & Hopman, 2002; Jongbloed, 1986). Outcomes are also influenced by the person's psychological characteristics (such as personality, motivation) and social circumstances (Osborne, 1998; West, Hill, Hewison, Knapp, & House, 2010). For example, it has been identified that culture and religious beliefs may influence the recovery of a person with stroke (Carlsson, Moller, & Blomstrand, 2009; Omu & Reynolds, 2012). However, such psychosocial and cultural factors are seldom considered in the health-care process (Angeleri, Angeleri, Foschi, Giaquinto, & Nolfe, 1993; Osborne, 1998). Thus, stroke recovery is a complex phenomenon with various interrelated factors contributing to the need for complex management strategies.

Currently, no drug treatments are available to reverse neuronal death; hence, recovery following the acute stage in stroke is largely due to natural recovery aided by neuroplasticity. Neuroplasticity is the process by which there is structural reorganization in the central nervous system, and there is some evidence that plasticity can be modulated by the rehabilitation interventions used with these patients (Johansson, 2000). It is recommended that rehabilitation should commence in the acute stages following the stroke in order to capitalize on the natural recovery process and also to prevent the development of secondary complications (Cumming et al., 2011).

Stroke rehabilitation involves multiple health professionals working together in a multidisciplinary team (MDT) in order to optimize the patient's potential in life after stroke (Department of Health, 2001a; Schwamm et al., 2005; Wade, 1999a). Guidelines suggest that such teams will normally consist of a combination of the following professionals:

physicians, nurses, physiotherapists, occupational therapists, speech and language therapists, dieticians, social workers, care assistants, administrative staff, pharmacists, radiologists, recreation therapists, clinical psychologists and specialist medical professionals as required (Department of Health, 2001b; Duncan et al., 2005; Lindsay et al., 2010). The family and caregivers are also considered part of the team in some guidelines, whereas other guidelines do not include them in the team, but advocate a close working relationship with the family and/or carer. It is important that this team delivers coordinated care in order to improve the patient's health and quality of life outcomes. A growing body of evidence suggests that stroke-specific multidisciplinary care can lead to an increase in the number of stroke patients who are alive, independent and living at home a year after stroke (Strasser et al., 2005). Despite these benefits, if multidisciplinary care is not coordinated, then there is a possibility of fragmentation of care delivery which can lead to compromised outcomes (Schwamm et al., 2005).

A key function of the MDT is to assess the needs of the patient and determine individualized goals for the care and future health of the patient (Department of Health, 2001b; Royal College of Physicians [RCP], 2012). Stroke rehabilitation which is directed by the goals set by the MDT has been recommended by most clinical guidelines (Duncan et al., 2005; Lindsay et al., 2010; RCP, 2008; Scottish Intercollegiate Guideline Network, 2008). In the United Kingdom, RCP guidelines recommend goal setting as an integral process in the management of stroke, and this is audited nationally at regular intervals. In the United States, the Veterans Health Administration, Department of Defense (Management of Stroke Rehabilitation Working Group, 2010), has recommended that rehabilitation programmes are guided by common goals set by the patient, his or her family and the MDT. Therefore, formal weekly team conferences are conducted in order to discuss, revise and document goals for each patient (Conroy, DeJong, & Horn, 2009). In Sweden, goal setting based on patient needs and fulfilment of goals has been a key marker for quality of healthcare and health professionals are held responsible for this quality assurance (Wressle, Oberg, & Henriksson, 1999). The Canadian best practice recommendation (Lindsay et al., 2010) for *advance care planning* involves a process of helping the patient to consider their goals, values and preferences. Goal setting therefore becomes the central point around which the whole rehabilitation process is built. A key principle for goal setting in rehabilitation is that the goals should be negotiated and agreed with the patient (Duncan et al., 2005; Lindsay et al., 2010). This principle of collaborating with the patient in rehabilitation processes is fundamental to the currently emphasized patient-centred approach to health care (Department of Health, 2005; World Health Organization, 2007).

The variety of forms and approaches to goal setting indicates a need to review the goal-setting process, discussing its relevance and making recommendations for its use in stroke rehabilitation. However, as research in goal setting for stroke is limited, evidence from neurological rehabilitation areas which included stroke patients has also been widely used in this chapter. This chapter intends to achieve the following objectives:

- Discuss psychological theories related to goal setting in stroke literature
- Briefly describe structures and processes involved in goal-setting practices which are currently employed in stroke rehabilitation
- Examine potential benefits of implementing goal-setting practices in stroke
- Propose methods for effective goal-setting practices within stroke rehabilitation

18.2 Psychology of Goal Setting: Relevance of Theory to Practice

In the field of psychology, much work has been done on the exploration of the cognitive, emotional, behavioural and motivational processes involved in setting goals. Knowledge of psychological theories relevant to behaviour and behavioural change (Antonovsky, 1988; Bandura, 1998; Carver & Scheier, 1990; Deci & Ryan, 1985; Locke & Latham, 1990; Powers, 1973) aids understanding of how patients' emotions, behaviour and thoughts may be influenced during the process of setting goals for rehabilitation (Scobbie, Dixon, & Wyke, 2011).

Some psychological theories and concepts referred to in the scientific literature in relation to stroke goal setting will be discussed in this section. There is a widespread assumption that goal setting is beneficial based on the goal-setting theory of Locke and Latham (1990). Changes in intrinsic motivation achieved in setting and achieving goals, especially personal goals for a patient, may be particularly relevant in stroke patients (Deci & Ryan, 1985). Intrinsic motivation is influenced by emotions which are in turn related to patient values. Thus, a consideration of patient values is pertinent when setting up goals for rehabilitation (Emmons, 1996; McClain, 2005; Parks & Guay, 2009). However, evidence of the usefulness of these psychological concepts (intrinsic motivation and patient values) in goal setting for stroke patients is anecdotal and inadequately researched. Further insights into these theories can be gained from reading Chapters 3 and 11 in this book.

Although the use of the aforementioned psychological theories in the stroke literature has been largely anecdotal, a small number of studies have made more detailed use of specific theories as a means to better understand patient's response and engagement in the goal-setting process in stroke rehabilitation. The following section will look at how some of these theories have been applied as a framework for discussion of findings in studies of stroke rehabilitation.

18.2.1 Perception Control Theory

Powers (1973) proposed, in his perception control theory, that people working towards goals function on the basis of a negative feedback loop, that is, they compare their performance to an intended performance and then try to modify behaviour to reduce discrepancy in order to draw closer to the goal. Such goals are reported to depend on a set of arbitrary hierarchical values ranging from an idealized self-image through to principles and values such as honesty and concrete actions (Powers, 1973). Extrapolating this theory to studies in stroke, it has been found that patients tend to strive for goals aimed towards, or actions that are congruent with, their life principles. These principles usually conform to what they visualize as their idealized self. If one were to idealize oneself as self-made through hard work, then it is possible that one's goal, and ensuing activity, will be oriented towards getting back to work. An example of this, commonly seen in the literature, is a patient's expression of the desire to regain pre-stroke status as their primary goal for rehabilitation (Carlsson et al., 2009; Wressle et al., 1999), regardless of the severity of their stroke. However, professionals are usually of the view that these patient goals are unrealistic and they work towards modifying such goals to those that they perceive to be more achievable.

Building on perception control theory, Carver and Scheier (1990) proposed a meta-monitoring process, which is a cognitive process that monitors 'the rate of discrepancy reduction' (p. 22) between the intended goal and current performance over a period of time. The outcome of this meta-monitoring, that is, the rate of reduction of discrepancy, influences the resulting affect or emotions of the person. For example, if a person perceives that he or she is approaching an intended goal more rapidly than expected, that is, the discrepancy reduces faster, then that person will experience positive emotions. Conversely, when progress towards their goals is perceived to be slow or impossible, there is a risk of emotional distress for the patient. This is demonstrated in a study conducted by McGrath and Adams (1999) where patients with stroke or other neurological disorders frequently described negative emotions such as frustration, sadness, fear and confusion when they perceived that the rate of achievement of goals was slower or was unachievable in contrast to their original expectations. However, it was found that these emotions could be modified through implementation of a patient-centred goal-setting process. This involved setting and approaching goals with a realistic timeline which reduced discrepancies in expected rate of goal achievement with consequent alleviation of the negative emotions.

However, Bandura and Locke (2003) criticized the aforementioned theory, stating that negative feedback mechanisms can only play a role in adjustment of the person's effort to achieve desired outcomes. They argued that humans do not just respond to discrepancies but are primarily capable of forethought and have anticipatory control which can lead to desired motivation and goal-directed behaviour. In other words, goals are capable of directing attention and producing positive action without people being first required to experience negative performance in relation to a goal.

18.2.2 Self-Efficacy Theory

Self-efficacy is a person's belief or confidence in their abilities to perform activities. Self-efficacy beliefs contribute to the level of motivation and performance and predict behavioural functioning in individuals over time and in different situations (Bandura, 1998). The theory predicts that where an individual perceives an increase in self-efficacy, their performance will improve (Bandura, 1997).

Dixon, Thornton, and Young (2007) explored various factors that could influence the self-efficacy beliefs of patients and identified that goal setting could play a major role in improving perceived self-efficacy. Goal-setting process served as a source of information and feedback which enhanced a patient's motivation towards goal achievement. The feedback given during these interactions included information about achievements or the progress they were making in relation to their goals. According to the theory, achievements or task mastery must be self-recognized in order to improve one's self-efficacy beliefs. However, these patients suggested that they relied on the help of rehabilitation specialists rather than self-recognition to identify their progress. Hence, feedback during goal-setting interactions could help with recognition of successes and therefore improve self-efficacy beliefs. The goal-setting process may also facilitate social persuasion, that is, influence of outside agents such as a professional providing encouragement in order to improve self-efficacy. If professionals collaborate with patients in information sharing, determination and achievement of goals, social persuasion techniques can be employed to achieve desired outcomes. Further, theory suggests that raised self-efficacy beliefs can help with coping. However, if a patient is anxious, the protective effect of self-efficacy is lessened (Bandura & Locke, 2003). Therefore, the process of goal setting could effectively incorporate strategies to improve self-efficacy while adopting measures to alleviate anxiety for better coping.

18.2.3 Sense of Coherence Model

Andreassen and Wyller (2005) conducted a study to explore patients' experiences of a self-referral programme of rehabilitation for stroke and multiple sclerosis patients. They found that in the acute phase of conditions such as stroke, patients tried to comprehend their circumstances and made attempts to manage their situation. They attempted this by seeking person-specific information and education, in common with the patients reported in Dixon et al.'s (2007) study. They also perceived a need for psychological support and physical strengthening as pragmatic strategies to manage their condition. Patients whose illness was more chronic and disabling reported looking for inspiration and seeking meaningfulness in their life, while trying to make sense of their situation. These findings were explained based on Antonovsky's sense of coherence model (1988) which is a proposed model of how we make sense of illness and health and build coping strategies. The model comprises three components:

1. Comprehensibility (interpreting the world as rational and ordered)
2. Manageability (a belief about having the resources to cope with problems)
3. Meaningfulness (making sense of the problem and taking efforts to cope with problems arising due to illness)

When people go through major stress, their sense of coherence directs them to a choice of strategy to help them cope. Antonovsky (1988) suggested that this trait is fairly stable in individuals' personality. However, there is an alternate view that this sense of coherence is flexible and tends to shift after major stress such as stroke (Geyer, 1997). This flexibility is evident from Andreassen and Wyller's (2005) study which found that patients with different disease onset (sudden or gradual), and in different stages of their disease, adopted different strategies to influence their sense of coherence. Professionals therefore may need to consider the stroke onset or the chronicity of a condition to understand patients' choice of strategies that best help them cope. Knowledge of the sense of coherence model may help the professional to better understand how patients make sense of their situation, influencing the mutual goals set for rehabilitation.

18.2.4 Hope Theory

One of the frequently reported psychological challenges of stroke is the high incidence of depression (Hackett, Yapa, Parag, & Craig, 2005). Depression can have a negative effect on physical functioning and participation in rehabilitation processes (Herrmann, Black, Lawrence, Szekely, & Szalai, 1998; Teoh, Sims, & Milgrom, 2009). It has been hypothesized that hopeful thinking is associated with lower levels of depression and hence better participation. This was investigated by Gum, Snyder, and Duncan (2006) who measured levels of hope in stroke patients using hope scales (Snyder, Irving, & Anderson, 1991). They found that mild to moderately disabled patients, with *low hope* scores, had a tendency to become depressed especially if they were low in motivation and determination (considered as agency components). Patients who had mild to moderate disability with *high hope* scores were able to maximize their abilities in physical functioning, memory and communication and achieved better participation. However, in severely disabled patients, *high hope* was negatively associated with participation in social activities (Gum et al., 2006). This may be due to these people continually attempting to pursue impossible goals, while concurrently neglecting reachable goals, thus failing to undertake activities that were within their reach. However, given that prior research has generally found hope to be positively associated with better function, Gum et al. were cautious about reading too much into this finding until it had been replicated in other studies.

Findings from Gum et al.'s (2006) study have been explained based on hope theory, which defines hope as a 'positive motivational state that is based on interaction between pathways thinking (planning to meet goals) and agency thinking (goal directed energy)' (Snyder et al. (1991) cited in Snyder, 2002, p. 250). Thinking focused on finding routes to achieve goals is defined as *pathways thinking*. *Agency thinking* refers to the motivational energy that enables the use of these pathways to reach goals. Thus, both pathways and agency thinking are interactive and iterative in goal pursuits. People with *high hope* can invoke both components in order to find ways to overcome obstacles to pursue goals. They can be decisive and flexible; therefore, they will be able to find alternate pathways as needed. On the other hand, in people with *low hope, pathways thinking* is not very strong and pathways are less flexible with no alternate routes. Thus, knowledge of hope theory enables professionals to support positive hopeful thinking in the process of goal setting in order to reduce levels of depression, improve motivation and therefore function (Gum et al., 2006).

Psychological theories shed light on the psychological responses in people following a stroke, demonstrating the value of goal setting specifically with the involvement of the patient in the process. An understanding of these aspects could potentially help facilitate patients' capability to engage in the rehabilitation processes of goal setting. However, research has not adequately evaluated the direct application of psychological models to inform optimal goal-setting practices with more work needing to be done in this field.

18.3 Aspects of Goal-Setting Practices in Stroke Rehabilitation

The interdisciplinary team or MDT* faces the challenge of delivering effective rehabilitation to the person who is left with multiple consequences as a result of stroke. A key aspect of this challenge is to formulate common rehabilitation goals and work towards their achievement (Wade, 1999a). The methods by which goals are set within MDTs vary around the world reflecting geographical, cultural and economic variability (Faux et al., 2009; Slingsby, 2006; Teasell et al., 2009). For example, in countries like India, an elderly stroke patient would rely more on the family for care than the state-funded social support system which is non-existent there. Hence, goals set in this context would be influenced to a large extent by the family. The situation in Japan is also similar in that goal-setting practices tend to devolve more power to the family and decision making is described as family-centred (Slingsby, 2006). Moreover, national variability arising from factors such as health-care policies, care pathways and economic resources has given rise to national guidelines and recommendations that also help to shape local goal-setting practices. The following section will discuss some common goal setting practices described in the literature while simultaneously exploring the evidence supporting their use. The discussion will also highlight potential barriers that may get in the way of the goal setting process.

18.3.1 Goal-Setting Processes in Different Phases of Rehabilitation

As mentioned earlier, rehabilitation following stroke is designed to occur in multiple phases, following the pattern of recovery, with each stage being formally mapped out in certain guidelines. For example, in England, patients tend to move from acute stroke units

---

* For differences between these two team approaches, refer to Cifu and Stewart (1999).

and stroke rehabilitation wards to intermediate care (services that enable independence either at home, short stay facilities or community facilities like a care home) and then to community-based rehabilitation services with 6 week and 6 month reviews in place (Department of Health, 2007). In the United States and Canada, the phases are broadly classified as acute, post-acute (where the patient is medically stable and hence suitable for focused rehabilitation) and community care.

Regardless of the organization of rehabilitation across the continuum of stroke recovery, it is generally accepted that collaborative decision making is a vital part of the rehabilitation programme. This initial step of planning for rehabilitation is usually followed by a period of intervention, then reviews to assess progress and goal achievement.

18.3.2 Role of Assessment and Professional Team Meetings in Setting Goals

The RCP guidelines (2012) recommend that the patient should be assessed by key professionals in the team within 24–48 h of admission to stroke care in order to perform profession-specific assessments. Sometimes, joint assessments by professionals from more than one discipline might be carried out to enable patients to benefit from different professional expertise as seen in a Swedish study by Wressle et al. (1999). These assessments form the basis on which the professionals set goals to inform their treatments (Duncan et al., 2005; Health and Care Professions Council, 2012). However, assessment-based goal setting tends to focus on pathology, impairment and disability (focusing mainly on functional ability and discharge) neglecting other contextual and psychosocial factors as recommended by the World Health Organization (2001); therefore, such an approach frequently leads to the formulation of professionally owned goals (Playford et al., 2000; Wressle et al., 1999).

It is recommended that the professionals use the MDT meeting as a forum to discuss their individual assessments in order to set collaborative goals (Lindsay et al., 2010; National Institute for Health and Clinical Excellence, 2008). However, evidence suggests that these weekly team meetings, originally intending to discuss the condition, life situation and professional goals for the rehabilitation of the patient, have not been exactly fit for these purposes (Baxter & Brumfitt, 2008; Gibbon, 1999). Rather, they have tended to serve as a forum for dissemination of information within the team (Gibbon, 1999) and resulted in minimal decision making, focusing on authorizing decisions made previously in informal meetings (Baxter & Brumfitt, 2008). Gibbon observed that in stroke rehabilitation team conferences, the decisions that were made focused largely on discharge destinations and timelines for discharge or transfers and included limited discussions on current alternate planning and rehabilitation goal setting. Further, Wressle et al.'s (1999) study identified that previously set goals had not been reviewed. This suggests there is a risk that team meetings do not serve the purpose of collaborative team working for goal setting (Levack, Dean, Siegert, & McPherson, 2011) and related issues for the patient, paying lip service in some cases to the multiprofessional approach to goal setting.

18.3.3 Documentation

The guidelines and professional standards of practice recommend documentation of care processes such as goal setting for communication, auditing, clinical governance, quality improvement and legal purposes (Duncan et al., 2005; Health and Care Professions Council, 2012; RCP, 2012). Structured and standardised documents, either locally developed or selected from recommendations in the literature, can be used for documenting and reviewing goals (Harwood et al., 2011; Monaghan, Channell, McDowell, & Sharma, 2005;

Rentsch et al., 2003; Wade, 2009). One example of a locally developed document is the assessment and goal setting document developed by Rentsch et al. (2003). This documentation contained a checklist based on the International Classification of Functioning, Disability and Health (ICF) (World Health Organization, 2001) to categorize issues with body structure and functions, activities, participation and contextual barriers and facilitators, which was used for assessment by the interdisciplinary team. Goals from patient and family were identified at the beginning of the process. These goals, along with a summary of needs identified by the assessment, were the basis on which goals were derived for rehabilitation. The documentation was further used to review goals in team meetings. A preliminary evaluation of this structure showed that since the documentation was holistic, it shifted the focus from impairment-based goals and interventions to more patient-focused outcomes. An added benefit was that, as the process of documentation was collaborative, there was improvement in interprofessional communication (Rentsch et al., 2003). The documents also served as a better tool to review the progress of the patient and modify goals based on the change in circumstances reported at successive weekly meetings. Furthermore, the use of collaborative documents for setting and reviewing goals could ensure that referrals are made to other health and social care professionals who are not a part of the core team such as the clinical psychologist.

18.3.4 Nature and Type of Goals Set

The scope of goals set, in terms of levels of function and time length, seems to vary dependent on certain contextual factors. Due to the lengthy nature of the rehabilitation process, goals are usually expressed as long-term goals and short-term goals by health professionals (Wade, 2009). In the inpatient rehabilitation stage, short-term goals are targeted towards impairment-based outcomes and discharge (Playford et al., 2000). This is driven by the finite length of stay allowable in the stroke rehabilitation unit, 6 weeks being reported in one study (Playford et al., 2000). The stage between hospital-based rehabilitation and independent community living is bridged by day hospital rehabilitation or intermediate care in some countries (Department of Health, 2007; Duncan et al., 2005; Hershkovitz, Gottlieb, Beloosesky, & Brill, 2003). Since this stage of health care usually occurs after the initial period of recovery, or when the recovery is clearly slowing down, the goals for patients in this stage are focused on extended activities of daily living, social integration and overall well-being and less focused on impairment or disability (Hershkovitz et al., 2003). In the chronic phase of rehabilitation, goals tend to be set for a longer period of time, based on the potential for recovery extending up to 18 months (Playford et al., 2000). The patients' goals move from a focus on improving physical ability in the acute stage to gaining increased independence, establishing roles and relationships, focusing on achievement of more meaningful activities for the patient in the later stage (Wood, Connelly, & Maly, 2010). Patients generally try to restructure their lives in this phase and hence their goals tend to be more personalized, broader and life oriented (Reed, Harrington, Duggan, & Wood, 2010). However, therapy professionals mostly defined goals in this chronic phase based on their assessment of activities of daily living and participation based on scales such as the Nottingham Extended Activities of Daily Living and Barthel Index (Playford et al., 2000). These measures are not suitable for assessing the patient's life situation and higher-level meaningful activities which are broader and personalized to the individual. Thus, assessment of needs and goal setting in the long-term or chronic phase must be made more sensitive to the person's unique or individual social context (Roman, 2008).

Wressle et al. (1999) reported that professionals recorded goals of a discipline-specific nature in their own discipline-specific documents. For example, physiotherapy-specific goals commonly focused on developing independence in functional activities (Wressle et al., 1999). The rehabilitation goals for patients were usually set at the disability level by the therapists. Safety of the patient was stressed as a primary concern where mobility was identified as a physiotherapy goal (Wressle et al., 1999). Occupational therapy goals tended to focus on improving activities of daily living, communication, personal care and recommendations for home modifications. Home assessments helped to get a better understanding of the patient's context for rehabilitation and family expectations (Playford et al., 2000; Wressle et al., 1999). Thus, goals could be more relevant to the patient's living context following home visits (Playford et al., 2000) rather than being based on the disability issues.

18.3.5 Patient and Family Involvement

It has been suggested that the patient and their family/carer should be seen as part of the MDT, being involved in collaborative decision making in the goal setting process (Duncan et al., 2005; Lindsay et al., 2010; RCP, 2008). Additionally, as goal setting has been identified as one key element to improve patients' self-efficacy and motivation (Dixon et al., 2007), there is a need for involvement of the patient and their family in the process. However, involvement of the patient and family in an acute setting is often limited due to the focus on gaining medical stability and also the limited length of stay. Patient or family involvement seems more feasible and relevant in a post-acute rehabilitation setting due to the time and effort required for coordination with the family and the longer period of contact with the MDT. One study reported that collaboration with patients and families can occur through health-care teams running group meetings involving professionals and patients' families in order to set or modify goals (Ferguson, Worrall, & Sherratt, 2009). These *family conferences* may include the patient, where the patient is able to participate. However, Barnard, Cruice, and Playford (2010) reported that such meetings were limited in that professionals tended to present information in a stepwise manner and moved on quickly from one step to the other so that the patient was not necessarily able to dissent or negotiate in such meetings. Professionals made their authority very clear by agreeing with other professionals and moved on despite the patient's resistance. Hence, a patient's presence in the goal setting meeting did not always mean that the patient was really empowered to participate in the process. These family conferences were a means to convey the decisions made by the team to the families rather than actively seeking the family's perspective on setting goals. Thus, there is a clear power imbalance observed between professionals and patients during these collaborative sessions. This dominance of professionals in the goal setting process is incongruent with the empowerment and power sharing principle of a patient-centred approach to health care (Mead & Bower, 2000).

18.3.6 Contextual Factors

The early stage of rehabilitation is carried out in the hospital setting where contextual factors often impede the effectiveness of goal setting. For example, the environment itself was not found to be conducive to patients being able to formulate personalized goals (van Koch, Wottrich, & Widén-Holmquist, 1998). In some centres, during the inpatient phase, MDT meetings were conducted in a room distant to the patient, further separating them from involvement in the goal setting process (McGrath & Adams, 1999). By contrast, patients who were receiving rehabilitation at home following an early supported discharge programme were better able to formulate goals relevant to their situation (Langhorne & Widen-Holmqvist, 2007; van Koch et al., 1998). In some cases, local hospital policies influenced practice. For example, some hospitals in Sweden had local policies that affected the clinical autonomy of the practitioners limiting their ability to influence the patient's length of stay (Langhorne & Widen-Holmqvist, 2007). Thus, external environmental and contextual factors such as hospital policies may significantly influence the goal setting process, overriding factors related to clinical and patient need.

18.3.7 Communication

Professionals frequently used informal methods of questioning when communicating with patients about their goals that lacked a specific structure (McClain, 2005). Since these informal methods relied heavily on the communication skills of the professional involved, patient priorities were not always established effectively (Neistadt, 1995). Further evidence of a communication barrier in setting goals was evident from a conversational analysis of goal setting sessions reported by Parry (2004). The study found that patient problems were derived from a structured assessment process. Goals were set for these previously identified problems without asking open-ended questions; patients rarely had the ability to influence this closed process. Therapists proposed goals that patients very briefly agreed with. Patients did have the capacity to seek clarification or express dissent; however, patient views were frequently overlooked and the original goals were rarely revised by the professional.

Stroke nurses by contrast appeared to be less profession-centred in their approach. In a study exploring goal setting in the community, stroke nurses have been reported to perceive that the terminology related to goal setting was misunderstood by patients as *hard to get* rather than *that which can be achieved* (Lawler, Dowswell, Hearn, Forster, & Young, 1999). So they asked for problems, solutions and actions and recorded them as goals in their documents (Lawler et al., 1999; Playford et al., 2000). Therefore, the professionals set goals for the purposes of recording clinical plans of action rather than focusing on the needs identified by individual patients.

It is clear from the aforementioned examples that communication is a key skill for rehabilitation professionals. It involves gaining the participation of patients in order to elicit relevant goals, through negotiation and definition of realistic goals. Parry (2004) offered some strategies for effective use of communication skills in goal setting sessions. She suggested that the clinician must offer an opportunity for a patient to discuss a wide range of problems, guiding this in a prioritised manner. Once generic problems are derived, then questioning can become more focused, with questions specific to the individual's problems and formulated from the patient responses. Even problems that may not be amenable to treatment should still be discussed to clarify the scope of treatment. The reluctance or resistance of the patient in responding can be gently overcome with probing and focused questions. The therapist, on identification of a patient priority, should propose goals with a time limit, justify the goal based on patient's current status and clarify the appropriateness of the goal with the patient. This might sometimes result in a renegotiation of a goal and rewriting some goals in the patient's own words. Further problems are brought up and goals proposed, negotiated and reformulated. Since the unstructured, open-ended questioning method raises issues of communication skills, structured goal assessment protocols are increasingly being used and will be discussed later in this chapter.

18.3.8 Professional Prejudices

Though professional prejudices have been not discussed explicitly as a barrier in the literature, they can limit effective establishment of goals. For example, it has been reported that professionals use the bereavement model to discuss the stages of coping for a patient post-stroke. They predict that patients following stroke have to pass through different stages of coping similar to the journey which follows bereavement or grief (Wade, Langton, Skilbeck, & David, 1985; Western, 2007). These authors suggested that patients are most often stuck in one of the stages of coping which then leads them to develop unrealistic expectations. However, Alaszewski, Alaszewski, and Potter (2004) revealed the patients themselves do not refer to being stuck in these stages. Rather, patients in Alaszewski et al.'s study were dynamically planning and working towards achieving goals they had set for themselves. It was the professional's perspective that the patients were stuck in the stage of *non-acceptance* or *denial* when there was incongruence in goals between the patient and health professional. This led to the patients' goals being classified as *unrealistic*, and hence patients were branded as unmotivated or *stuck* within bereavement stages. Therefore, a reflective awareness of one's prejudices or assumptions is essential for a practitioner. Moreover, awareness that the application of conceptual models may not be generalizable to all patients is essential to maintain the individualistic therapeutic relationship when working towards goal establishment and achievement.

18.3.9 Need for Novel Strategies for Goal Setting for Stroke Rehabilitation

Conducting the goal setting process in stroke rehabilitation has been shown to be complex with multiple challenges (Wressle et al., 1999). Being aware of these challenges can help health professionals make the process more fit for purpose. However, it has been recommended that health professionals need to improvise on current methods or develop new strategies, such as a structured method of information elicitation, for goal setting to be effective (McClain, 2005). Some novel methods have been developed and are discussed in this section.

A dedicated care pathway with predetermined goals based on severity of the condition, functional ability following stroke, predicted prognosis, pre-stroke health status and support of the carers was developed by Sulch, Perez, Melbourn, and Kalra (2000). The predetermined short-term goals, with timeline specifications, were implemented with patients and discussed in team meetings. This predetermined pathway enabled better documentation of routine impairment-based goals for the patient. However, the lack of flexibility and adaptability in this process potentially caused a significant reduction in identification of patient-centred higher-level goals (leisure and occupation) when compared to the conventional method of MDT goal setting. Carer needs were also not fully addressed in this process.

Attempts have been made to improve standards of goal setting based on national frameworks in the United Kingdom (Monaghan et al., 2005). This method involved weekly MDT meetings at each patient's bedside and exploration of patient and carer views on their goals. A document that listed patient problems, prompted involvement of patient and carers and recorded the collaborative goals set was used in these meetings. This method was found to improve documentation of treatment goals and the team members' understanding of the common goals. Further, it improved patient and carer involvement in the process and documented individual patient views on the goals. Thus, this method helped achieve standards prescribed by the national service framework in the United Kingdom (Department of Health, 2001b; Monaghan et al., 2005). However, it is not clear whether the original goals had been modified to accommodate patient views as a result of the discussions with the patient and carer by the bedside.

A large-scale, block, randomized controlled trial (Holliday, Cano, Freeman, & Playford, 2007) evaluated the use of an improved participation structure using a goal setting workbook. The patients were asked to identify the problem areas they wanted to improve in and their priorities within the rehabilitation time frame. Families or key workers were permitted to help in the process. The goals were then refined collaboratively, classifying the goals as long-term and short-term goals, and documented, with a copy given to the patient and the family who attended the goal setting meeting. This approach enabled effective patient participation that resulted in documentation of a smaller number of goals, but these goals were perceived as the patient's own choice and thus more relevant. The derived goals were focused on higher levels of participation such as in life roles. There was no difference in the functional outcomes between the group with higher participation and the limited participation group, but overall, the patients in the higher participation group felt more satisfied with the rehabilitation process.

Another approach has been to use the structure provided by the ICF (World Health Organization, 2001) to organize and document the goal planning process (Alguren, Lundgren-Nilsson, & Sunnerhgen, 2010; Geyh et al., 2004; Rentsch et al., 2003). This approach has been described in detail in Chapter 9 of this textbook, but one example of its application to stroke rehabilitation in particular has been provided by Gustafsson and McLaughlin (2009). These researchers used the ICF framework to classify goals of stroke patients from inpatient and outpatient rehabilitation facilities. The majority of inpatients (78%) in this study designated functional goals such as walking, driving and spending time with family which were *activities and participation* (ICF) goals. However, patients from outpatient rehabilitation identified impairment goals such as movement return, physical well-being and speech and participatory goals such as work and walking. Thus, the use of the ICF framework for classification of goals identified that patients who had been discharged were more aware of the impairments resulting from stroke, whereas patients with acute stroke had focused on higher level of functioning. The authors explain this contradiction by suggesting that patients had to overcome their initial shock of stroke and engage with reality in normal life situations in order to realize the impact of impairments on participation (van Veenendaal, Grinspun, & Adriaanse, 1996; Wressle et al., 1999). This suggests that professionals should be aware of how patients' needs may evolve during the transition from inpatient to outpatient settings and be able to accommodate a refocusing of goals to ensure that they remain relevant to patients' evolving needs. Despite these proposed uses of the ICF framework for goal setting, the need for knowledge regarding the ICF, time required for comprehensive coverage of all aspects and training to use the tools are factors that need to be considered when such tools are developed and implemented in stroke goal setting services.

18.4 Evidence on the Effects of Goal Setting for People with Stroke

Goal setting has been acknowledged as a key element of rehabilitation and is recommended by various guidelines. However, evidence for the effects of goal setting in stroke must be examined to understand the efficiency of goal setting for practice. Further proposals for future research and practice can be built based on this understanding. The limited evidence related to evaluation of goal setting in stroke is summarized in the following sections, concentrating on the psychological effects, functional effects and social benefits of goal setting.

18.4.1 Psychological Effects

An early study by McGrath and Adams (1999), which involved a modified goal setting process, demonstrated positive effects on the psychological status of patients. Self-reported fear and anxiety measured using the Hospital Anxiety and Depression Score were reportedly reduced when the Rivermead Life Goals Questionnaire was used to structure collaborative goal setting (McGrath & Adams, 1999). This improvement potentially arose as a result of patients' improved knowledge about the plans for their rehabilitation, the relevance of the rehabilitation goals to their life goals and due to patients gaining an increased sense of control over the management of their situation. These positive changes in the psychological status of a patient can feed into their sense of self-determination and self-efficacy and therefore can potentially improve motivation (Carlsson et al., 2009; Dixon et al., 2007). Improved motivation could lead to increased participation in the entire rehabilitation process resulting in better outcomes.

Health-care quality assessment, based on patient reports about the care they received, was measured following implementation of a method of goal setting that involved increased patient participation (Holliday, Cano et al., 2007). The outcome measures in this study included patient participation, relevance of goals to the patient, patient satisfaction and physical, social and psychological outcomes. Patients with increased involvement in the goal setting process showed slight improvements in psychological well-being (measured by the General Health Questionnaire). They also agreed that they were enabled to choose their own goals (with more participatory life goals) and hence their goals were more relevant to them. If the goals were personally relevant, the patients seemed to develop an increased sense of purpose, improved confidence and greater self-belief (Reed et al., 2010) – attributes which support effective engagement in the rehabilitation processes.

Patient satisfaction feedback is becoming increasingly important in current health service evaluation. Patients in Holliday, Cano et al. (2007) study who experienced increased involvement in the goal setting process reported higher satisfaction with rehabilitation. Satisfaction with rehabilitation was also enhanced when patients received better information about the rehabilitation process prior to setting goals (Dixon et al., 2007). Thus, appropriate strategies for increasing patient involvement and improved information provision, as a part of goal setting, could improve the overall experience of hospitalization and rehabilitation.

Coping strategies (ability to cognitively and emotionally handle stress) following stroke have been found to be an important determinant of quality of life in stroke survivors (Darlington et al., 2007; Donnellan, Hevey, Hickey, & O'Neill, 2006). The process of setting goals has been identified as a possible mechanism to help patients improve their ability to cope with the consequences of stroke (Carlsson et al., 2009; Dixon et al., 2007). Further research has indicated that patients who adopted coping strategies that included a tendency towards *flexible goal adjustment* (i.e. accepting the consequences of stroke and adjusting their goals at discharge accordingly) experienced significantly better quality of life at 9–12 months after stroke (Darlington et al., 2009). Patients with a *tenacious goal pursuit* tendency as a coping strategy (i.e. who tried to maintain life post-stroke as it was before stroke) also showed a good quality of life in the same time period; however, the association between tenacious goal pursuit tendencies and quality of life was not statistically significant (Darlington et al., 2007). Thus, coping tendencies appear to be predictive of quality of life for patients with stroke and could potentially be a useful factor to target through the creation of new goal setting processes.

18.4.2 Functional Effects

Specific goals that are based on patient preferences and meaningful function can influence performance of tasks (van Vliet, Sheridan, Kerwin, & Fentern, 1995). A functional goal of taking a drink from a cup (with a preferred drink), compared to a less functional goal of reaching and grasping a cup, was tested in stroke patients. The higher functional goal incorporating personal preferences improved movement time and reaction times (van Vliet et al., 1995; Wu, Wong, Lin, & Chen, 2001). More recently, a self-directed rehabilitation programme based on patient identified problem areas and goals with the support of a facilitator in identifying problems and the use of documentation to record and review these goals has shown to significantly improve health-related quality of life (Physical Component Summary of the Short Form 36) and reduce dependency (Rankin Scale scores) at 12 months post-intervention (Harwood et al., 2011). Thus, setting more specific goals that are functional and personally relevant appears to enable gains in goal achievement.

Based on Locke and Latham's (1990) goal setting theory, patients could have been more focused by goal specificity and might have worked harder for challenging and personally relevant goals. However, goal specificity and relevance did not seem to influence outcomes in more complex activities in certain studies (Holliday, Cano et al., 2007; Trombly & Wu, 1999). Patients in Holliday, Cano et al.'s (2007) study did not show significant improvement in functional outcomes even though rehabilitation goals were deemed to be more relevant to the patients. Therefore, effective methods to translate these psychological attributes into better participation in therapy and further functional outcomes need to be investigated.

18.4.3 Social Effects and Team Function

Goal setting has been shown to improve collaborative teamwork so that the team accomplishes common goals (Playford et al., 2000; Wade, 1999b). Further, when carried out by a coordinated team, goal setting has been shown to improve motivation for the team and helps them to deliver patient-centred care (McGrath & Adams, 1999; Suddick & De Souza, 2006). With a modified ward round method of goal setting, team functions (such as documentation of patient goals, team member communication and involvement of patients with the team) can be improved, although these activities do require additional team time for implementation (Monaghan et al., 2005). It can also be noted that goal setting appears to satisfy the team members' aspirations for team cohesiveness. However, somewhat ironically, it has been suggested that there is a risk that greater team cohesion around goal setting has the potential to further alienate the patient from the team process, if their involvement is not actively encouraged (Playford et al., 2000).

18.5 Improving the Effectiveness of Goal Setting in Stroke Rehabilitation

The discussion thus far has explored the benefits of goal setting within stroke rehabilitation. Improvements to current processes have also been identified with a view towards developing more efficient and effective methods of goal setting. A universal method of goal setting for stroke is not practicable due to the variability in culture, systems and guidelines across different countries. Moreover, the shifting needs and attitudes of patients during recovery following stroke cannot be reliant on a rigidly structured goal setting process. Therefore, this section will summarize the principles of best practice for goal setting derived from stroke and related health literature. It will outline some structures and mechanisms which can be adapted to suit local practice, practitioners and the patient to optimize the goal setting process in stroke rehabilitation.

Rehabilitation aims to bring about behavioural change in a patient (Wade, 1999b, 1999c). Rehabilitation processes must consider the relevance of patient goals in order to drive the behavioural change (Bendz, 2000). Thus, goal setting should define rehabilitation needs and the consequential behavioural change following stroke. As each individual has their unique problems and expectations, behaviour modification for the person becomes effective only if the goals focus on their particular needs. Therefore, in order to identify individual problems and set goals that will support a change in the behaviour of the patient, involvement of the patient is crucial, enabling agreement about what change they are willing to participate in.

Additionally, the psychological benefits brought about by patient involvement, such as increased motivation and sense of control in an otherwise alienating hospital environment, could enhance participation in rehabilitation interventions and ownership of health in the long term. Furthermore, involving patients in health-care decision making is seen as respect for the *patient as a person* (Mead & Bower, 2000; Ozer & Kroll, 2002) and thus can result in improved patient satisfaction with stroke rehabilitation. Such patient involvement in setting goals is a key aspect of a patient-centred approach to rehabilitation. Contrary to this logic, professionals have been found repeatedly to not explore the individual needs of the patient. Where health professionals seem to focus primarily on physical, functional aspects and discharge, patients appear to desire goals related to returning to their pre-stroke status (Doolittle, 1992; Rosewilliam, Roskell, & Pandyan, 2011; Wressle et al., 1999). Patients' desire for pre-stroke status is often perceived as unrealistic by professionals based on their own knowledge and experience, and this difference in expectation may contribute to the differences in the types of goals that patients and professionals wish to focus on.

However, this lack of congruence in goals between the provider and the patient could also be due to professionals practising within a largely biomedical model of health care. An alternative to this model is the biopsychosocial model of health care which involves a far more holistic perspective on health and well-being in all care processes (Engel, 1977). The following discussion presents one approach to goal setting for stroke rehabilitation that is built on principles of patient-centred practice within a biopsychosocial framework (Department of Health, 2005; Leplege et al., 2007; Mead & Bower, 2000; NHS Next Stage Review Implementation Team, 2009; Ozer & Kroll, 2002). The proposed patient-centred strategies could counterbalance the challenge of unrealistic expectations by plugging the knowledge and communication gap between patients and professionals.

Goals set during the acute phase of stroke recovery are usually short term, looking at investigating and stabilizing a patient's condition if they are medically unstable, with further referrals based on presenting problems (Wade, 1999b). However, as stroke has long-term consequences, goal setting should adopt a long-term perspective right from the acute stage. Such a long-term perspective requires an understanding of the patient's medical condition and life situation; it is crucial that attempts are made to engage the patient and their family in the process of goal setting even in the early stages (Turner-Stokes, Williams, Abraham, & Duckett, 2000; World Health Organization, 2003).

It is sometimes suggested that patients are too fragile to participate in the goal setting process due to medical instability in the early stages of a stroke. Other reasons such as cognition, communication problems and psychological problems such as depression can be barriers to greater patient involvement in goal setting (Rosewilliam et al., 2011). Hence, goal setting is done predominantly by professionals, in collaboration with the family, until the patient recovers the ability to contribute to the process. As the patient progresses, the responsibility for goal selection should be gradually devolved to the patient as a strategy to enhance their coping and motivation (Bandura & Locke 2003; Darlington et al., 2009; Dixon et al., 2007).

Evidence suggests that many patients do want to get involved in decisions made about their care (Ferguson et al., 2009). They want providers to understand their individual situation and tailor goals to their specific needs (Cott, 2004). Some patients, by contrast, feel inferior to professionals and therefore do not want to contribute to the process (Holliday, Ballinger et al., 2007; Levinson, Kao, Kuby, & Thisted, 2005). Considering these two contrasting patient attitudes, good practice would involve exploring patient preferences towards engagement in decision making as well as evaluation of their emotional status in the first few days of their admission to the hospital. This early assessment of affective and cognitive functioning would give the professional an idea of the patient's ability and willingness to participate in the process. Furthermore, such an assessment could lead to goals and interventions pertaining to these functions sooner (e.g. resulting in goals to improve cognitive and communicative functioning and to therapies involving psychiatrists or clinical psychologists). An improvement in psychological functioning has been identified as contributing to achievement of other more physical and practically oriented goals later on in the stroke recovery process (Prigatano & Wong, 1999).

Another key principle of good goal setting is effective communication (Parry, 2004), which is an essential skill for professionals interacting with patients in a patient-centred way. Communication regarding a patient's condition, the process of goal setting, who the key players are, what their roles are and what is expected of the patient in the goal setting process in various stages all need to be discussed with the patient. The professional should be aware that jargon can be exclusive and even threatening to patients (Lawler et al., 1999) and hence phrases that are simple and used in everyday life such as *problems*, *needs* and *expectations following the hospital stay* are recommended. Information leaflets can be provided for supplementary training but should not be provided in the absence of personal communication with patients.

One consideration when communicating expectations to patients in the early days of stroke is that health professionals have only a limited ability to estimate the potential recovery for any individual with stroke. In these circumstances, it is better to communicate this knowledge gap to the patient and then empower the patient to make realistic goals within the constraints of the information available. It must be remembered that goal setting is a two-way process involving interaction and negotiation with the patient. Hence listening, negotiating and not ignoring patient opinions are further communication skills that will encourage the two-way flow of information (Parry, 2004).

Yet another form of collaborative communication involves the use of written guides and documents to encourage patient engagement in the goal planning process. One example of this described earlier was in the study by Holliday, Ballinger et al. (2007) in which a workbook was given to patients, requiring them to (1) learn about the goal setting practice in rehabilitation, (2) consider their priorities for rehabilitation and (3) define their goals, in their own time, shortly after admission. Further information about this particular approach is presented in Chapter 5.

In addition to the strategies described earlier, it is also useful to formally identify an individual from the team to act as the key worker of the goal setting process for each patient (Barnard et al., 2010; Baxter & Brumfitt, 2008; Harwood et al., 2011; Playford et al., 2000; Strasser et al., 2005). This person can steer the goal setting meetings and coordinate information from the various people involved in the patient's rehabilitation. They can also liaise with the patient and their family before any goal planning meeting to introduce the notion of rehabilitation goals; to find out about the patient's particular personal, emotional and social situation; and to develop rapport with the patient and his or her family. In the goal setting meetings, this person can also take responsibility for running the meeting and for ensuring that the patient's needs and preferences remain prominent in any goal-related discussion.

Further principles of effective goal setting described in the literature include setting long-term goals, encompassing discharge planning and the construction of short-term goals that lead to long-term goals (Playford et al., 2000; Wade, 1999a). Goals pertinent to the patient can be set and broken down into short-term goals (based on activity limitations) working towards higher-level goals (Playford et al., 2000). These short-term and long-term goals are provided with a specified time limit for achievement by the concerned professionals (Sulch et al., 2000).

The process of goal setting can be broken down into several logical steps that can be adopted within a routine care pathway. Of note, however, these steps do overlap, so it cannot necessarily be implemented in an entirely linear manner:

1. Goal exploration
2. Goal discussion
3. Goal documentation and communication
4. Goal review

18.5.1 Goal Exploration

The first step to setting goals is the identification of needs. Though assessments play an important role to derive patient's needs, exploring patient-specific goals may or may not be based on these assessments. The literature describes several methods for exploration of potential goals, ranging from simple unstructured interviews to more formal and tested goal setting tools. As an unstructured approach to goal exploration, an informal conversation between patients and therapists can sometimes suffice, where the therapist simply asks questions regarding possible goals for rehabilitation. This is potentially the most common method for establishing goals in rehabilitation services. However, the goals that are eventually selected on the basis of this discussion may have in fact been predetermined by the professional following their clinical assessments and broached as goals during these informal discussions.

Some practices identify patient-prioritized need areas by asking about typical problem areas and by deriving goals based on the patients' current abilities and what they need to do to function more independently (Holliday, Cano, Freeman, & Playford, 2007; Parry, 2004; Playford et al., 2000). A pre-specified list of problems in stroke can be used to formulate goals in this context. The ICF core sets for stroke provide a good foundation in this regard since they are comprehensive and holistic and cover the majority of domains of health and functioning commonly related to stroke (Alguren et al., 2010; Geyh et al., 2004). Another example of a checklist approach to goal setting is the modification of the

Occupational Performance History Interview (Culler, 1993), which covers patient interests, life routines, life roles and values.

Even though these informal methods have been criticized for their dependence on interviewing skills, their lack of structure (and thus low reliability) and the time it takes to implement them (Kamioka et al., 2009; Neistadt, 1995), these approaches have certain advantages. The interaction between patient and professional, being open-ended, allows the professional to gain a better understanding of the patient's perspectives as a basis for establishing greater rapport. This might include clarifying a patient's usual roles and responsibilities enabling the negotiation of realistic and relevant goals.

As goals are more meaningful to patients when they are set at the level of higher-order life goals, knowledge of a patient's values or motivations in this regard can be beneficial (Siegert & Taylor, 2004). For example, a 72-year-old man who cannot walk after a stroke might have a higher-order life goal related to maintaining his role as the husband and intimate partner to his spouse. If, for this patient, a goal of walking with the spouse to help with shopping is not realistic (due the length of time since stroke onset and other predictive variables), then an alternative goal of mobilizing with a wheelchair in the community can be formulated instead, as it might be the companionship that matters to the patient and not community walking per se. Such higher values or motives can probably be best explored using informal unstructured methods.

In addition to an informal approach, many structured tools have been developed to systematically explore and record goals for rehabilitation. However, there has been limited reliability and validity testing for the use of these tools in a stroke context. The most common tools that are being used for clinical or research purposes, and which have been described in stroke rehabilitation, are goal attainment scaling (GAS) and the Canadian Occupational Performance Measure (COPM). More information on these approaches to goal setting is provided in Chapters 7 and 10 of this textbook.

The Rivermead Life Goals Questionnaire is yet another structured and patient-focused method for the exploration of goals that has been frequently used in practice. In particular, it has been shown to have clinical utility in neurorehabilitation services (McGrath & Adams, 1999). Though it has not been evaluated for reliability in a rigorous research study, it is multidisciplinary, centres on patient values and helps rank areas of stroke patients' lives in an order of personal importance so that goals can be focused in these areas (McGrath & Adams, 1999; Nair & Wade 2003).

18.5.2 Goal Discussion

The next step following the identification of goals is to discuss how feasible they are and to create an action plan for their achievement. It is important that the goals are understood and agreed on by all involved in the rehabilitation of the patient and, importantly, by the patients themselves. This can occur in case conferences in the presence of the patient. Monaghan et al. (2005) have identified that ward rounds by the bedside, instead of a case conference away from the patient, enabled better patient involvement and hence more patient-oriented goals. However, if sensitive issues are to be discussed, it is advisable to leave those issues for later, perhaps to be discussed between the patient and key worker. Issues such as privacy in a common ward, space for meetings, lengthened times and organizing the meeting to facilitate the family's attendance need to be considered if such a method is implemented. This method of involving patients in care planning by the bedside seems to improve communication and relationships with patients, helps patients to realize the professionals' roles and can improve satisfaction and compliance (Laws & Amato, 2010).

Goal discussion with the patient can be complicated by professionals' beliefs regarding their need to protect the patient from experiencing goal failure or loss of hope. Professionals sometimes do not want to make transparent a patient's areas of weakness or to give them any false expectations by discussing goals for areas that may not benefit from intervention (Parry, 2004). Instead, good communication skills must be employed by the professional to explicitly discuss their situation without destroying hope (Gum et al., 2006). Smaller subgroups within teams caring for specific patients can also have their set days for goal setting meetings. The advantage of this will be a smaller number of patients to discuss on that particular day and hence attention to detail and time given for the individual patients (Newman, Ellis, Foley, & Hendricks, 2005).

18.5.3 Goal Documentation and Communication

Documentation of rehabilitation goals is a professional, legal requirement in many countries, including the United Kingdom, for certain health-care professionals (Health and Care Professions Council, 2012). Professionals either document in separate sections of the case notes or use specific goal setting forms. However, in order to comprehensively capture all facets of health issues in a stroke patient (a biopsychosocial approach), various documentation tools based on the ICF have been developed in recent years (Rentsch et al., 2003). It is suggested that these documents are made available to the patient and their family as a motivational and communication tool and not just retained by the professionals (Harwood et al., 2011).

It may not be possible for all team members or all the professionals caring for the patients to be present in the goal setting meetings, and hence an effective system of communication about the goals amongst all members is essential. The National Rehabilitation Hospital model uses coordinators who have the responsibility to communicate the team's goals to all nursing professionals in the team (Newman et al., 2005). Visibility of the documentation is another factor that can improve communication of goals to relevant team members working with the patient.

18.5.4 Goal Review

Reviews of goals should be conducted at regular intervals (Lindsay et al., 2010). Every patient contact session should include a reiteration and review of the current goals. Achievements must be applauded, progressive goals established, any alterations made must be discussed in the meetings and documentation updated. Barriers to achievement of goals need to be identified and discussed. Furthermore, if the intention is to use goals to motivate patients to higher levels of affect in therapy sessions, the patient themselves need to be aware of how they are progressing with regard to their goal, so that they can alter their behaviour and activities accordingly (Locke & Latham, 2002).

Achievement of goals will feed into the self-efficacy beliefs and can contribute to higher levels of affect in ongoing rehabilitation activities (Brock et al., 2009). Hence, goals should be evaluated periodically, either using subjective questioning (self-reported) such as is employed in the COPM or with structured tools like GAS (Turner-Stokes, 2009). Evaluation of goal achievement can be followed up with review and resetting of goals.

Review of goals can however sometimes cause patients to feel dissatisfied with their level of goal achievement since the onset of rehabilitation (Lawler et al., 1999). Their focus may be more on what they are unable to do rather than what they can do. The documentation that provides a timeline of the initial goals and the reviewed goals, along with the achievements to date, can help patients be aware of and perhaps even celebrate their progress. Thus, transparency and visibility of goal setting documents should support patients' and families' motivation by charting progress. This may reduce dissatisfaction with services due to differing goal expectations (Playford et al., 2000).

In inpatient rehabilitation, a review of goals will often benefit from a home visit. The two main reasons for conducting a home visit from a goal setting perspective are (1) to prompt the patient to consider goals relevant to the environment that he or she will be returning to after discharge and (2) to enhance the professionals' understanding of their patient's home context, allowing professionals to initiate activities earlier in the rehabilitation process that will facilitate achievement of goals related to their transition home (e.g. home adaptations).

Closer to discharge home, goals should again be reviewed, with attention towards the patient's next phase of rehabilitation. Long-term goals can be revised at this stage in light of improvements made in the inpatient environment. Here, if the patient is progressing on to another rehabilitation or health-care service, it is advisable to have a representative from that service attend the goal review or case conference meeting in order to help with continuity in the goal setting process across contexts of care. Secondary prevention of stroke and risk factor management need to be built into the goals with relevant actions such as referrals and patient education at this late stage of rehabilitation planning. Most importantly, as goals post-stroke have a bearing on the rest of the patient's life, it is recommended that the patients are given a named contact for future goal-oriented support.

18.6 Summary

This chapter has discussed methods of goal setting prevalent in current stroke rehabilitation practice and suggests methods to improve aspects of goal setting, advocating for a patient-centred approach. However, these recommendations are not based on high-level evidence as the research of goal setting in stroke rehabilitation, especially from a patient-centred perspective, is still in its infancy. As stroke is a condition where rehabilitation is focused on maximizing potential for recovery, all possible methods for enhancing the rehabilitation process should be explored. While substantial challenges exist in the implementation of goal setting, the development of more patient-focused processes appears essential to the delivery of effective and meaningful rehabilitation programmes after stroke.

References

Alaszewski, A., Alaszewski, H., & Potter, J. (2004). The bereavement model, stroke and rehabilitation: A critical analysis of the use of a psychological model in professional practice. *Disability and Rehabilitation, 26*(18), 1067–1078.

Alguren, B., Lundgren-Nilsson, A., & Sunnerhgen, K. S. (2010). Functioning of stroke survivors – A validation of the ICF core set for stroke in Sweden. *Disability and Rehabilitation, 32*(7), 551–559.

Andreassen, A., & Wyller, T. B. (2005). Patients' experiences with self-referral to in-patient rehabilitation: A qualitative interview study. *Disability and Rehabilitation, 27*(21), 1307–1313.

Angeleri, F., Angeleri, V. A., Foschi, N., Giaquinto, S., & Nolfe, G. (1993). The influence of depression, social activity, and family stress on functional outcome after stroke. *Stroke, 24*, 1478–1483.

Antonovsky, A. (1988). *Unraveling the mystery of health: How people manage stress and stay well.* San Francisco, CA: Jossey-Bass.

Bagg, S., Pombo, A. P., & Hopman, W. (2002). Effect of age on functional outcomes after stroke rehabilitation. *Stroke, 33,* 179–185.

Bandura, A. (1997). *Self-efficacy: The exercise of control.* New York, NY: Freeman.

Bandura, A. (1998). Health promotion from the perspective of social cognitive theory. *Psychology Health, 13,* 623–649.

Bandura, A., & Locke, E. A. (2003). Negative self-efficacy and goal effects revisited. *Journal of Applied Psychology, 88*(1), 87–99.

Barnard, R. A., Cruice, M. N., & Playford, E. D. (2010). Strategies used in the pursuit of achievability during goal setting in rehabilitation. *Qualitative Health Research, 20,* 239–250.

Baxter, S. K., & Brumfitt, S. M. (2008). Once a week is not enough, evaluating current measures of team working in stroke. *Journal of Evaluation in Clinical Practice, 14,* 241–247.

Bendz, M. (2000). Rules of relevance after a stroke. *Social Science and Medicine, 51,* 713–723.

Brock, K., Black, S., Cotton, S., Kennedy, G., Wilson, S., & Sutton, E. (2009). Goal achievement in the six months after inpatient rehabilitation for stroke. *Disability and Rehabilitation, 31*(11), 880–886.

Carlsson, G. E., Moller, A., & Blomstrand, C. (2009). Managing an everyday life of uncertainty – A qualitative study of coping in persons with mild stroke. *Disability and Rehabilitation, 31*(10), 773–782.

Carver, C. S., & Scheier, M. F. (1990). Origins and functions of positive and negative affect: A control-process view. *Psychological Review, 97*(1), 19–35.

Cifu, D. X., & Stewart, D. G. (1999). Factors affecting functional outcome after stroke: A critical review of rehabilitation interventions. *Archives of Physical Medicine and Rehabilitation, 80*(5 Suppl. 1), S35–S39.

Conroy, B. E., DeJong, G., & Horn, S. D. (2009). Hospital-based stroke rehabilitation in the United States. *Topics in Stroke Rehabilitation, 16*(1), 34–43.

Cott, C. A. (2004). Client centred rehabilitation: Client perspectives. *Disability and Rehabilitation, 26*(24), 1411–1422.

Culler, K. H. (1993). Home and family management. In H. L. Hopkins & H. D. Smith (Eds.), *Willard and Spackman's occupational therapy* (8th ed.) (pp. 207–269). Philadelphia, PA: Lippincott.

Cumming, T. B., Thrift, A. G., Collier, J. M., Churilov, L., Dewey, H. M., Donnan, G. A., and Bernhardt, J. (2011). Very early mobilization after stroke fast-tracks return to walking further results from the phase II AVERT randomized controlled trial. *Stroke, 42,* 153–158.

Darlington, A. S. E., Dippel, D. W. J., Ribbers, G. M., van Balen, R., Passchier, J., & Busschbach, J. J. V. (2007). Coping strategies as determinants of quality of life in stroke patients: A longitudinal study. *Cerebrovascular Diseases, 23,* 401–407.

Darlington, A.-S. E., Dippel, D. W. J., Ribbers, G. M., van Balen, R., Passchier, J., & Busschbach, J. J. V. (2009). A prospective study on coping strategies and quality of life in patients after stroke, assessing prognostic relationships and estimates of cost effectiveness. *Journal of Rehabilitation Medicine, 41,* 237–241.

Deci, E., & Ryan, R. (1985). *Intrinsic motivation and self determination in human behavior.* New York, NY: Plenum.

Department of Health. (2001a). *National service framework for older people. Standard 5-stroke.* London, U.K.: Department of Health.

Department of Health. (2001b). *National service framework for older people. Modern standards and service models.* London, U.K.: Department of Health.

Department of Health. (2005). *The national service framework for long term conditions.* London, U.K.: Department of Health.

Department of Health. (2007). *Impact assessment of national stroke strategy.* London, U.K.: Department of Health.

Dixon, G., Thornton, E. W., & Young, C. A. (2007). Perceptions of self-efficacy and rehabilitation among neurologically disabled adults. *Clinical Rehabilitation, 21,* 230–240.

Donnellan, C., Hevey, D., Hickey, A., & O'Neill, D. (2006). Defining and quantifying coping strategies after stroke: A review. *Journal of Neurology, Neurosurgery & Psychiatry, 77*, 1208–1218.

Doolittle, N. D. (1992). The experience of recovery following lacunar stroke. *Rehabilitation Nursing, 17*, 122–125.

Duncan, P. W., Zorowitz, R., Bates, B., Choi, J. Y., Glasberg, J. J., Graham, J. D., … Reker, D. (2005). Management of adult stroke rehabilitation care: A clinical practice guideline. *Stroke, 36*, e100–e114.

Emmons, R. A. (1996). Striving and feeling: Personal goals and subjective well-being. In P. M. Gollwitzer & J. A. Bargh (Eds.), *The psychology of action linking cognition and motivation to behavior*. New York, NY: Guilford Press.

Engel, G. L. (1977). The need for a new medical model: Challenge for biomedicine. *Science, 196*(4286), 129–136.

Faux, S., Ahmat, J., Bailey, J., Kesper, D., Crotty, M., Pollack, M., & Olver, J. (2009). Stroke rehab down under: Can Rupert Murdoch, Crocodile Dundee, and an Aboriginal Elder expect the same services and care? *Topics in Stroke Rehabilitation, 16*(1), 1–10.

Ferguson, A., Worrall, L., & Sherratt, S. (2009). The impact of communication disability on interdisciplinary discussion in rehabilitation case conferences. *Disability and Rehabilitation, 31*(22), 1795–1807.

Geyer, S. (1997). Some conceptual considerations on the sense of coherence. *Social Science and Medicine, 44*, 1771–1779.

Geyh, S., Cieza, A., Schouten, J., Dickson, H., Frommelt, P., Omar, Z., … Stucki, G. (2004). ICF core sets for stroke. *Journal of Rehabilitation Medicine*, (Suppl. 44), 36(S44), 135–141.

Gibbon, B. (1999). An investigation of interprofessional collaboration in stroke team conferences. *Journal of Clinical Nursing, 8*, 246–252.

Gum, A., Snyder, C. R., & Duncan, P. W. (2006). Hopeful thinking, participation, and depressive symptoms three months after stroke. *Psychology & Health, 21*(3), 319–334.

Gustafsson, L., & McLaughlin, K. (2009). An exploration of clients' goals during inpatient and outpatient stroke rehabilitation. *International Journal of Therapy and Rehabilitation, 16*(6), 324–328.

Hackett, M. L., Yapa, C., Parag, V., & Craig, S. (2005). Anderson frequency of depression after stroke: A systematic review of observational studies. *Stroke, 36*, 1330–1340.

Harwood, M., Weatherall, M., Talemaitoga, A., Barber, P. A., Gommans, J., Taylor, W., … McNaughton, H. (2011). Taking charge after stroke: Promoting self-directed rehabilitation to improve quality of life – A randomized controlled trial. *Clinical Rehabilitation, 26*(6), 493–501.

Health and Care Professions Council. (2012). *Standards of proficiency for physiotherapists*. London, U.K.: Health and Care Professions Council.

Herrmann, N., Black, S. E., Lawrence, J., Szekely, C., & Szalai, J. P. (1998). The sunnybrook stroke study: A prospective study of depressive symptoms and functional outcome. *Stroke, 29*, 618–624.

Hershkovitz, A., Gottlieb, D., Beloosesky, Y., & Brill, S. (2003). Programme evaluation of a geriatric rehabilitation day hospital. *Clinical Rehabilitation, 17*, 750–755.

Holliday, R. C., Ballinger, C., & Playford, E. D. (2007). Goal setting in neurological rehabilitation: Patients' perspectives. *Disability and Rehabilitation, 29*(5), 389–394.

Holliday, R. C., Cano, S., Freeman, J. A., & Playford, E. D. (2007). Should patients participate in clinical decision making? An optimised balance block design controlled study of goal setting in a rehabilitation unit. *Journal of Neurology Neurosurgery and Psychiatry, 78*, 576–580.

Horn, S. D., DeJong, G., Smout, R. J., Gassaway, J., James, R., & Conroy, B. (2005). Stroke rehabilitation patients, practice, and outcomes: Is earlier and more aggressive therapy better? *Archives of Physical Medicine & Rehabilitation, 86*(12 Suppl. 2), S101–S114.

Indredavik, B., Bakke, F., Slørdahl, S. A., Rokseth, R., & Håheim, L. L. (1999). Treatment in a combined acute and rehabilitation stroke unit: Which aspects are most important? *Stroke, 30*, 917–923.

International Stroke Trial (IST)-3 Collaborative Group. (2012). The benefits and harms of intravenous thrombolysis with recombinant tissue plasminogen activator within 6 h of acute ischaemic stroke (the third international stroke trial [IST-3]): A randomised controlled trial. *The Lancet, 379*(9834), 2352–2363.

Johansson, B. B. (2000). Brain plasticity and stroke rehabilitation: The Willis Lecture. *Stroke, 31,* 223–230.

Jongbloed, L. (1986). Prediction of function after stroke: A critical review. *Stroke, 17,* 765–776.

Kamioka, Y., Yoshino, T., Sugaya, K., Saito, H., Ohashi, Y., & Iijima, S. (2009). Goal setting method and goal attainment measures in physical therapy for stroke patients: A systematic review. *Journal of Physical Therapy Science, 21,* 399–415.

Langhorne, P., & Widén-Holmquist, L. (2007). Early supported discharge after stroke. *Journal of Rehabilitation Medicine, 39,* 103–108.

Lawler, J., Dowswell., G., Hearn, J., Forster, A., & Young, J. (1999). Recovering from stroke: A qualitative investigation of the role of goal setting in late stroke recovery. *Journal of Advanced Nursing, 30,* 401–409.

Laws, D., & Amato, S. (2010). Incorporating bedside reporting into change-of-shift report. *Rehabilitation Nursing, 35*(2), 70–74.

Levack, W. M. M., Dean, S. G., Siegert, R. J., & McPherson, K. M. (2011). Navigating patient-centered goal setting in inpatient stroke rehabilitation: How clinicians control the process to meet perceived professional responsibilities. *Patient Education & Counseling, 85*(2), 206–213.

Levinson, W., Kao, A., Kuby, A., & Thisted, R. A. (2005). Not all patients want to participate in decision making. *Journal of General Internal Medicine, 20*(6), 531–535.

Lindsay, M. P., Gubitz, G., Bayley, M., Hill, M. D., Davies-Schinkel, C., Singh, S., & Phillips, S. (2010). *Canadian best practice recommendations for stroke care* (Update 2010). On behalf of the Canadian Stroke Strategy Best Practices and Standards Writing Group. Ottawa, Ontario, Canada: Canadian Stroke Network.

Locke, E. A., & Latham, G. P. (1990). *A theory of goal setting and task performance.* Englewood Cliffs, NJ: Prentice-Hall.

Locke, E. A., & Latham, G. P. (2002). Building a practically useful theory of goal setting and task motivation: A 35-year odyssey. *American Psychologist, 57*(9), 705–717.

Leplege, A., Gzil, F., Cammelli, M., Lefeve, C., Pachoud, B., & Ville, I. (2007). Person-centredness: Conceptual and historical perspectives. *Disability and Rehabilitation, 29*(20–21), 1555–1565.

Management of Stroke Rehabilitation Working Group. (2010). *VA/DoD clinical practice guideline for the management of stroke rehabilitation.* Washington, DC: Veterans Health Administration, Department of Defense.

McClain, C. (2005). Collaborative rehabilitation goal setting. *Topics in Stroke Rehabilitation, 12*(4), 56–60.

McGrath, J. R., & Adams, L. (1999). Patient centered goal planning: A systemic psychological therapy? *Topics in Stroke Rehabilitation, 6*(2), 43–50.

Mead, M., & Bower, P. (2000). Patient-centredness: A conceptual framework and review of the empirical literature. *Social Sciences and Medicine, 51,* 1087–1110.

Monaghan, J., Channell, K., McDowell, D., & Sharma, A. K. (2005). Improving patient and carer communication, multidisciplinary team working and goal setting in stroke rehabilitation. *Clinical Rehabilitation, 19,* 194–199.

Nair, K. P. S., & Wade, D. T. (2003). Changes in life goals of people with neurological disabilities. *Clinical Rehabilitation, 17,* 797–803.

National Institute for Health and Clinical Excellence. (2008). *NICE clinical guideline 68 stroke: Diagnosis and initial management of acute stroke and transient ischaemic attack (TIA).* London, U.K.: National Institute for Health and Clinical Excellence.

Neistadt, M. E. (1995). Methods of assessing clients' priorities: A survey of adult physical dysfunction settings. *American Journal of Occupational Therapy, 49*(5), 428–436.

Newman, E., Ellis, C., Foley, M., & Hendricks, J. (2005). A new approach to patient-centered care. *Topics in Stroke Rehabilitation, 12*(2), 57–64.

NHS Next Stage Review Implementation Team. (2009). *High quality care for all: Our journey so far.* London, U.K.: Department of Health.

Omu, O., & Reynolds, F. (2012). Health professionals' perceptions of cultural influences on stroke experiences and rehabilitation in Kuwait. *Disability and Rehabilitation, 34*(2), 119–127.

Osborne, J. R. (1998). Psychological behavioural and environmental influences on stroke recovery. *Topics in Stroke Rehabilitation, 5*(2), 45–53.

Ozer, M. N., & Kroll, T. (2002). Patient-centered rehabilitation: Problems and opportunities. *Critical Reviews in Physical and Rehabilitation Medicine, 14*(3–4), 273–289.

Parks, L., & Guay, R. P. (2009). Personality, values and motivation. *Personality and Individual Differences, 47,* 675–684.

Parry, R. H. (2004). Communication during goal setting in physiotherapy treatment sessions. *Clinical Rehabilitation, 18,* 668–682.

Playford, E. D., Dawson, L., Limbert, V., Smith, M., Ward, C. D., & Wells, R. (2000). Goal setting in rehabilitation: Report of a workshop to explore professionals' perceptions of goal setting. *Clinical Rehabilitation, 14,* 491–496.

Powers, W. T. (1973). *Behavior: The control of perception.* Chicago, IL: Adine.

Prigatano, G. P., & Wong, J. L. (1999). Cognitive and affective improvement in brain dysfunctional patients who achieve inpatient rehabilitation goals. *Archives of Physical Medicine and Rehabilitation, 80,* 77–84.

Reed, M., Harrington, R., Duggan, A., & Wood, V. A. (2010). Meeting stroke survivors' perceived needs: A qualitative study of a community-based exercise and education scheme. *Clinical Rehabilitation, 24,* 16–25.

Rentsch, H. P., Bucher, P., Nyffeler, I. D., Wolf, C., Hefti, H., Fluri, E., ... Boyer, I. (2003). The implementation of the 'International Classification of Functioning, Disability and Health' (ICF) in daily practice of neurorehabilitation: An interdisciplinary project at the Kantonsspital of Lucerne, Switzerland. *Disability and Rehabilitation, 25*(8), 411–421.

Roman, M. W. (2008). Lessons learned from a school for stroke recovery. *Topics in Stroke Rehabilitation, 15*(1), 59–71.

Rosewilliam, S., Roskell, C. A., & Pandyan, A. D. (2011). A systematic review and synthesis of the quantitative and qualitative evidence behind patient-centred goal setting in stroke rehabilitation. *Clinical Rehabilitation, 25*(6), 501–514.

Royal College of Physicians (RCP) — The Intercollegiate Working Party for Stroke. (2012). *National clinical guidelines for stroke* (3rd ed.). London, U.K.: Royal College of Physicians.

Schwamm, L. H., Pancioli, A., Acker, J. E., III, Goldstein, L. B., Zorowitz, R. D., Shephard, T. J., ... Adams, R. J. (2005). Recommendations for the establishment of stroke systems of care: Recommendations from the American Stroke Association's Task Force on the Development of Stroke Systems Task Force Members. *Stroke, 36,* 690–703.

Scobbie, L., Dixon, D., & Wyke, S. (2011). Goal setting and action planning in the rehabilitation setting: Development of a theoretically informed practice framework. *Clinical Rehabilitation, 25,* 468–482.

Scottish Intercollegiate Guideline Network. (2002). *Management of patients with stroke – Rehabilitation, prevention and management of complications, and discharge planning.* Edinburgh, Scotland: Scottish Intercollegiate Guideline Network.

Siegert, R., & Taylor, W. J. (2004). Theoretical aspects of goal setting and motivation in rehabilitation. *Disability and Rehabilitation, 26*(1), 1–8.

Skilbeck, C. E., Wade, D. T., Hewer, R. L., & Wood, V. A. (1983). Recovery after stroke. *Journal of Neurology, Neurosurgery, and Psychiatry, 46,* 5–8.

Slingsby, B. T. (2006). Professional approaches to stroke treatment in Japan: A relationship-centred model. *Journal of Evaluation in Clinical Practice, 12*(2), 218–226.

Snyder, C. R. (2002). Hope theory: Rainbows in the mind. *Psychological Inquiry, 13*(4), 249–275.

Snyder, C. R., Irving, L., & Anderson, J. R. (1991). Hope and health: Measuring the will and ways. In C. R. Snyder & D. R. Forsyth (Eds.), *Handbook of social and clinical psychology: The health perspective* (pp. 285–305). Elmsford, NY: Pergamon Press.

Strasser, D. C., Falconer, J. A., Herrin, J. S., Bowen, S. E., Stevens, A. B., & Uomoto, J. (2005). Team functioning and patient outcomes in stroke rehabilitation. *Archives of Physical Medicine and Rehabilitation, 86,* 403–409.

Suddick, K. M., & De Souza, L. (2006). Therapists' experiences and perceptions of teamwork in neurological rehabilitation: Reasoning behind the team approach, structure and composition of the team and team working processes. *Physiotherapy Research International, 11*(2), 72–83.

Sulch, D., Perez, I., Melbourn, A., & Kalra, L.(2000). Randomized controlled trial of integrated (managed) care pathway for stroke. *Stroke, 31*, 1929–1934.

Teasell, R., Meyer, M. J., McClure, A., Pan, C., Murie-Fernandez, M., Foley, N., & Salter, K. (2009). Stroke rehabilitation: An international perspective. *Topics in Stroke Rehabilitation, 16*(1), 44–56.

Teoh, V., Sims, J., & Milgrom. J.(2009). Psychosocial predictors of quality of life in a sample of community-dwelling stroke survivors: A longitudinal study. *Topics in Stroke Rehabilitation, 16*(2), 157–166.

The Stroke Unit Trialists' Collaboration (SUT). (1997). A collaborative systematic review of the randomised trials of organised inpatient (stroke unit) care after stroke. *British Medical Journal, 314*, 1151–1159.

Trombly, C. A., & Wu, C. Y. (1999). Effect of rehabilitation tasks on organization of movement after stroke. *American Journal of Occupational Therapy, 53*(4), 333–344.

Turner-Stokes, L. (2009). Goal attainment scaling (GAS) in rehabilitation: A practical guide. *Clinical Rehabilitation, 23*(4), 362–370.

Turner-Stokes, L., Williams, H., Abraham, R., & Duckett, S. (2000). Clinical standards for inpatient specialist rehabilitation services in the UK. *Clinical Rehabilitation, 14*, 468–480.

van Koch, L., Wottrich, A. W., & Widén-Holmquist, L. (1998). Rehabilitation in the home versus the hospital: The importance of the context. *Disability and Rehabilitation, 20*(10), 367–372.

van Veenendaal, H. V., Grinspun, D. R., & Adriaanse, H. P. (1996). Educational needs of stroke survivors and their family members, as perceived by themselves and by health professionals. *Patient Education and Counselling, 28*, 1089–1103.

van Vliet, P., Sheridan, M., Kerwin, D. G., & Fentern, P. (1995). The influence of functional goals on the kinematics of reaching following stroke. *Neurology Report, 19*, 11–16.

Wade, D. T. (1999a). Goal planning in stroke rehabilitation: What? *Topics in Stroke Rehabilitation, 6*(2), 8–15.

Wade, D. T. (1999b). Goal planning in rehabilitation: Why? *Topics in Stroke Rehabilitation, 6*(2), 1–7.

Wade, D. T. (1999c) Goal planning in stroke rehabilitation: Evidence. *Topics in Stroke Rehabilitation, 6*(2), 37–42.

Wade, D. T. (2009). Goal setting in rehabilitation: An overview of what, why and how. *Clinical Rehabilitation, 23*, 291–295.

Wade, D. T., Langton, H. R., Skilbeck, C. E., & David, R. M. (1985). *Stroke: A critical approach to diagnosis, treatment and management.* London, U.K.: Chapman and Hall Medical.

West, R., Hill, K., Hewison, J., Knapp, P., & House, A. (2010). Psychological disorders after stroke are an important influence on functional outcomes. *Stroke, 41*, 1723–1727.

Western, H. (2007). Altered living: Coping, hope and quality of life after stroke. *British Journal of Nursing, 16*(20), 1266–1270.

Wood, J. P., Connelly, D. M., & Maly, M. R. (2010). Getting back to real living: A qualitative study of the process of community reintegration after stroke. *Clinical Rehabilitation, 24*, 1045–1056.

World Health Organization. (2000). *The world health report 2000.* Geneva, Switzerland: World Health Organization.

World Health Organization. (2001). *International classification functioning, disability and health (ICF).* Geneva, Switzerland: World Health Organization.

World Health Organization. (2003). *Key policy issues in long term care.* Geneva, Switzerland: World Health Organization.

World Health Organization. (2007). *People centred care: A policy frame work.* Geneva, Switzerland: World Health Organization.

Wressle, E. B., Oberg, B., & Henriksson, C. (1999). The rehabilitation process for the geriatric stroke patient – An exploratory study of goal setting and interventions. *Disability and Rehabilitation, 21*(2), 80–87.

Wu, C., Wong, M.-K., Lin, K.-C., & Chen, H.-C. (2001). Effects of task goal and personal preference on seated reaching kinematics after stroke. *Stroke, 32*, 70–76.

Section IV

Conclusion

19

Concluding Comments, Current Trends and Future Directions

Richard J. Siegert and William M.M. Levack

CONTENTS

19.1 Introduction

As avid consumers of the goal-setting research literature, we have on more than one occasion been rather critical of the evidence in support of its effectiveness. However, this book and the many fine chapters comprising it demonstrate unequivocally that goal setting is flourishing in rehabilitation and that strenuous efforts are being made by researchers and clinicians around the world to develop better theory and stronger evidence to underpin its practice. Indeed, one of the most striking features of the book is the sheer diversity evident across its chapters. This diversity extends to the purposes goal setting is used for, the conditions or disorders with which it is applied and the actual ways of *goal setting* with patients or clients. In closing this book, we wish to speculate a little about just where the future developments in rehabilitation goal setting might lie and to make some recommendations about how rehabilitation teams might think about their own goal-setting practice.

We suspect that, increasingly, goal setting, both in routine clinical practice and in the research literature, will be characterized by (1) greater diversity, (2) greater specificity and (3) greater sophistication. Diversity refers to increasing divergence in the many ways that goal setting will be practised in the future. Specificity refers to the notion that how we practise goal setting will be increasingly defined by the unique characteristics of the patient or client and the context in which goal setting happens. Sophistication refers to increasingly explicit application of robust theory to goal-setting practice and to a growing evidence base to support it. So, in the rehabilitation services of the future, we expect to see a diverse range of goal-setting approaches being employed to address specific aims in specific rehabilitation settings for specific people, with a clear theoretical statement as to the mechanism by which goal setting facilitates changes in the behaviour of patients or clinical teams.

19.2 Increasing Diversity, Specificity and Sophistication

19.2.1 Increasing Diversity

The current diversity of approaches to goal setting is exemplified in this book by advocates of goal attainment scaling (GAS); theory-based goal setting; goal setting based on the Canadian Occupational Performance Measure (COPM); goal setting based on the International Classification of Functioning, Disability and Health (ICF); and goal setting as *shared decision making*, to give just a few examples. Moreover, these approaches are not mutually exclusive, for example, goal setting based on the ICF (see Chapter 9) or on the COPM (see Chapter 10) may also be integrated with the use of GAS goals (see Chapters 7 and 8) to operationalize the goals being set. Indeed, any one person may benefit from a number of different approaches to goal setting during the course of their rehabilitation. Different approaches to goal setting may be more applicable or useful at different stages of recovery from an acquired illness or injury and at different stages of life.

Different approaches to goal setting may also be usefully employed concurrently. For example, a person may benefit from an approach to goal setting based on principles of shared decision making (see Chapter 5) or goal setting with *meaning* (see Chapter 6) to help structure the overall plan for their rehabilitation. At the same time, they might also have specific, challenging goals set for them by a physiotherapist in the gym such as making specific gains on a particular physical exercise. Ideally, these specific and challenging goals will be linked to the achievement of higher-order, more personally meaningful life goals established in the rehabilitation plan – in accord with Locke and Latham's goal setting theory (see Chapter 3). Here, the different approaches to goal setting have different purposes: some are being used to enhance patient involvement in clinical decision making and to provide an overall framework for the clinician–patient relationship – others are being used to help motivate patients undertaking strenuous and repetitive therapeutic exercise.

We suspect that this pluralistic approach to goal setting will continue and the array of goal-setting techniques will continue to grow. Rather than this being viewed as a problem in rehabilitation, with concerns being raised about lack of standardization of practice, we believe that greater diversification in approaches to goal setting should be considered as a positive development especially if the diverse approaches used are grounded in theory and rigorously researched for their clinical effectiveness.

Unfortunately, given the limited evidence for goal setting, especially the absence of published trials comparing different approaches, it is difficult at present for rehabilitation teams to make evidence-based decisions on how best to implement or modify their own goal-setting approach. Consequently, we recommend that rehabilitation teams intending to implement or improve their goal setting should start this process with careful reflection on their fundamental aims. This should include exploring the team members' individual and shared assumptions and beliefs about goal setting in rehabilitation. Team discussions might involve revisiting some fundamental issues such as the following:

- Why do we think goal setting in rehabilitation is important?
- What do we consider to be the primary and secondary purposes or functions of goal setting *in our service*, that is, what do we hope to achieve by using goal setting in practice? Is it to improve outcomes, to engage and empower clients or to better coordinate team activities towards shared outcomes?

- If goal setting serves more than one function, how compatible are these, and how are tensions between functions addressed in practice?

- How should goal setting be conducted? Do we all agree on what is best practice in goal setting?

- What moral responsibilities do we believe we share regarding goal-setting practice?

- How do patients respond to goal setting and how are we as a service helping them to understand, to engage in and to own the process?

- What research evidence exists to support these assumptions, beliefs and practices? Have we considered the original, empirical research underpinning these claims to an evidence base, or are these beliefs based on second-hand reports on the research?

While the state of our knowledge on goal setting in rehabilitation is still rudimentary and precludes a simple *cookbook* approach to goal planning, the future of rehabilitation is likely to see more options opening up for approaches to goal setting, not fewer. Clinicians need to develop the skills required to distinguish between these approaches and to decide at an individual service level which approach is best for their patients or clients. Increasing diversity in goal setting is a positive trend as it will provide rehabilitation clinicians with greater opportunities to adapt their practice to best meet the personal needs of the people receiving their services.

19.2.2 Increasing Specificity

The diverse range of approaches to goal setting in rehabilitation allows for much greater specificity in how goal setting can be practised for specific problems associated with specific conditions. This is clearly evident in this book in which we see specific goal setting approaches advocated for children (see Chapters 8 and 15), for older adults in the community (see Chapter 16), for adults with aphasia (see Chapter 17), for adults living with long-term conditions (see Chapter 14), in adult neurorehabilitation (see Chapters 7, 13 and 18) and so on. Increasingly, as the evidence base develops, we expect to see greater advances in the specification of which types of patients respond best to which types of goal setting. For instance, it might be that patients with problems with executive functioning due to brain injury might respond well to approaches to goal setting that are based on theories of self-regulation (see Chapters 3 and 6). In contrast, elite athletes in sports rehabilitation, who already have self-regulation skills, might be better served by other approaches to goal setting, for example, an approach emphasizing the selection of specific and challenging goals (i.e. derived from Locke and Latham's goal-setting theory). These are just two of many plausible hypotheses about people and their responses to different goal-setting processes. Further research is now required to map out and test hypotheses such as these.

This specification of goal setting could, as suggested earlier, be developed for particular health conditions and particular rehabilitation services. However, it is important to avoid assuming that two people with the same condition in the same rehabilitation service will necessarily respond to one approach to goal setting in similar ways. So perhaps just as we have seen a rise in interest in personalized medicine (Hamburg & Collins, 2010), so too might we see the development of personalized goal setting. Here, the emphasis is not so much on the individualization of the actual goals being set but rather on the individualization of the goal-setting process itself.

The idea of people having a personal disposition towards certain types of goals and goal setting is one that has been explored extensively in sport psychology through the application of *achievement goal theory* (Duda, 2001). Two central goal dispositions according to achievement goal theory are a *task orientation* and an *ego orientation*. People who score highly on measures of task orientation tend to define success in sports in terms of their personal learning and effort, whereas people with an ego orientation define success more in terms of publicly demonstrated achievement in comparison to others (Duda, 2007). Goal orientations are said to be orthogonal or uncorrelated. In other words, some individuals score high in both task and ego orientations, others score low in both, and others can be high on one and low on the other (Duda, 2007). The value of achievement goal theory is that it can be used to explain people's intrinsic motivation in sports and to predict how they might respond to certain external factors, such as different types of obstacles to progress in skill acquisition. Further research has gone on to explore other type of goal disposition in sports environments, such as the influence of socially motivated goal setting in the context of competitive sport for older adults (Hodge, Allen, & Smellie, 2008).

It is interesting to consider whether patients might also enter the rehabilitation environment with individual orientations towards different types of goals. Certainly qualitative research on goal setting in rehabilitation suggests that patients (1) bring different attitudes towards goal setting with them based on individual life experiences, (2) have different levels of interest in goal setting and (3) differ in terms of the willingness with which they share their personal goals with the health professionals who provide their care (Brown et al., 2013; Holliday, Antoun, & Playford, 2005; Laver, Halbert, Stewart, & Crotty, 2010; Parry, 2004; Young et al., 2008). While it might seem less relevant to test achievement goal theory in rehabilitation environments, as it is hard to conceptualize how an ego orientation would translate in a hospital setting, further exploration of goal dispositions in clinical populations might well be of value. Future research could be conducted to see if patients can be categorized in terms of individual differences associated with goal orientation and whether it would be possible to develop more specific approaches to goal planning that were individualized to personality types.

19.2.3 Increasing Sophistication

The Oxford Online Dictionary notes that when referring to a system or technique, *sophisticated* means 'developed to a high degree of complexity' (Sophisticated, n.d.). With increased diversity and specificity in goal setting, it is inevitable that this rehabilitation technique will become more complex. However, increased complexity is not a virtue in itself and could be a real disadvantage if the process of goal setting becomes more time-consuming or laborious for patients and clinical teams. In our opinion, the key element in the development of a more sophisticated approach to goal setting is the establishment of a clear outline of the theoretical basis for a particular approach to goal setting for clients in a particular situation. A sound theoretical basis will generate more hypotheses that can be empirically examined in relation to certain approaches to goal setting. In this regard, we encourage teams to reflect on the theoretical basis for the approach to goal setting that they employ.

To take just one example, Locke and Latham's (2002) goal-setting theory has often been cited to support or justify the use of goal setting in rehabilitation. However, as already discussed in Chapter 3, it is not uncommon to see this theory (or the research underpinning it) being cited in rehabilitation publications where the details of the actual model are ignored and with little attention to the notion of how this model from industrial-organization psychology exactly fits with the rehabilitation context. Typically the finding that people perform better when set specific, challenging goals is mentioned, but while this finding has been extensively replicated, it is still only one part of the full model. For example, Locke and Latham posit a number of mediators (e.g. persistence) and moderators (e.g. goal commitment) that can affect performance in their model. However, these are rarely if ever considered when this model is cited to support rehabilitation goal setting. Thus, a more sophisticated approach to goal setting in rehabilitation based on goal-setting theory would be explicit about issues such as the following: How does this well-developed and evidence-based approach to goal setting translate into a rehabilitation setting? How is the clinical rehabilitation context fundamentally different from the factory or company setting in which this model was first developed? What adaptations are necessary and why? Which components in the *high-performance cycle* of Locke and Latham are most relevant (or not relevant) to people in rehabilitation programmes (as opposed to workers in a company)?

Another aspect of taking a more sophisticated approach to goal setting would be to include consideration of the whole social system within which rehabilitation goals are selected and used. Rather than considering rehabilitation goals as cognitive tools to influence only patient behaviour, we ought to begin considering (from both a clinical and research perspective) the influence that goals and goal setting can or might have on the individual and collective behaviour of rehabilitation team members as well as on other people and social systems involved in a person's recovery from illness or injury. These other people might include family members, whose involvement in goal setting for rehabilitation is at times marginalized or treated in a token manner (Levack, Siegert, Dean, & McPherson, 2009), or health funders, insurance providers and policy makers, who can directly or indirectly influence the type of goals being set for people receiving rehabilitation services. A systems approach to goal setting in rehabilitation is reminiscent of King's (1981) goal attainment theory for nursing (see Chapter 1) but also raises a number of new questions for policy, research and clinical practice. These questions include how the goals of individuals can be best integrated into the goals of a group, how conflict around the goals of these various stakeholders might be resolved and how goal setting could be altered to positively influence the motivation and engagement of rehabilitation providers in creative clinical decision making.

19.3 Conclusions

Since the 1960s and 1970s when goal setting was first introduced to clinical rehabilitation, there has been a proliferation of academic articles, research studies and published clinical guidelines on how to apply goal setting to clinical practice. For a time, goal setting was, arguably, viewed as a rather simple but effective way of facilitating teamwork within rehabilitation services and a way of better engaging patients in the uptake of rehabilitation interventions. It was described as an essential feature of good rehabilitation practice (Barnes & Ward, 2000; Schut & Stam, 1994; Wade, 1998). Since 2000, there has been a dramatic growth in our appreciation of some of the complexities surrounding the application of goal setting to clinical rehabilitation. This has included the following:

- Increasing recognition that goal-setting practice differs from one clinical environment to the next (e.g. Playford et al., 2000; Playford, Siegert, Levack, & Freeman, 2009).

- Increasing evidence that goal setting in the *real world* of rehabilitation is not always consistent with some of the ideology around person-centred practice, including the level of patient participation in goal section (e.g. Baker, Marshak, Rice, & Zimmerman, 2001; Barnard, Cruice, & Playford, 2010; Nijhuis et al., 2008).

- Increasing suggestions that this mismatch between practice and ideology results in part from factors in the *real world* of clinical practice that impact on goal selection. This includes factors such as organizational pressures, perceptions of professional obligations and sociological influences on clinical interactions (Barnard et al., 2010; Levack, Dean, Siegert, & McPherson, 2011; Parry, 2004).

- Increasing recognition that an atheoretical approach to goal setting had proliferated and that current approaches to clinical practice do not always match goal theory or have yet to be substantiated in rehabilitation contexts (Scobbie, Wyke, & Dixon, 2009; Siegert, McPherson, & Taylor, 2004; Siegert & Taylor, 2004).

- The recent emergence of theory-based research on goal setting in rehabilitation (e.g. McPherson, Kayes, & Weatherall, 2009; Scobbie et al., 2009; Siegert et al., 2004), which is still in its infancy but which will be an area of considerable growth in the near future.

In this book, we have *not* provided a prescriptive list of instructions about how to apply goal setting to clinical practice nor have we provided an algorithm for deciding which type of goal or goal-setting approach to use and when. Rather, we have presented a range of different approaches to goal setting, advocated by various rehabilitation leaders internationally, and have provided a text that will help to guide how clinicians *think* about goal setting: clinically, scientifically, philosophically and critically. Above all, we hope that this book provides a snapshot of the state of the art of rehabilitation goal setting in the early twenty-first century and the foundations for the next century of clinical practice and scientific research on this vital topic for rehabilitation professionals and people with disabilities.

References

Baker, S. M., Marshak, H. H., Rice, G. T., & Zimmerman, G. J. (2001). Patient participation in physical therapy goal setting. *Physical Therapy*, *81*(5), 1118–1126.

Barnard, R. A., Cruice, M. N., & Playford, E. D. (2010). Strategies used in the pursuit of achievability during goal setting in rehabilitation. *Qualitative Health Research*, *20*(2), 239–250.

Barnes, M. P., & Ward, A. B. (2000). *Textbook of rehabilitation medicine*. Oxford, U.K.: Oxford University Press.

Brown, M., Levack, W., McPherson, K. M., Dean, S. G., Reed, K., Weatherall, M., & Taylor, W. J. (2013). Survival, momentum, and things that make me 'me': Patients' perceptions of goal setting after stroke [Early Online]. *Disability & Rehabilitation*, 1–7. Posted online 20 August 2013. Accessed 25.02.14, DOI: 10.3109/09638288.2013.825653.

Duda, J.L. (2001). Achievement goal research in sport: Pushing the boundaries and clarifying some misunderstandings. In G.C. Roberts (Ed.), *Advances in Motivation in Sport Exercise Science*, pp. 129–182, Champagne, IL: Human Kinetics Books.

Hamburg, M. A., & Collins, F. S. (2010). The path to personalized medicine. *New England Journal of Medicine*, *363*(4), 301–304.

Hodge, K., Allen, J. B., & Smellie, L. (2008). Motivation in Masters sport: Achievement and social goals. *Psychology of Sport and Exercise, 9,* 157–176.

Holliday, R. C., Antoun, M., & Playford, E. D. (2005). A survey of goal-setting methods used in rehabilitation. *Neurorehabilitation and Neural Repair, 19*(3), 227–231.

King, I. M. (1981). *A theory for nursing: Systems, concepts, process.* New York, NY: Wiley.

Laver, K., Halbert, J., Stewart, M., & Crotty, M. (2010). Patient readiness and ability to set recovery goals during the first 6 months after stroke. *Journal of Allied Health, 39*(4), e149–e154.

Levack, W. M. M., Dean, S. G., Siegert, R. J., & McPherson, K. M. (2011). Navigating patient-centered goal setting in inpatient stroke rehabilitation: How clinicians control the process to meet perceived professional responsibilities. *Patient Education & Counseling, 85*(2), 206–213.

Levack, W. M. M., Siegert, R. J., Dean, S. G., & McPherson, K. M. (2009). Goal planning for adults with acquired brain injury: How clinicians talk about involving family. *Brain Injury, 23*(3), 192–202.

Locke, E. A., & Latham, G. P. (2002). Building a practically useful theory of goal setting and task motivation: A 35-year odyssey. *American Psychologist, 57*(9), 705–717.

McPherson, K. M., Kayes, N., & Weatherall, M. (2009). A pilot study of self-regulation informed goal setting in people with traumatic brain injury. *Clinical Rehabilitation, 23,* 296–309.

Nijhuis, B. J. G., Reinders-Messelink, H. A., de Blécourt, A. C. E., Boonstra, A. M., Calamé, E. H. M., Groothoof, J. W., … Postema, K. (2008). Goal setting in Dutch paediatric rehabilitation. Are the needs and principal problems of children with cerebral palsy integrated into their rehabilitation goals? *Clinical Rehabilitation, 22,* 348–363.

Parry, R. H. (2004). Communication during goal-setting in physiotherapy treatment sessions. *Clinical Rehabilitation, 18*(6), 668–682.

Playford, E. D., Dawson, L., Limbert, V., Smith, M., Ward, C. D., & Wells, R. (2000). Goal-setting in rehabilitation: Report of a workshop to explore professionals' perceptions of goal-setting. *Clinical Rehabilitation, 14*(5), 491–496.

Playford, E. D., Siegert, R. J., Levack, W., & Freeman, J. (2009). Areas of consensus and disagreement about goal-setting in rehabilitation: A conference report. *Clinical Rehabilitation, 23,* 334–344.

Schut, H. A., & Stam, H. J. (1994). Goals in rehabilitation teamwork. *Disability & Rehabilitation, 16*(4), 223–226.

Scobbie, L., Wyke, S., & Dixon, D. (2009). Identifying and applying psychological theory to setting and achieving rehabilitation goals. *Clinical Rehabilitation, 23,* 321–333.

Siegert, R. J., McPherson, K. M., & Taylor, W. (2004). Toward a cognitive-affective model of goal-setting in rehabilitation: Is self-regulation theory a key step? *Disability & Rehabilitation, 26*(20), 1175–1183.

Siegert, R. J., & Taylor, W. J. (2004). Theoretical aspects of goal-setting and motivation in rehabilitation. *Disability & Rehabilitation, 26*(1), 1–8.

Sophisticated. (n.d.). Oxford Dictionaries. Oxford University Press. Retrieved 12 October 2013, from http://oxforddictionaries.com/definition/english/sophisticated?q=sophisticated.

Wade, D. T. (1998). Evidence relating to goal planning in rehabilitation. *Clinical Rehabilitation, 12*(4), 273–275.

Young, C. A., Manmathan, G. P., Ward, J. C., Young, C. A., Manmathan, G. P., & Ward, J. C. R. (2008). Perceptions of goal setting in a neurological rehabilitation unit: A qualitative study of patients, carers and staff. *Journal of Rehabilitation Medicine, 40*(3), 190–194.

Index